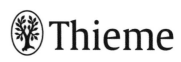

Biological Approaches to Spinal Disc Repair and Regeneration for Clinicians

Roger Härtl, MD
Professor of Neurological Surgery
Director of Spinal Surgery
Director, Weill Cornell Medicine Center for Comprehensive Spine Care
Attending Neurosurgeon
Weill Cornell Medicine, New York-Presbyterian Hospital
New York, New York

Lawrence J. Bonassar, PhD
Professor
Meinig School of Biomedical Engineering
Sibley School of Mechanical and Aerospace Engineering
Cornell University
Ithaca, New York

82 illustrations

Thieme
New York • Stuttgart • Delhi • Rio de Janeiro

Executive Editor: Timothy Hiscock
Managing Editor: Sarah Landis
Director, Editorial Services: Mary Jo Casey
Editorial Assistant: Nikole Connors
Production Editor: Naamah Schwartz
International Production Director: Andreas Schabert
International Marketing Director: Fiona Henderson
International Sales Director: Louisa Turrell
Director of Sales, North America: Mike Roseman
Senior Vice President and Chief Operating Officer: Sarah Vanderbilt
President: Brian D. Scanlan

Library of Congress Cataloging-in-Publication Data

Names: Härtl, Roger, editor. | Bonassar, Lawrence J., editor.
Title: Biological approaches to spinal disc repair and regeneration
    for clinicians / [edited by] Roger Härtl, Lawrence J. Bonassar.
Description: New York : Thieme, [2017] | Includes bibliographical
    references and index.
Identifiers: LCCN 2016057426| ISBN 9781626232501 (hardback) |
    ISBN 9781626232518 (eISBN)
Subjects: | MESH: Intervertebral Disc Degeneration–complications |
    Intervertebral Disc–physiopathology | Intervertebral Disc
    Degeneration–therapy | Low Back Pain–etiology | Low Back
    Pain–therapy |
    Total Disc Replacement–methods
Classification: LCC RD771.B217 | NLM WE 740 | DDC 617.564–dc23
LC record available at https://lccn.loc.gov/2016057426

© 2017 Thieme Medical Publishers, Inc.

Thieme Publishers New York
333 Seventh Avenue, New York, NY 10001 USA
+1 800 782 3488, customerservice@thieme.com

Thieme Publishers Stuttgart
Rüdigerstrasse 14, 70469 Stuttgart, Germany
+49 [0]711 8931 421, customerservice@thieme.de

Thieme Publishers Delhi
A-12, Second Floor, Sector-2, Noida-201301
Uttar Pradesh, India
+91 120 45 566 00, customerservice@thieme.in

Thieme Publishers Rio de Janeiro, Thieme Publicações Ltda.
Edifício Rodolpho de Paoli, 25º andar
Av. Nilo Peçanha, 50 – Sala 2508
Rio de Janeiro 20020-906 Brasil
+55 21 3172 2297 / +55 21 3172-1896

Cover illustration: Thomas Graves
Typesetting by DiTech Process Solutions

Printed in India by Replika Press Pvt. Ltd.   5 4 3 2 1

ISBN 978-1-62623-250-1

Also available as an e-book:
eISBN 978-1-62623-251-8

Important note: Medicine is an ever-changing science undergoing continual development. Research and clinical experience are continually expanding our knowledge, in particular our knowledge of proper treatment and drug therapy. Insofar as this book mentions any dosage or application, readers may rest assured that the authors, editors, and publishers have made every effort to ensure that such references are in accordance with **the state of knowledge at the time of production of the book.**

Nevertheless, this does not involve, imply, or express any guarantee or responsibility on the part of the publishers in respect to any dosage instructions and forms of applications stated in the book. **Every user is requested to examine carefully** the manufacturers' leaflets accompanying each drug and to check, if necessary in consultation with a physician or specialist, whether the dosage schedules mentioned therein or the contraindications stated by the manufacturers differ from the statements made in the present book. Such examination is particularly important with drugs that are either rarely used or have been newly released on the market. Every dosage schedule or every form of application used is entirely at the user's own risk and responsibility. The authors and publishers request every user to report to the publishers any discrepancies or inaccuracies noticed. If errors in this work are found after publication, errata will be posted at www.thieme.com on the product description page.

Some of the product names, patents, and registered designs referred to in this book are in fact registered trademarks or proprietary names even though specific reference to this fact is not always made in the text. Therefore, the appearance of a name without designation as proprietary is not to be construed as a representation by the publisher that it is in the public domain.

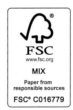

Contents

Foreword

Disc degeneration and regeneration is an important contemporary medical issue of concern for the vast majority of physicians that manage patients on a daily basis with the ubiquitous complaint of low back discomfort. We understand that a healthy lifestyle of avoiding excessive weight gain and exposure to nicotine products as well as getting daily exercise is beneficial for intervertebral disc homeostasis. We have also made tremendous gains over the last decade in understanding the genetics of disc degeneration and the potential for disc regeneration. Research has allowed us to understand that the disc itself harbors stem cells that may be activated with appropriate cues and promoted to proliferate with the correct cocktail of growth factors yet to be determined. We have recently understood the importance of the intervertebral endplate and its ability to allow and regulate stress transfer as well as nutritional support to the disc. We have so much further to go in understanding methods to replenish the disc with viable cells in an innocuous fashion not to cause iatrogenic discal injury.

The background for understanding the complex intervertebral disc milieu is wonderfully laid out in this book by Dr. Roger Härtl and Dr. Lawrence Bonassar. Great thought was placed in organizing a book that introduces not only the novice but also the expert in the lab on the anatomy, pathophysiology and biomechanics of the intervertebral disc. Interesting insight is provided in understanding the applicability of chosen animal models that have been validated as analogous to the human intervertebral disc. An exploration into our failed attempts in the past of substituting mechanical disc replacements of the human disc is discussed in detail and potential avenues for treatment in the future are explored.

The editors' list of authors is a "Who's Who" in the study of the intervertebral disc. The book is captivating, as the subject matter is well thought out, the format is easy to read, and the illustrations are striking. This textbook will certainly be a staple in all educational venues such as colleges, universities, medical schools, clinical residencies and fellowship programs and, most importantly, the basic science world. I congratulate Dr. Härtl, Dr. Bonassar, all of the well-known contributing authors throughout the world, and especially the publisher for allowing such an insightful book to be created for the benefit of those who suffer from low back pain.

Alexander R. Vaccaro, MD, PhD, MBA
Richard H. Rothman Professor and Chairman,
Department of Orthopaedic Surgery
Professor of Neurosurgery
Co-Director, Delaware Valley Spinal Cord Injury Center
Co-Chief of Spine Surgery
Sidney Kimmel Medical Center at Thomas Jefferson University
President, Rothman Institute
Philadelphia, Pennsylvania

Preface

This book was written to shed light on one of the most puzzling problems we are facing in medicine today: our approach to low back pain (LBP) that originates from degenerative disc disease (DDD). LBP is a leading cause of disability worldwide and has been linked directly and indirectly to DDD. LBP has a global lifetime prevalence of almost 40% and a large socioeconomic impact with estimated annual indirect and direct costs exceeding $100 billion in the United States alone. There is a genetic component that puts individuals with a family history of DDD at greater risk of developing low back or neck pain themselves.

Today we know that prevention of and treatment for any type of back, neck, or leg pain should always begin with the adaptation of basic rules of healthy living: weight control, healthy food, exercises to strengthen core, flexibility and stretching, and physical activity or therapy. We are successful in treating patients who suffer from pain caused by nerve root compression: neurogenic claudication, for example, can be treated successfully with minimally invasive ambulatory surgery. Radicular pain due to disc herniations can be relieved with outpatient procedures. What we consider "mechanical back pain" due to mechanical instability of the spine can be treated with sometimes complex spinal reconstruction and stabilization procedures. However, there are two sources of pain and suffering that we are struggling to understand, adequately diagnose, and treat: muscle and intervertebral disc (IVD). Whereas muscle physiology has been studied extensively for decades, by comparison, relatively little is known about the physiology of IVD.

This book focuses on pain caused by DDD, which we characterize broadly as "discogenic back pain." The contributors include the scientific and clinical leaders in the field. The current surgical treatment options for back pain resulting from DDD are associated with risks and undesirable long-term effects, and they are clearly unsatisfactory. Fusion surgery or disc arthroplasty procedures are only partially successful and probably not better than, for example, physical therapy and cognitive behavioral interventions. Finding effective treatments for pain stemming from DDD has been difficult due to its complicated pathophysiology and our incomplete knowledge of the underlying processes leading to degeneration of the IVD. Many factors work together to initiate, exacerbate, and maintain the degenerative process; these include genetic predisposition, decreased nutrient transport, abnormal biomechanics, smoking, and the normal wear and tear of the IVD associated with aging. Whereas the relative importance of each risk factor in initiating DDD is uncertain, these factors initiate a cascade of molecular mechanisms, leading to the breakdown of the disc and possibly back pain.

This book is dedicated to the practitioners who treat patients with back pain and who want to learn about what is being done at the forefront of basic and translational science to solve the challenges associated with DDD. We do not have final answers, but this book will highlight and explain the many exciting and promising approaches that are being explored to better understand, diagnose, and treat pain and disability deriving from DDD. Ultimately, the successful approach to the management of back and neck pain will likely involve a combination of preventive measures such as healthy lifestyle modifications and exercises to address muscular origin, and minimally invasive surgical and biological treatment interventions to address more advanced stages related to DDD.

Lawrence J. Bonassar, PhD
Roger Härtl, MD

Contributors

Fahad H. Abduljabbar, MBBS, FRCSC
Spine Fellow
McGill Scoliosis and Spine Centre
McGill University Health Centre
Montreal, Quebec, Canada
Orthopaedic Teaching Assistant
Department of Orthopedic Surgery
King Abdulaziz University
Jeddah, Saudi Arabia

H. Davis Adkisson, PhD
Chief Scientific Officer
Isto Biologics
St. Louis, Missouri

Mauro Alini, PhD
Head, Musculoskeletal Regeneration Program
AO Research Institute Davos
Davos, Switzerland

Howard An, MD
The Morton International Professor
Director of Spine Fellowship
Department of Orthopaedic Surgery
Rush University Medical Center
Chicago, Illinois

Lorin Michael Benneker, MD
Head of Spine Unit
Associate Professor
Department of Orthopaedic Surgery
Inselspital
University of Bern
Bern, Switzerland

Edward C. Benzel, MD
Chairman, Department of Neurosurgery
Neurological Institute
Cleveland Clinic
Cleveland, Ohio

Lawrence J. Bonassar, PhD
Professor
Meinig School of Biomedical Engineering
Sibley School of Mechanical and Aerospace Engineering
Cornell University
Ithaca, New York

Robby D. Bowles, PhD
Assistant Professor
Department of Bioengineering
University of Utah
Salt Lake City, Utah

Jason Pui Yin Cheung, MBBS (HK), MMedSc
Clinical Assistant Professor, Division of Spine Surgery
Department of Orthopaedics & Traumatology
The University of Hong Kong
Pokfulam, Hong Kong

Kenneth M.C. Cheung, MBBS(UK), MD (HK), FRCS, FHKCOS, FHKAM(Orth)
Jessie Ho Professor in Spine Surgery,
Head, Department of Orthopaedics and Traumatology
The University of Hong Kong
Hong Kong, SAR, China

Michelle A. Cruz, BS
MD, PhD Candidate
Case Western Reserve University School of Medicine
Cleveland, Ohio

Niloofar Farhang, BS
Graduate Research Assistant
Department of Bioengineering
University of Utah
Salt Lake City, Utah

Fabio Galbusera, PhD
Head of the Laboratory of Biological Structures Mechanics
IRCCS Istituto Ortopedico Galeazzi
Milan, Italy

Timothy Ganey, PhD
Director of Orthopaedic Research
Atlanta Medical Center
Atlanta, Georgia

Tony Goldschlager, MBBS, PhD, FRACS
Professor, Neurosurgeon
Department of Surgery
Monash University
Melbourne, Victoria, Australia

Sibylle Grad, PhD
Principal Scientist
Musculoskeletal Regeneration Program
AO Research Institute Davos
Davos, Switzerland

Elliott A. Gruskin, PhD
Life Sciences Consultant
Malvern, Pennsylvania

Peter Grunert, MD
Spine Fellow
Swedish Neuroscience Institute
Seattle, Washington

Lisbet Haglund, PhD
Associate Professor, Surgery
The Orthopaedic Research Laboratory
Montreal General Hospital
Montreal, Quebec, Canada

Colin M. Haines, MD
Fellow
Center for Spine Health
Neurological Institute
Cleveland Clinic
Cleveland, Ohio

Roger Härtl, MD
Professor of Neurological Surgery
Director of Spinal Surgery
Director, Weill Cornell Medicine Center for Comprehensive
  Spine Care
Attending Neurosurgeon
Weill Cornell Medicine, New York-Presbyterian Hospital
New York, New York

Andrew C. Hecht
Chief, Spine Surgery Mount Sinai Health System
Director, Spine Center
Leni and Peter W. May Department of Orthopaedics
Icahn School of Medicine at Mount Sinai
New York, New York

Christian Hohaus, MD
Consultant Neurosurgeon
Department of Neurosurgery
BG Klinikum Bergmannstrost
Halle, Germany

William C. Horton, MD
Vice President of Research & Development
Franchise Medical Leader, Spine
DePuy Synthes Spine
Adjunct Professor of Orthopaedic Surgery
The Emory Spine Center
Emory University
Atlanta, Georgia

Ibrahim Hussain, MD
Spine Fellow
Weill Cornell Brain and Spine Center
Department of Neurological Surgery
Weill Cornell Medicine, New York-Presbyterian Hospital
New York, New York

James C. Iatridis, PhD
Professor & Vice Chair for Research
Mount Sinai Endowed Chair in Orthopaedic Research
Director, Spine Research Program
Leni and Peter W. May Department of Orthopaedics
Icahn School of Medicine at Mount Sinai
New York, New York

Kenji Kato, MD, PhD
Postdoctoral Fellow
Department of Orthopaedic Surgery
University of California, San Diego
La Jolla, California

Gernot Lang, MD
Spine Fellow
Weill Cornell Brain and Spine Center
Department of Neurological Surgery
Weill Cornell Medical College
New York, New York

Brandon Lawrence, MD
Associate Professor
Department of Orthopaedic Surgery
University of Utah
Salt Lake City, Utah

Victor Y. Leung, PhD
Research Assistant Professor
Department of Orthopaedics & Traumatology
The University of Hong Kong
Hong Kong, SAR, China

Zhen Li, PhD
Research Scientist, Musculoskeletal Regeneration
AO Research Institute Davos
Davos, Switzerland

William Omar Contreras Lopez, MD, PhD
Professor
Department of Functional Neurosurgery & Spine Surgery
NEMOD International Neuromodulation Center
UNAB University
Bucaramanga, Colombia

Jeffrey C. Lotz, PhD
Professor and Vice Chair of Research
David S. Bradford, MD, Endowed Chair of Orthopaedic Surgery
Department of Orthopaedic Surgery
University of California San Francisco
San Francisco, California

Keith D.K. Luk, MBBS, MCh(Orth), FRCSE, FRCSG, FRACS, FHKAM(Orth)
Tam Sai-kit Professor in Spine Surgery
Chair Professor and Division Chief, Division of Spine Surgery
Department of Orthopaedics & Traumatology
The University of Hong Kong
Pokfulam, Hong Kong

John T. Martin, PhD
Postdoctoral Researcher
Department of Orthopaedic Surgery
Duke University
Durham, North Carolina

Koichi Masuda, MD
Professor
Department of Orthopaedic Surgery
University of California San Diego
La Jolla, California

Robert L. Mauck, PhD
Mary Black Ralston Professor of Orthopedic Surgery
Professor of Bioengineering
Director, McKay Orthopaedic Research Laboratory
Department of Orthopaedic Surgery
University of Pennsylvania
Philadelphia, Pennsylvania

Hans Jörg Meisel, MD, PhD
Director Centre of Neurosciences
Chair Department of Neurosurgery
BG Klinikum Bergmannstrost
Halle, Germany

Yu Moriguchi, MD, PhD
Research Fellow
Weill Cornell Brain and Spine Center
Department of Neurological Surgery
Weill Cornell Medicine, New York-Presbyterian Hospital
New York, New York

Rodrigo Navarro-Ramirez, MD
Neurosurgeon
Weill Cornell Brain and Spine Center
Department of Neurological Surgery
Weill Cornell Medicine, New York-Presbyterian Hospital
New York, New York

Jean Ouellet, MD, FRCSC
Chair of McGill Scoliosis and Spine Centre
Deputy Chief of Shriners Hospital
Professor of Pediatric Surgery
McGill University Health Centre
Montreal, Quebec, Canada

Brenton Pennicooke, MD, MS
Neurological Surgery Resident
Weill Cornell Brain and Spine Center
Department of Neurological Surgery
Weill Cornell Medicine, New York-Presbyterian Hospital
New York, New York

Marianna Peroglio, PhD
Senior Research Scientist Musculoskeletal Regeneration
AO Research Institute Davos
Davos, Switzerland

Hollis G. Potter, MD
Chairman, Department of Radiology & Imaging
The Coleman Chair, MRI Research
Hospital for Special Surgery
Weill Medical College of Cornell University
New York, New York

Steven Presciutti, MD
Assistant Professor
Orthopaedic Surgery
Emory University
Atlanta, Georgia

Michaela H. Purcell
Vice President, Clinical Affairs
Isto Biologics
St. Louis, Missouri

Timothy T. Roberts, MD
Fellow
Center for Spine Health
Neurological Institute
Cleveland Clinic
Cleveland, Ohio

Dike Ruan, MD
Chair Professor
Department of Orthopaedics
Vice Chairman
Navy General Hospital
Beijing, China

Jaime Arias Ruiz, MD
NEMOD International Neuromodulation Center
UNAB University
Bucaramanga, Colombia

Daisuke Sakai, MD, PhD
Associate Professor
Tokai University School of Medicine
Department of Orthopaedic Surgery
Surgical Science
Isehara, Kanagawa, Japan

Jordy Schol, BS
Tokai University School of Medicine
Department of Orthopaedic Surgery
Surgical Science
Isehara, Kanagawa, Japan

Hassan Serhan, PhD
Distinguished Engineering Fellow, DePuy Synthes Spine
Prestige Adjunct Professor
Department of Bioengineering
University of Toledo
Toledo, Ohio

Stephen R. Sloan, Jr., BS
PhD Candidate
Meinig School of Biomedical Engineering
Cornell University
Ithaca, New York

Harvey E. Smith, MD
Assistant Professor
Department of Orthopaedic Surgery
University of Pennsylvania School of Medicine
Hospital of the University of Pennsylvania
Veteran's Administration Medical Center
Philadelphia, Pennsylvania

Lachlan J. Smith, PhD
Assistant Professor of Neurosurgery and Orthopaedic
    Surgery
Department of Neurosurgery
University of Pennsylvania
Philadelphia, Pennsylvania

Darryl B. Sneag, MD
Assistant Attending Radiologist
Department of Radiology & Imaging, Hospital for
    Special Surgery
Assistant Professor of Radiology
Weill Medical College of Cornell University
New York, New York

Joshua Stover
University of Utah
Salt Lake City, Utah

Claudius Thomé, MD
Professor and Chairman
Department of Neurosurgery
Medical University Innsbruck
Innsbruck, Austria

Olivia M. Torre
PhD Candidate
Leni and Peter W. May Department of Orthopaedics
Icahn School of Medicine at Mount Sinai
New York, New York

Julien Tremblay Gravel, MSc
Research Assistant
McGill Scoliosis and Spine Centre
McGill University Health Centre
Montreal, Quebec, Canada

Luiz Vialle, MD, PhD
Professor of Orthopedics, School of Medicine
Catholic University
Spine Unit
Curitiba, Brazil

Penny J. White
Vice President Emeritus, Regulatory and Quality Affairs
Isto Biologics
St. Louis, Missouri

Hans-Joachim Wilke, MD
Co-Director
Head of Spine Research
Institute of Orthopaedic Research and Biomechanics
Trauma Research Center Ulm
University Hospital Ulm
Ulm, Germany

Micaella Zubkov, BS
Student Researcher
Weill Cornell Brain and Spine Center
Department of Neurological Surgery
Weill Cornell Medical College
New York, New York

Part I

Basics

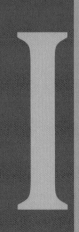

1 The Human Spinal Disc: Relevant Anatomy and Physiology

Julien Tremblay Gravel, Fahad H. Abduljabbar, Jean Ouellet, and Lisbet Haglund

Abstract

The intervertebral disc (IVD) is a well-engineered avascular fibrocartilaginous organ designed to unite two adjacent vertebral bodies. Its anatomical and physiological properties provide constrained motion and force dissipation while maintaining the mechanical stability of the spine. The IVD is divided into two main sections: the annulus fibrosus (AF) and the nucleus pulposus (NP). The NP's structure is of gelatinous consistency and has a high concentration of aggrecan and water that enable it to resist compression. As the spine is axially loaded, the forces are dissipated via the NP and the lamina of the AF.

Keywords: anatomy, biomechanics, intervertebral disc, spine

1.1 The Vertebral Column

The vertebral column is part of the axial skeleton; it is composed of 33 vertebral bodies that connect the skull base to the pelvis. It is divided into five regions: cervical (7 vertebrae), thoracic (12 vertebrae), lumbar (5 vertebrae), sacral (5 vertebrae), and coccygeal (4 vertebrae). The vertebral bodies are named in the cervical region C1–C7, in the thoracic region T1–T12, and in the lumbar region L1–L5. In the coronal plane the spine is straight, yet in the sagittal plane the spine has primary and secondary curves (► Fig. 1.1). The primary curvatures consist of the thoracic and sacral kyphosis. As we learn to sit and stand, the secondary curves take shape, giving rise to the cervical and lumbar lordosis. These curves are important for absorbing forces, maintaining balance, and allowing a range of motion throughout the vertebral column. Motion within the vertebral column varies between each spinal segment. The greatest freedom of motion is found in the cervical and lumbar segments and the most restrained motion is found in the thoracic and sacral segments as they are constrained by the ribs and pelvis. Each vertebra is composed of the vertebral body anteriorly and vertebral arch posteriorly. Each vertebral segment has a spinal canal and two intervertebral foramina, formed by the bony structures of the posterior arch. These structures provide a protected passage for the spinal cord and nerve roots, respectively. The vertebrae also serve as anchor points for the rib cage posteriorly, which helps protect the thoracic cavity organs. The vertebral arches have, posteriorly, two articulating synovial diarthrodial joints called facet joints. The facet joints' surfaces are covered with articular cartilage and are enclosed by a synovial capsule. The facets prevent two adjacent vertebrae from translating during spinal motion, avoiding damage to the nerve roots and spinal cord. IVDs separate the upper 24 vertebral bodies, whereas the lower 9 are fused in adults. The IVDs and the facet joints provide the capacity for flexion and extension and to a lesser extent, rotation and lateral bending. Moreover, these facets share the load transmitted through the spine with the IVDs. The IVD is a fibrocartilaginous organ uniting two adjacent vertebral bodies, contributing to the spine's height and function (► Fig. 1.2). The discs are named according to the upper and lower vertebrae they join. For example, the disc situated between the thoracic vertebra T12 and the lumbar vertebra L1 is called T12–L1. The discs, in aggregate, make up approximately one fourth of the height of the spinal column excluding the sacrum and coccyx.[1] The human spinal disc is essential for maintaining posture and for protecting delicate neural tissue and rigid structures of the vertebrae and skull during locomotion.

1.2 Development of the Intervertebral Disc

The internal structure of the disc has distinct anatomical regions of different developmental origin. These structures are traditionally separated into the central, gelatinous NP, the outer, fibrous AF, and the cartilaginous end plates.

Structures of the spinal column originate from the notochord and from the sclerotome of the mesodermal somites. There are four developmental stages to the formation of the vertebrae and discs. First, the notochord is formed from the mesoderm

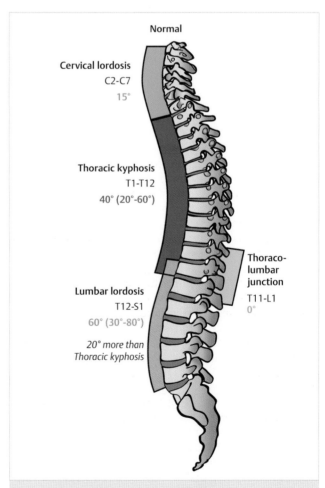

Fig. 1.1 Schematic representation and anatomical regions of the human spine.

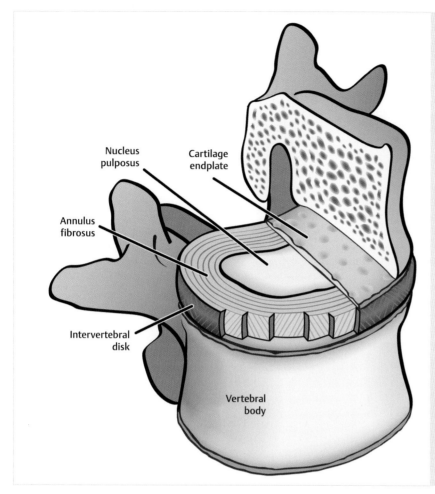

Fig. 1.2 Schematic representation and structure of the human intervertebral disc and position within the human vertebral segment. Note the concentric arrangement of the annulus' lamellae.

Nucleus pulposus

Cartilage endplate

Annulus fibrosus

Intervertebral disk

Vertebral body

during gastrulation. It is positioned in the dorsal region of the embryo, along the anteroposterior axis. The notochord consists of a flexible core of glycoprotein with high osmotic potential surrounded by a sheath of fibrous connective tissue.[2] During the second stage, at the 4th week of development, cells of the sclerotome migrate around the notochord forming the vertebrae, cartilaginous end plate, AF, and ribs. In the ventromedial region, the notochord is segmented. Some sections are remodeled to make way for the forming vertebral bodies, whereas others expand to form the NP, the gelatinous portion of the IVD.[3] The annulus is formed by a condensation of sclerotomal cells surrounding the remaining sections of notochord. The condensation of these cells makes way for the expansion of the notochordal tissue, forming the NP.[4] During the third stage, at 6 weeks, the vertebral parts of the spine undergo chondrogenesis and become cartilaginous (► Fig. 1.3). The fourth and final stage is ossification, which begins during the 8th week of the embryonic period and is completed around 25 years of age.

During fetal/early natal life, blood vessels penetrate the disc to the inner annulus. By the juvenile stage, the blood vessels resorb to the outer annulus and the cartilaginous end plates.[5] In the nondegenerate adult disc, blood vessels are only seen in the connective tissue surrounding the AF and budding in the cartilaginous end plates. This lack of vascularity limits the flow of nutrients reaching the central region of the disc. Nerves follow

a similar pattern, penetrating only the outer AF in nondegenerate adult discs (► Fig. 1.4, ► Fig. 1.5).

1.3 Cells in the Intervertebral Disc

The overall cell density of the disc is fairly high in the fetal stage but decreases significantly with age, especially in the regions furthest from the periphery.

Cells of the NP are notochordal in origin.[6,7] Notochordal cells are large (> 15 μm) and contain large vacuoles,[8] whereas mature NP cells are relatively small (10 um diameter) and display a rounded chondrocyte-like morphology. Multiple studies have demonstrated that cells of the mature human NP express distinct notochordal markers, such as brachyury, further establishing the notochord as the developmental origin of NP cells.[8,9] The vacuoles of notochord cells carry a multitude of anabolic factors suggested to induce matrix synthesis in neighboring cells. Notochordal cells disappear with age and are no longer visible by the age of 4 in humans.[2] Loss or terminal differentiation of these cells may therefore contribute to age-related tissue deterioration. NP cells are situated in lacunae and do not contain vacuoles.[3] They are sparsely and randomly distributed within the tissue, with a cell density of about 4,000 cells per mm[3] in the adult.[10]

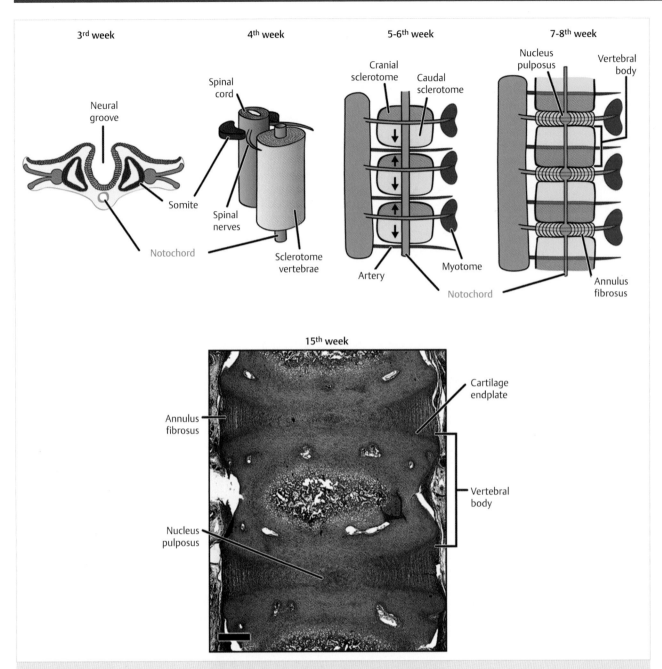

Fig. 1.3 Schematic representation of intervertebral disc development. At *22 days postconception* the notochord forms on the ventromedial aspect of the embryo, elongating along its craniocaudal axis. The neural groove closes to form the early spinal cord, positioned dorsally to the notochord along the same axis. These structures are flanked on each side by a row of somites. At *30 days postconception* sclerotomal cells of the somites separate from myotomal cells and migrate around the notochord toward the midline. At the *4th to 6th embryonic week* sclerotomal cells aggregate around the notochord and spinal cord. Segments of alternating high and low sclerotomal cell density form, giving rise to the early annulus fibrosus and vertebral bone, respectively. At the *7th to 9th embryonic week* sclerotomal cells of the early vertebral bone expand, pushing away the notochord from the center of the vertebral body. Simultaneously, cells of the early annulus condense to allow space for the notochordal tissue exiting the vertebral body, giving rise to the nucleus pulposus region.

Annulus cells originate from the sclerotome, and are elongated and spindle shaped. They are arranged following the lamellae's orientation. Their diameter varies between 15 and 30 μm.[11] The AF is more densely cellularized, with about 9,000 cells per mm[3] in the adult human.[10]

The cells in the end plate cartilage are chondrocytes of mesenchymal origin. Like in the deep layers of articular cartilage, the chondrocytes are situated in lacunae arranged in a columnar fashion. The end plate has the highest cell density of any disc tissue, with approximately 15,000 cells/mm[3].[10] Their average diameter is 20 μm[12] (▶ Fig. 1.6).

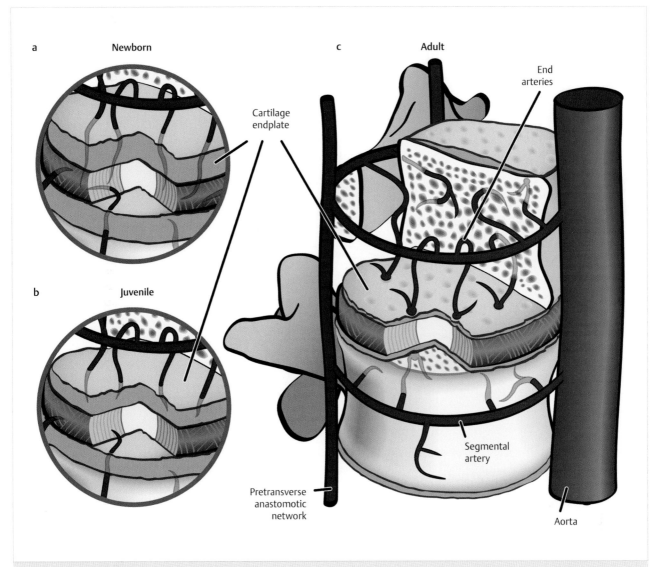

Fig. 1.4 **(a)** Vascular network of the vertebral body and intervertebral disc in the *newborn*; vessels reach into the inner region of the annulus fibrosus (AF). **(b)** *Juvenile* vessels recede to the outer region of the AF. **(c)** *Adult* vessels are restricted to the end plate and connective tissue surrounding the AF.

NP, AF, and cartilage end plate cells are, in addition to matrix synthesis, responsible for maintenance and turnover of the extracellular matrix (ECM), a process that is in balance in the young and nondegenerate disc.

1.4 Intervertebral Disc Organization and Composition

The disc's distinct anatomical regions have different mechanical and biological properties. The AF and NP regions are clearly distinguishable in fetal and juvenile discs but the clear demarcations diminish in the adult. The NP region expands in the adult disc into a transition region called the inner AF, and it can be difficult to establish where one region begins and the other ends (▶ Fig. 1.2). The tissue regions contain similar matrix elements, albeit in widely differing concentrations.[13] The disc's

ECM is rich in collagen and proteoglycan. Collagen is a ubiquitous protein in mammalian connective tissue. Different types of collagen are present in varying amounts within the disc, but the most prominent by far are types I and II. Other collagens present within the mature, nondegenerate disc are types III, V, VI, IX, XI, XII, and XIV.[14] Collagen provides attachment to disc cells and a three-dimensional (3D) mesh confining other matrix elements, such as proteoglycans. Proteoglycans exist in two forms within the disc, either bound to hyaluronic acid or unbound. The most abundant proteoglycan within the disc is aggrecan. In early development stages, most aggrecan within the disc is bound to hyaluronan, with a shift toward unbound forms in later stages of development. Other proteoglycans found in the disc's ECM are versican and members of the small leucine rich protein (SLRP) family: chondroadherin, decorin, fibromodulin, and lumican.[15] The SLRPs have many defined functions in the tissue and most of them carry

5

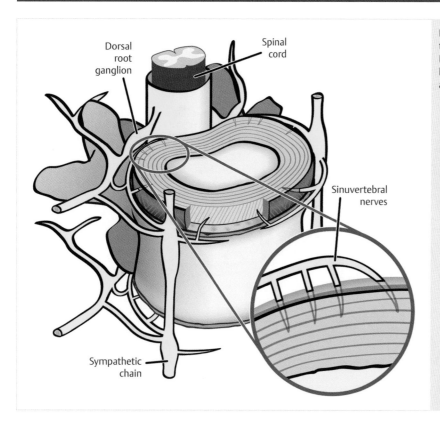

Fig. 1.5 The sinuvertebral nerve originates near the vertebral segment to innervate the disc. Nerve endings rarely penetrate beyond the outer layer of the annulus fibrosus in a nondegenerate adult disc.

glycosaminoglycan (GAG) chains. Chondroadherin is one of the few without GAG chains; it anchors the cells to the ECM via integrin and syndecan receptors.[16,17,18] Decorin, fibromodulin, and lumican carry GAG chains. Decorin cross-links collagen fibers, whereas fibromodulin and lumican have highly negative sulfated tyrosine domains that bind cytokines and matrix metalloproteinases.[18,19,20] Proteoglycans are made up of a core protein to which one or more GAG chains of highly sulphated repeating disaccharide units are covalently attached. Most proteoglycans have 1 or 2 GAG chains, whereas aggrecan has up to 150.

1.4.1 Nucleus Pulposus

The NP's structure is gelatinous and has high aggrecan content. This molecule's many GAG chains contribute to water retention and provide swelling pressure through their fixed negative charges. Aggrecan is the greatest contributor to NP function by enabling it to resist compression. Aggrecan concentration is highest in the central portion of the NP and declines throughout the AF. The other matrix molecule primarily responsible for the mechanical function of the NP is collagen type II. Collagen provides a scaffold entrapping aggrecan and other molecules and provides tensile properties to the tissue. Collagen and aggrecan make up 20% and 50% of the NP's dry weight, respectively.[21] The same molecules are responsible for the mechanical properties of cartilage. However, the ratio of aggrecan to collagen is 2:1 in cartilage, whereas it is 27:1 within the NP.[22] Although aggrecan represents 50% of the dry weight, 70 to 90% of the NP's wet volume is occupied by water bound to

aggrecan.[23] The high proteoglycan content with its negative charge is also thought to be a major factor preventing nerve ingrowth into the largely aneural and avascular mature, nondegenerate IVD.[24,25] Peripherally, the NP is encircled by the AF.

1.4.2 Annulus Fibrosus

The function of the AF is to restrict lateral motion, as well as to prevent extrusion, of the nuclear material. To accomplish this, the collagen fibers of the mature annulus are arranged in up to 25 concentric lamellae wrapped around the NP. The lamellae are parallel to one another traversing between adjacent vertebrae at an angle of 60 degrees to the axis of the spine (▶ Fig. 1.2). The collagen fibers within a single annular lamella are organized in a parallel fashion, whereas the fibers in adjacent layers differ by 30 degrees.[26] The concentration of collagen type I is highest in the annulus and decreases radially toward the NP. Collagen type II follows an inverse pattern with the highest concentration in the NP.[21]

Proteoglycans, such as aggrecan, are present throughout the AF but at a concentration much lower than in the NP. Collagen makes up 50 to 70% of annular tissue dry weight and proteoglycans only 10 to 20% of dry weight.[27] Elastin fibers, arranged in a network between the lamellae, contribute to the structure and mechanical functions of the AF.[28]

1.4.3 Vertebral End Plate

The vertebral end plate has a dual function. It anchors the disc to the vertebrae and provides the main avenue for nutrient and

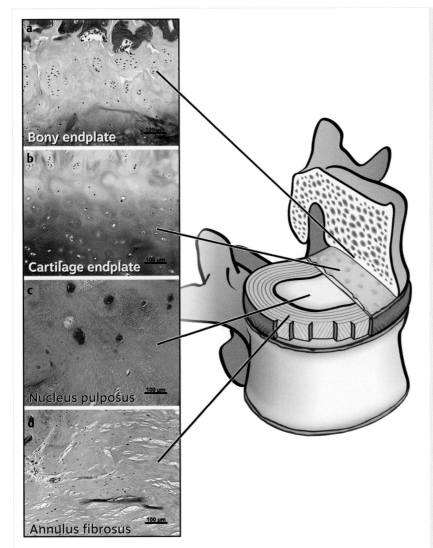

a

Bony endplate 100 μm

b

Cartilage endplate 100 μm

c

Nucleus pulposus 100 μm

d

Annulus fibrosus 100 μm

Fig. 1.6 Human intervertebral disc histology. **(a,b)** Human bony and cartilaginous end plates of a 15 year old. Note the unfused bony end plate, containing hypertrophic cartilage. **(c,d)** The nucleus pulposus and annulus fibrosus of a 52 year old. Staining performed with Safranin-O for proteoglycans, fast green FCF as counterstain, and Weigert's hematoxylin as nuclear stain.

waste exchange for the disc. Hence, it must be both resilient and porous. To achieve this, it is made up of two layers, the cartilage end plate consisting of hyaline cartilage and the bony end plate consisting of cortical bone. The main components of the cartilage end plate are water, type II collagen, and proteoglycans. Water makes up to 80% of tissue weight after birth, but lowers to below 70% after 15 years of age.[21] The ratio between proteoglycans and collagens within the cartilaginous end plate is 2:1, which is similar to that of articular cartilage.[22] The collagen fibers of the annulus' lamellae clearly extend into the cartilage end plate, whereas integration is comparatively less organized in the NP region.[29] Along the outermost region of the disc, the end plate is absent and the AF integrates directly with the vertebral bodies.[30] The collagen fibers of the bony end plate are not connected to those of the cartilaginous layer.[31]

The thickness of the cartilage varies across the end plate and at various spinal levels, from 0.1 to 2.0 mm. The thickness of the cartilage end plate is higher in upper spinal levels than in lower spinal levels. Cartilage thickness is higher in the periphery of the disc and is thinner in the central region.[32] The thickness of the bony layer, like that of the cartilaginous layer, varies between spinal levels and within each end plate. It is thicker at higher spinal levels and in the outer ring of each end plate.[33] The bony end plate on the cranial surface of each spinal segment is also thicker and has higher bone mineral density overall than the one covering the caudal surface.[34]

With age, there is a decrease in aggrecan content and an increase in collagen and calcification of the cartilage end plate.[35] This participates to the end plate's gradual loss of permeability with age, reducing nutrient exchange.[36]

Microfractures within the end plate also become more common, leading to bulges of nuclear tissue into the end plate later in life. This decompresses the nuclear tissue, transferring the biomechanical load to the annulus.[37] Nuclear extrusions into the end plate will progressively become calcified, forming Schmorl's nodes.

1.5 Vascularization and Innervation of the Intervertebral Disc

Vascularization of the end plate is supplied by the basivertebral vessel bundles, which enter the vertebral body through the posterior basivertebral foramen and capillary branches from the segmental artery arising from the anterior spinal artery.[38] Early in postnatal life, the vascular density of the end plate decreases, reducing nutrient supply to the disc. The nondegenerate adult disc is largely avascular and the capillaries form an intricate "mesh" throughout the porous bony end plate and bud in the superficial cartilage layer, providing nutrient delivery and waste exchange with the disc tissue (▶ Fig. 1.4). The density of this network is greatest in the region adjacent to the NP.[39]

Following a similar pattern to vascularization, the nondegenerate adult human disc is largely aneural. The nerve fibers surrounding the discs are branches of the sinuvertebral nerve, or derived from the ventral rami or gray rami communicantes.[38] A meningeal branch of the spinal nerve, known as the recurrent sinuvertebral nerve, nerve of Luschka, or ramus meningeus, originates near the disc space. This nerve exits from the dorsal root ganglion and enters the foramen, where it then divides into a superior and an inferior branch to supply two IVD spaces. The posterolateral aspects of the discs receive branches from adjacent ventral primary rami and from the gray rami communicantes near their junction with the ventral primary rami. The lateral aspects of the discs receive other branches from the rami communicantes.[40] Nerve endings rarely penetrate beyond the outer layer of the AF in a nondegenerate adult disc (▶ Fig. 1.5). However, nerve fibers deep inside the disc have been demonstrated in painful degenerate samples, often accompanying blood vessels.[13] Innervation is an important distinction between the diseased and aged disc. More information on the physiology of degenerative discs is available in Chapter 2.

1.6 Disc Mechanical Properties

The unique structure of the IVD facilitates the capacity to absorb shock and transmit high forces from different vectors around the spine. Yang and King reported that between 75 and 97% of the compressive load applied to the lumbar spine is carried by the IVDs.[41] The tensile and elastic properties of different components of the disc allow a state of equilibrium between stability and flexibility. The fluid in the NP is distorted by compression forces from the vertebral bodies and redistributes them radially to the AF. In turn, the AF is distorted by the pressure imparted by the NP which allows the disc to be compressed, and the resilience of the AF allows it to recover its shape after the pressure has been removed (▶ Fig. 1.7).

The disc benefits from moderate, dynamic loading because it promotes the exchange of nutrients with the end plate.[42,43] It has been demonstrated that physiological strain can regenerate tissue following matrix damage induced by trypsin injection.[44] Strain will affect a variety of factors such as nutrient and waste-product transport in and out of the disc. Disc cells are tethered to the ECM and will be stretched and deformed by strain applied to it. This will directly transmit a signal from the matrix to the inside of the cell trough; for example, integrin receptors will also cause mechanically sensitive ion channels to open and close, initiating signaling cascades with direct effects on cell metabolism, viability, and phenotype. Mechanical strain of the disc has a number of effects on the extracellular environment as well, which indirectly affects disc cells. For example, strain will change disc water content, pressure, and pH.[45] Chronic overloading and traumatic loads damage matrix elements, affecting disc integrity, and can cause herniation or annular tears.[46] These lead to disc decompression and therefore jeopardize disc elasticity after load.

Adverse load leads to an increase in secretion of catabolic enzymes by disc cells, as well as apoptotic and inflammatory factors, negatively affecting surrounding cells and ECM.[46,47] Biomechanical factors are therefore essential to disc function, but adverse loading events will initiate the process of disc degeneration. With age, the water content of the NP decreases and the collagen content increases, causing it to decompress. The AF then becomes the main load-bearing structure of the disc.[48]

1.7 Matrix Homeostasis and Repair

A balance in synthesis and degradation of matrix components maintains homeostasis in the nondegenerate disc. Metalloproteinases are enzymes involved in this process. They cleave specific matrix substrates during remodeling. The two groups of metalloproteinases present within the disc are matrix metalloproteinases (MMPs) and the disintegrin-like metalloproteases with thrombospondin type 1 motif (ADAMTS).[49,50] MMPs are secreted in an inactive form into the ECM and are activated by processing of their N-terminal domain. Whereas MMPs are inactive at the moment of secretion, ADAMTS are secreted in an active form. Remodeling activity is most prominent in early years of life, as the tissue matures from a fluid to a more fibrous state.[51]

When disc tissue is damaged, secretion of these enzymes is increased to drive matrix degradation.[49] Certain metalloproteinases are much more specialized and efficient than others at degrading specific substrates. ADAMTS-4 and ADAMTS-5 (known as the aggracanases), for example, are highly specific to aggrecan[52] and are 10 times more efficient than enzymes of the MMP family at degrading it.[53] Collagen also has enzymes that are specialized in its breakdown. In the disc, these are MMP-1 and MMP-13.[54] This however occurs at a much slower rate than for aggrecan. The half-life of aggrecan is around 12 years within the disc,[55] whereas for collagen it is much longer, at more than 100 years.[56,57] Due to the low cell density of the IVD, remodeling and repair occurs more slowly than in most other tissues.[58,59] The types of MMPs

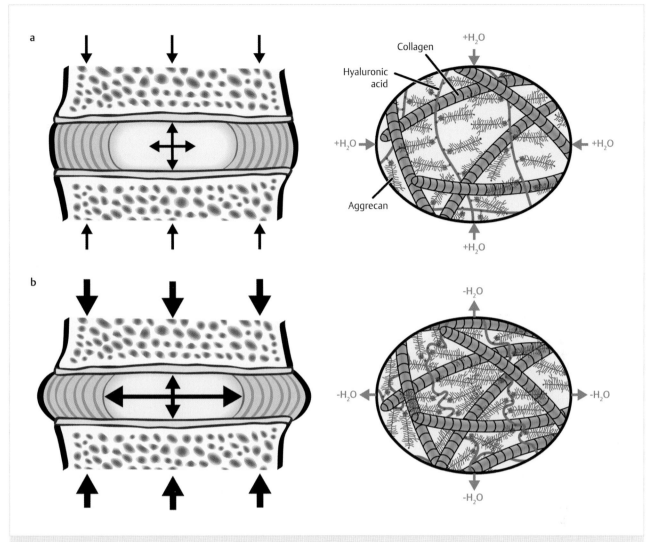

Fig. 1.7 (a) The fluid in the nucleus pulposus is distorted by compression forces from the vertebral bodies and redistributes them radially to the AF. Distortion of the AF by the pressure of the NP will result in disc compressibility, and its resilience provides elasticity. **(b)** Mechanical strain of the disc changes its water content. Water leaves the disc when it is compressed and returns when compression is released.

secreted changes as the tissue ages, most likely in response to the changes occurring in the nature of the matrix itself.[60]

1.8 Conclusion

The anatomical and biochemical properties of the IVD illustrate the complex and high demands the spine puts on this fibrocartilaginous complex. Despite its inherent properties, degenerative processes lead to loss of its internal structure and mechanical failure. In the hope to regenerate the disc, one must be able to regenerate both its anatomical characteristics and its mechanical properties.

Acknowledgment

The authors would like to thank Guylaine Bédard for the artwork in the figures.

1.9 References

[1] Herkowitz HN. Rothman-Simeon The Spine. Vol 1. 6th ed. PA: Elsevier-Saunders; 2011

[2] Pazzaglia UE, Salisbury JR, Byers PD. Development and involution of the notochord in the human spine. J R Soc Med. 1989; 82(7):413–415

[3] Rodrigues-Pinto R, Richardson SM, Hoyland JA. An understanding of intervertebral disc development, maturation and cell phenotype provides clues to direct cell-based tissue regeneration therapies for disc degeneration. Eur Spine J. 2014; 23(9):1803–1814

[4] Peacock A. Observations on the postnatal structure of the intervertebral disc in man. J Anat. 1952; 86(2):162–179

[5] Nerlich AG, Schaaf R, Wälchli B, Boos N. Temporo-spatial distribution of blood vessels in human lumbar intervertebral discs. Eur Spine J. 2007; 16 (4):547–555

[6] McCann MR, Tamplin OJ, Rossant J, Séguin CA. Tracing notochord-derived cells using a Noto-cre mouse: implications for intervertebral disc development. Dis Model Mech. 2012; 5(1):73–82

[7] Choi KS, Cohn MJ, Harfe BD. Identification of nucleus pulposus precursor cells and notochordal remnants in the mouse: implications for disk degeneration and chordoma formation. Dev Dyn. 2008; 237 (12):3953–3958

[8] Minogue BM, Richardson SM, Zeef LA, Freemont AJ, Hoyland JA. Transcriptional profiling of bovine intervertebral disc cells: implications for identification of normal and degenerate human intervertebral disc cell phenotypes. Arthritis Res Ther. 2010; 12(1):R22

[9] Risbud MV, Schaer TP, Shapiro IM. Toward an understanding of the role of notochordal cells in the adult intervertebral disc: from discord to accord. Dev Dyn. 2010; 239(8):2141–2148

[10] Maroudas A, Stockwell RA, Nachemson A, Urban J. Factors involved in the nutrition of the human lumbar intervertebral disc: cellularity and diffusion of glucose in vitro. J Anat. 1975; 120(Pt 1):113–130

[11] Poiraudeau S, Monteiro I, Anract P, Blanchard O, Revel M, Corvol MT. Phenotypic characteristics of rabbit intervertebral disc cells. Comparison with cartilage cells from the same animals. Spine . 1999; 24(9):837–844

[12] Ross MH, Reith EJ, Romrell LJ. Histology: A Text and Atlas. Philadelphia, PA: Williams & Wilkins; 1989

[13] Humzah MD, Soames RW. Human intervertebral disc: structure and function. Anat Rec. 1988; 220(4):337–356

[14] Eyre DR, Matsui Y, Wu JJ. Collagen polymorphisms of the intervertebral disc. Biochem Soc Trans. 2002; 30(Pt 6):844–848

[15] Feng H, Danfelter M, Strömqvist B, Heinegård D. Extracellular matrix in disc degeneration. J Bone Joint Surg Am . 2006; 88 Suppl 2:25–29

[16] Camper L, Heinegård D, Lundgren-Akerlund E. Integrin alpha2beta1 is a receptor for the cartilage matrix protein chondroadherin. J Cell Biol. 1997; 138(5):1159–1167

[17] Haglund L, Ouellet J, Roughley P. Variation in chondroadherin abundance and fragmentation in the human scoliotic disc. Spine . 2009; 34(14):1513–1518

[18] Akhatib B, Onnerfjord P, Gawri R, et al. Chondroadherin fragmentation mediated by the protease HTRA1 distinguishes human intervertebral disc degeneration from normal aging. J Biol Chem. 2013; 288(26):19280–19287

[19] Heinegård D, Aspberg A, Franzén A, Lorenzo P. Chapter 4. Glycosylated matrix proteins. In: Royce PM, Steinmann B, eds. Connective Tissue and Its Heritable Disorders: Molecular, Genetic, and Medical Aspects. 2nd. ed. New York: Wiley-Liss; 2002

[20] Tillgren V, Onnerfjord P, Haglund L, Heinegård D. The tyrosine sulfate-rich domains of the LRR proteins fibromodulin and osteoadherin bind motifs of basic clusters in a variety of heparin-binding proteins, including bioactive factors. J Biol Chem. 2009; 284(42):28543–28553

[21] Pattappa G, Li Z, Peroglio M, Wismer N, Alini M, Grad S. Diversity of intervertebral disc cells: phenotype and function. J Anat. 2012; 221(6):480–496

[22] Mwale F, Roughley P, Antoniou J. Distinction between the extracellular matrix of the nucleus pulposus and hyaline cartilage: a requisite for tissue engineering of intervertebral disc. Eur Cell Mater. 2004; 8:58–63, discussion 63–64

[23] Buckwalter JA. Aging and degeneration of the human intervertebral disc. Spine. 1995; 20(11):1307–1314

[24] Johnson WE, Caterson B, Eisenstein SM, Hynds DL, Snow DM, Roberts S. Human intervertebral disc aggrecan inhibits nerve growth in vitro. Arthritis Rheum. 2002; 46(10):2658–2664

[25] Purmessur D, Cornejo MC, Cho SK, et al. Intact glycosaminoglycans from intervertebral disc-derived notochordal cell-conditioned media inhibit neurite growth while maintaining neuronal cell viability. Spine J. 2015; 15 (5):1060–1069

[26] Marchand F, Ahmed AM. Investigation of the laminate structure of lumbar disc anulus fibrosus. Spine . 1990; 15(5):402–410

[27] Johnstone B, Bayliss MT. The large proteoglycans of the human intervertebral disc. Changes in their biosynthesis and structure with age, topography, and pathology. Spine. 1995; 20(6):674–684

[28] Yu J, Winlove PC, Roberts S, Urban JP. Elastic fibre organization in the intervertebral discs of the bovine tail. J Anat. 2002; 201(6):465–475

[29] Wade KR, Robertson PA, Broom ND. A fresh look at the nucleus-endplate region: new evidence for significant structural integration. Eur Spine J. 2011; 20(8):1225–1232

[30] Nosikova, YS, Santerre, JP, Grynpas, M, Gibson, G, Kandel, RA. Characterization of the annulus fibrosus-vertebral body interface: identification of new structural features. J Anat. 2012; 221(6):577–589

[31] Balkovec C, Adams MA, Dolan P, McGill SM. Annulus fibrosus can strip hyaline cartilage end plate from subchondral bone: a study of the intervertebral disk in tension. Global Spine J. 2015; 5(5):360–365

[32] Roberts S, Menage J, Urban JP. Biochemical and structural properties of the cartilage end-plate and its relation to the intervertebral disc. Spine. 1989; 14 (2):166–174

[33] Wang Y, Owoc JS, Boyd SK, Videman T, Battié MC. Regional variations in trabecular architecture of the lumbar vertebra: associations with age, disc degeneration and disc space narrowing. Bone. 2013; 56(2):249–254

[34] Zhao FD, Pollintine P, Hole BD, Adams MA, Dolan P. Vertebral fractures usually affect the cranial endplate because it is thinner and supported by less-dense trabecular bone. Bone. 2009; 44(2):372–379

[35] Bernick S, Cailliet R. Vertebral end-plate changes with aging of human vertebrae. Spine. 1982; 7(2):97–102

[36] Rajasekaran S, Babu JN, Arun R, Armstrong BR, Shetty AP, Murugan S. ISSLS prize winner: a study of diffusion in human lumbar discs: a serial magnetic resonance imaging study documenting the influence of the endplate on diffusion in normal and degenerate discs. Spine. 2004; 29(23):2654–2667

[37] Holm S, Holm AK, Ekström L, Karladani A, Hansson T. Experimental disc degeneration due to endplate injury. J Spinal Disord Tech. 2004; 17(1):64–71

[38] Raj PP. Intervertebral disc: anatomy-physiology-pathophysiology-treatment. Pain Pract. 2008; 8(1):18–44

[39] Crock HV, Goldwasser M. Anatomic studies of the circulation in the region of the vertebral end-plate in adult Greyhound dogs. Spine. 1984; 9(7):702–706

[40] Bogduk N, Tynan W, Wilson AS. The nerve supply to the human lumbar intervertebral discs. J Anat. 1981; 132(Pt 1):39–56

[41] Yang KH, King AI. Mechanism of facet load transmission as a hypothesis for low-back pain. Spine. 1984; 9(6):557–565

[42] Wuertz K, Godburn K, MacLean JJ, et al. In vivo remodeling of intervertebral discs in response to short- and long-term dynamic compression. J Orthop Res. 2009; 27(9):1235–1242

[43] Chan SC, Ferguson SJ, Gantenbein-Ritter B. The effects of dynamic loading on the intervertebral disc. Eur Spine J. 2011; 20(11):1796–1812

[44] Gawri R, Moir J, Ouellet J, et al. Physiological loading can restore the proteoglycan content in a model of early IVD degeneration. PLoS One. 2014; 9(7):e101233

[45] McMillan DW, Garbutt G, Adams MA. Effect of sustained loading on the water content of intervertebral discs: implications for disc metabolism. Ann Rheum Dis. 1996; 55(12):880–887

[46] Alkhatib, B, Rosenzweig, DH, Krock, E, et al. Acute mechanical injury of the human intervertebral disc: link to degeneration and pain. Eur Cell Mater. 2014; 28:98–110, discussion 110–111

[47] Gawri R, Rosenzweig DH, Krock E, et al. High mechanical strain of primary intervertebral disc cells promotes secretion of inflammatory factors associated with disc degeneration and pain. Arthritis Res Ther. 2014; 16(1):R21

[48] Adams MA, Bogduk N, Burton K, Dolan P. The Biomechanics of Back Pain. 2nd ed. London, England: Churchill Livingstone; 2006

[49] Weiler C, Nerlich AG, Zipperer J, Bachmeier BE, Boos N. 2002 SSE Award Competition in Basic Science: expression of major matrix metalloproteinases is associated with intervertebral disc degradation and resorption. Eur Spine J. 2002; 11(4):308–320

[50] Apte SS. A disintegrin-like and metalloprotease (reprolysin-type) with thrombospondin type 1 motif (ADAMTS) superfamily: functions and mechanisms. J Biol Chem. 2009; 284(46):31493–31497

[51] Urban J, Roberts S, Ralphs J. The nucleus of the intervertebral disc from development to degeneration. Am Zool. 2000; 40:53–61

[52] Tortorella MD, Burn TC, Pratta MA, et al. Purification and cloning of aggrecanase-1: a member of the ADAMTS family of proteins. Science. 1999; 284 (5420):1664–1666

[53] Durigova M, Nagase H, Mort JS, Roughley PJ. MMPs are less efficient than ADAMTS5 in cleaving aggrecan core protein. Matrix Biol. 2011; 30 (2):145–153

[54] Le Maitre CL, Freemont AJ, Hoyland JA. Localization of degradative enzymes and their inhibitors in the degenerate human intervertebral disc. J Pathol. 2004; 204(1):47–54

[55] Sivan, SS, Tsitron, E, Wachtel, E, et al. Aggrecan turnover in human intervertebral disc as determined by the racemization of aspartic acid. J Biol Chem. 2006; 281(19):13009–13014

[56] Verzijl N, DeGroot J, Thorpe SR, et al. Effect of collagen turnover on the accumulation of advanced glycation end products. J Biol Chem. 2000; 275 (50):39027–39031

[57] Sivan, SS, Wachtel, E, Tsitron, E, et al. Collagen turnover in normal and degenerate human intervertebral discs as determined by the racemization of aspartic acid. J Biol Chem. 2008; 283(14):8796–8801

[58] Melrose J, Ghosh P, Taylor TK, et al. A longitudinal study of the matrix changes induced in the intervertebral disc by surgical damage to the annulus fibrosus. J Orthop Res. 1992; 10(5):665–676

[59] Adams MA, Dolan P. Could sudden increases in physical activity cause degeneration of intervertebral discs? Lancet. 1997; 350(9079):734–735

[60] Vo NV, Hartman RA, Yurube T, Jacobs LJ, Sowa GA, Kang JD. Expression and regulation of metalloproteinases and their inhibitors in intervertebral disc aging and degeneration. Spine J. 2013; 13(3):331–341

2 Pathophysiology of Disc Disease: Disc Degeneration

Niloofar Farhang, Joshua Stover, Brandon Lawrence, and Robby D. Bowles

Abstract

Disc degeneration describes the loss of disc height, loss of proteoglycan, disorganization of the extracellular matrix (ECM) architecture, development of annular tears, and herniation of intervertebral disc (IVD) fragments. Risk factors, such as genetic predisposition, decreased nutrient transport, abnormal biomechanics, smoking, and infection have been associated with degeneration of the IVD. These risk factors contribute to the loss of key ECM elements (most notably collagen and aggrecan), changes in disc composition, and loss of the disc tissue organization that is found in healthy IVDs. The breakdown of ECM components in the disc can activate signaling pathways that lead to increased expression of cytokines (e.g., interleukin [IL]-1β, tumor necrosis factor [TNF]-α, IL-6, IL-8, IL-17, and interferon [IFN]-γ). Increased cytokine levels in the degenerative IVD perpetuate disc tissue breakdown by upregulating expression of matrix degrading aggrecanases and proteases, and initiating a deleterious positive feedback loop leading to further expression of inflammatory cytokines in the disc tissue. Additionally, invading immune cells in the IVD contribute to the cascade of degenerative events by producing inflammatory factors in the disc. Furthermore, pathologically elevated cytokine levels promote neovascularization and neoinnervation of the IVD. It is through this complex combination of events, which includes inflammation, innervation, and altered mechanics, that discogenic pain is hypothesized to originate.

Keywords: Disc degeneration, degenerative disc disease, discogenic pain, back pain, intervertebral disc

2.1 Degenerative Disc Disease

Low back pain is the leading cause of disability worldwide[1] and has been linked directly and indirectly to degenerative disc disease (DDD).[2] Low back pain has a global lifetime prevalence of 38.9% and a large socioeconomic impact with estimated annual indirect and direct costs exceeding $100 billion in the United States alone.[3,4] Finding effective treatments for DDD has been difficult due to its complicated pathophysiology and our incomplete knowledge of the underlying processes leading to degeneration of the intervertebral disc (IVD). A number of deleterious factors work together to initiate, exacerbate, and maintain the degenerative process (▶ Fig. 2.1).

Several risk factors have been associated with disc degeneration and include genetic predisposition, decreased nutrient transport, abnormal biomechanics, smoking, and the normal wear and tear of the IVD associated with aging.[5,6,7,8,9] Although the relative importance of each risk factor in initiating DDD is uncertain, these factors initiate a known cascade of molecular mechanisms, described below, leading to the pathological breakdown of the IVD. This chapter discusses the key changes observed in the degenerative disc and the known underlying biological processes that drive those changes.

2.1.1 Composition Changes

Degeneration of the IVD varies with severity[10] and is typically diagnosed via magnetic resonance imaging (MRI),[11] utilizing the Thompson criteria,[12] to grade degeneration based on disc water content, bulging and narrowing of the disc, end plate sclerosis, and osteophyte formation (▶ Fig. 2.2 and ▶ Table 2.1).

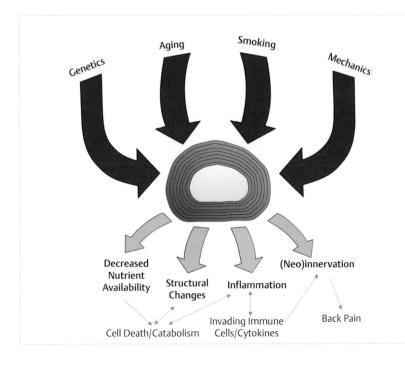

Fig. 2.1 Degenerative disc disease is a complicated process with many factors interacting to lead to the disc pathology that presents in the clinic. This figure demonstrates many of those factors and their interactions.

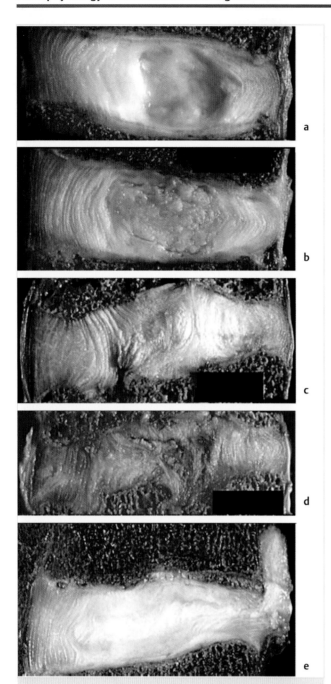

Fig. 2.2 Macroscopic images of the intervertebral disc (IVD) demonstrating multiple grades of disc degeneration.[10] **(a)** Healthy young adult disc with a defined nucleus pulposus (NP). **(b)** Middle age adult disc that is slightly aged but not yet degenerated. **(c)** Moderately degenerated young adult disc. **(d)** Severely degenerated young adult disc. **(e)** Prolapsed middle age adult disc.

Degenerative IVDs exhibit a loss of the transition zone between the nucleus pulposus (NP) and annulus fibrosus (AF) tissue partially caused by changes in collagen expression and synthesis within the disc. Early-stage disc degeneration can induce transient increases in expression of collagen type II,[13] but ultimately shifts to decreased collagen type II and increased collagen type I synthesis in the NP and the inner AF[14,15] as degeneration

progresses. In addition to changes in collagen content, there are also changes in proteoglycan (PG) content that occur with DDD.[16,17,18] PG content in the NP decreases as DDD progresses and results in the dehydration of the NP and formation of fissures beginning in the NP that extend into the AF. Furthermore, the AF of a degenerative IVD is characterized by collagen fiber reorganization,[19] scar/granulation tissue, fissure formation, neovascularization, and neoinnervation.[20,21,22] In addition to a general loss of PG content, there is a shift in the types of PGs found in the disc. Degenerative discs demonstrate increased synthesis of small PGs including versican, biglycan, and decorin,[15,19,23] along with increased degradation of aggrecan and versican, and decreased sulfation. The loss of PG and a shift toward expression of small PGs is linked to decreased hydrostatic pressure observed in degenerated discs. Additionally, the extracellular matrix (ECM) of degenerative discs exhibit increased fibronectin, increased elastin, collagen types X, VI, III, and amyloid.[24] Overall, these changes in matrix components in degenerative discs have deleterious effects on the discs' mechanical properties and ability to properly transmit load. These changes also alter the loads the encapsulated cells experience and have negative effects on the balance of ECM anabolism/catabolism.

2.1.2 Architectural and Mechanical Changes

The unique structure of the NP, AF, and end plates are adapted to perform specific mechanical functions. The interaction between these disc components allows the IVD to transmit mechanical loads while providing constrained flexibility between vertebrae. The NP of the healthy IVD is a hydrated, gel-like core that is constrained radially by the AF tissue and axially by the cartilaginous end plates (▶ Fig. 2.3). The NP is primarily composed of water, PGs, collagen type II, and other minor proteins.[25] The most abundant PG in the IVD, aggrecan,[26] contains keratin sulfate and chondroitin sulfate glycosaminoglycan (GAG) chains that are bound to the aggrecan core protein. This complex binds hyaluronic acid via a link protein to form large molecules that are contained within the type II collagen–rich network.[27] The negatively charged GAG chains of these molecules bind counter-ions, creating an imbalance of ions between the IVD and the surrounding tissue resulting in a large osmotic swelling pressure in the NP, which contributes 70 to 80% of the compressive strength of the IVD.[28] When the disc is compressed axially, water in the NP tissue pressurizes, resulting in a swelling of the NP that is contained axially by the end plates and radially by tension in fibers of the AF tissue[29] (▶ Fig. 2.3). In disc degeneration, aggrecan content in the NP is decreased and compromises the compressive properties of the NP.[18] These changes diminish the ability of the disc to hold water,[30] swell,[9] and subsequently results in reduced disc height. This loss in disc height results in increased strains in the axial direction and causes the compressive load to shift from the NP to the AF, which leads to buckling of the lamellae, an increased bulging of the AF tissue, and a loss of lamellae organization.[31] Furthermore, the loss of osmotic pressure leads to hypermobility of the IVD.[32]

Table 2.1 Thompson's description of the morphological grades of IVD degeneration (Reproduced with permission.[12])

Grade	NP	AF	End plate	Vertebral body
I	Bulging gel	Discrete fibrous lamellae	Hyaline, uniformly thick	Margins rounded
II	White fibrous tissue peripherally	Mucinous material between lamellae	Thickness irregular	Margins pointed
III	Consolidated fibrous tissue	Extensive mucinous infiltration, loss of AF–NP demarcation	Focal defects in cartilage	Early chondrophytes or osteophytes at margins
IV	Horizontal clefts parallel to end plate	Focal disruptions	Fibrocartilage extending from subchondral bone with irregularity and focal sclerosis in subchondral bone	Osteophytes < 2 mm
V	Clefts extend through NP and AF	Clefts extend through NP and AF	Diffuse sclerosis	Osteophytes > 2 mm

Abbreviations: AF, annulus fibrosus; IVD, intervertebral disc; NP, nucleus pulposus.

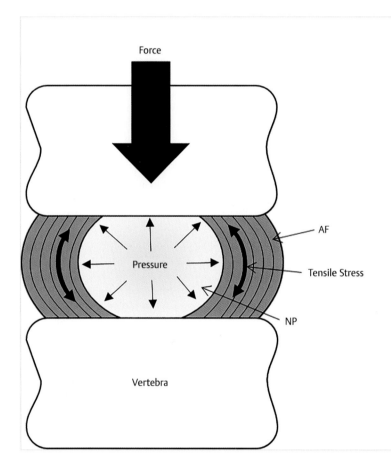

Fig. 2.3 The intervertebral disc (IVD) is a mechanical organ that must resist complex loading in compression, torsion, flexion, and bending. Here we demonstrate how the annulus fibrosus (AF) and nucleus pulposus (NP) interact in the IVD to provide the disc with its compressive mechanical function. When compressive forces are applied to the IVD, the NP becomes pressurized and bulges vertically and radially. This pressurization of the NP results in tensile stresses in the AF in the direction of the collagen organization, which is responsible for containing the NP during this pressurization.

AF tissue composition is similar to that of NP tissue in that its primary components are collagen and PGs; however, the percentage and organization of components differ.[33] The collagen fibers of the AF are organized into concentric lamellae that consist mainly of collagen type I. Moving toward the NP, collagen type II and PG increase in content with collagen type I decreasing. During physiological loading, the AF tissue is subjected to both compressive and tensile stresses, with more compressive loading toward the inner AF and more tensile loading toward the outer AF.[33] Both the collagen content, and the collagen architecture and lamellar organization allow the AF to handle the hoop stresses generated by the bulging of the NP tissue under loading. Collagen fibers of concentric lamellae surrounding the bulging NP are stretched and subjected to tension during loading. In degenerative discs, fissures, replacement of AF tissue with granulation and scar tissue, and loss of fiber orientation decrease the ability of the AF to resist tensile loading.[34,35] In addition, the loss of osmotic pressure, increased collagen cross-linking, and increased collagen type I levels[34] leads to stiffening of the AF. Furthermore, the changes in the NP leads to decreased disc height, a shift of compressive load to the AF, subsequent inward and outward buckling of the lamellae, and increased axial and tensile strains, which increases the likelihood of the AF tearing or rupturing. Overall, the hypermobility of the disc and propensity for herniation during the degenerative process provide a key component to pathology of the IVD and its role in back pain. A more in-depth look at the mechanics of healthy and degenerative IVD can be seen in Chapter 4.

2.1.3 Innervation

The healthy IVD is innervated primarily by afferent nerve fibers limited to the external lamellae[36] of the AF and consist primarily of small myelinated (A-δ) and unmyelinated (C) fibers[36] that are positive for the neuropeptides substance P and calcitonin gene-related peptide (CGRP), indicating that the disc is primarily innervated by small nociceptive fibers.[36] In the degenerative IVD, nerve fibers extend into typically aneural regions of the inner AF and NP tissue and, in some cases, are accompanied by neovascularization and granulation tissue.[37,38] In the degenerative disc, the increased expression of nerve growth factor (NGF) and loss of chondroitin sulfate create an environment conducive to neoinnervation.[39] Furthermore, degenerative discs exhibit increased levels of inflammatory cytokines, such as interleukin (IL)-1β, IL-6, and tumor necrosis factor (TNF)-α, which have been shown to sensitize nociceptive neurons to noxious stimuli including heating[40] and mechanical loading[41] in radiculopathy models. Furthermore, recent reports demonstrate that IL-6 released from degenerative discs sensitizes neurons to noxious stimuli,[42] suggesting cytokines from degenerative IVD may contribute to back pain by sensitizing nociceptive neurons to noxious stimuli. Overall, the interactions between these nociceptive neurons and the degenerative IVD are a key component for the development of discogenic back pain but are currently poorly understood and are a major area of ongoing research.

2.2 Underlying Biological Processes

2.2.1 IVD Cell Metabolism

The structural, mechanical, and morphological changes that result due to disc degeneration are regulated by cells in the disc, which respond to their environment to mediate the structural and compositional changes that are observed during disc degeneration. At birth, cells within the IVD are composed of fibroblast-like cells in the AF, chondrocyte-like cells in the end plate, and a mix of notochordal and chondrocyte-like cells in the NP.[43] As the disc matures over the first 10 years of life, the notochordal cells within the NP disappear and leave only chondrocyte-like cells.[44] This loss of notochordal cells has been speculated to have direct consequences on the ECM composition of the IVD. These notochordal cells have been linked to a number of anabolic activities, which include the synthesis of growth factors, the stimulation of IVD cell proliferation, the elevated synthesis of collagen type II and aggrecan,[45] and the decrease in matrix metalloproteinases (MMP)-3 and MMP-13 expression.[46,47] It has been hypothesized that the loss of notochordal cells leads to decreased cell proliferation, decreased production of PGs, decreased collagen type II production, and increased tissue catabolism.

The alterations in the PG and collagen content in the NP, that occur with aging and degeneration, lead to changes in the osmotic and hydrostatic pressure, which can have deleterious effects on cell function. For example, decreased hydrostatic pressure observed in the degenerative IVD leads to decreased (20–40%) NP PG production, increased MMP-3 production, and upregulated tissue inhibitors of matrix metalloproteinase (TIMP) production.[48] Similarly, the decreased osmotic pressure of degenerative IVDs leads to decreased PG production by NP cells.[49] The end plates respond to low hydrostatic pressure by entering hypertrophic conversion, which leads to type X collagen production and eventually end plate calcification.[50] This calcification can lead to a decreased supply of oxygen and nutrients to the NP and produce an increase in NP acidity, and ultimately a decrease in viable cells.[51] In addition to a decrease in cell viability being associated with DDD, an increase in the number of senescent cells has been found in the degenerative disc.[52] These senescent cells show a decrease in anabolism and no longer divide to replace the cells lost to apoptosis. Additionally, these senescent cells produce increased levels of cytokines and matrix-degrading enzymes.[53] Overall, changes that move the IVD away from its healthy state tend to decrease anabolism and increase catabolism in the IVD cell population.

2.2.2 Immune Cells and Inflammatory Cytokines

It has been well established that there is an elevated level of pro-inflammatory cytokines in degenerative and herniated discs.[38] These increased cytokine levels are a cellular response to decreased nutrient availability and the presence of invading immune cells.[37] The cells involved with the production and secretion of these pro-inflammatory molecules include NP cells, AF cells, macrophages, T cells, and neutrophils.[38] The pro-inflammatory molecules they secrete result in numerous pathological changes in the IVD, including cell senescence/apoptosis of IVD cells,[54,55] breakdown of ECM,[56] increased expression of cytokines, increased expression of neurotrophic factors,[21] recruitment of immune cells,[57] angiogenesis, neoinnervation of the disc, and sensitization of neurons to noxious stimuli.[42]

Many of these pathological changes are induced by the presence of immune cells in the IVD. Studies done on degenerative or herniated discs from patient samples have shown that there is a presence of invading CD 68 + macrophages, neutrophils, and T cells (CD 4+ and CD 8+) within the degenerative disc.[37,58] Concurrent with immune cell invasion, degenerative IVDs exhibit increased levels of the chemokines CCL2, CCL3, CCL4, CCL5, CCL7, CCL13, CXCL10, and IL-8,[38,57] which promote recruitment of macrophages, neutrophils, and T cells. The accompaniment of invading immune cells by angiogenesis suggests macrophages enter the herniated or degenerative IVD via blood vessels in an attempted healing response.[37,59] Consequently, these immune cells stimulate the expression of pro-inflammatory cytokines and NGF by NP cells.[60] NGF expression can lead to dorsal root ganglion (DRG) neurons expressing neuronal pain–associated cation channels, which may provide a link to disc degeneration and low back pain.[61,62] Overall, once these immune cells are recruited to the degenerative disc, they further elevate the level of inflammatory cytokines, which propagates a catabolic environment in the disc.

There are multiple cytokines that have been shown to propagate the inflammatory environment in the degenerative disc. The inflammatory cytokines that have been studied and associated with disc degeneration include TNF-α, IL-1α, IL-1β, IL-2, IL-4, IL-6, IL-10, IL-17, and interferon-γ (IFN-γ).[38] The two most commonly studied cytokines are TNF-α, and IL-1β, which both induce inflammatory signaling and cell apoptosis through their respective receptors, TNFR1 and IL1R1. Signaling through both of these receptors is known to cause activation of the transcription factor NF-κB, which induces the expression of a number of pro-inflammatory and catabolic target genes involved with the breakdown of IVD tissue (▶ Fig. 2.4).[63,64] It is believed that TNF-α and IL-1β play important roles in tissue breakdown mediated by NF-κB activity, as these cytokines have been linked to IVD degradation in numerous studies and blocking NF-κB activity has been shown to reduce degradation in rodent models of disc degeneration.[65,66,67] Although TNF-α and IL-1β have been heavily associated with disc

degeneration, in one study, increased levels of TNFR1 expression was only found in herniated discs, which indicates disease-specific roles for TNF-α and IL-1β in the degenerative process.[66] Additionally, this indicates that inflammatory signaling is being regulated by both the specific expression of cytokines and the expression of specific receptors. In addition to mediating tissue breakdown, TNF-α and IL-1β are also involved with production of chemokines that promote recruitment of immune cells. IVD cells cultured with these two cytokines exhibit increased expression of pro-inflammatory chemokines, (i.e., CCL3 and CCL5), shown to be elevated in degenerate discs.[57,68] Overall, the body of literature implicates TNF-α and IL-1β in the processes of catabolism, inflammation, angiogenesis, and neoinnervation that characterize DDD.

Additional cytokines that have shown prominent roles in disc degeneration are IL-6, IL-17, IFN-γ, and IL-8. In NP cells, it has been shown that IL-6 along with its soluble receptor sIL-6R potentiates the catabolic activity of TNF-α and IL-1β.[69] In addition, IL-6 has been shown to be predictive of pain sensitivity in a model of neuropathy and IL-6 produced by degenerative disc tissue has been implicated in the sensitization of nociceptive neurons to noxious stimuli.[42,70] Therefore IL-6 is not only tied

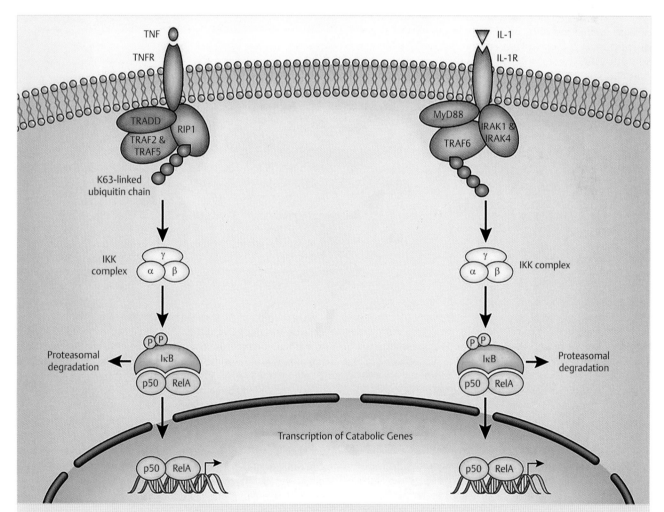

Fig. 2.4 Signaling pathway of TNFR1 and IL1R1 demonstrating how activation of NF-κB occurs through the proteasomal degradation of IκB. This allows NF-κB to translocate to the nucleus where it activates catabolic target genes, which include inflammatory cytokines, aggrecanases, and proteases. (Adapted with permission from Macmillan Publishers Ltd: [Nat Immunol][63] copyright [2011].)

to catabolic activity but also to nociception within the degenerative IVD. IL-17 is involved with the recruitment of monocytes and neutrophils to the inflamed disc by increasing the secretion of chemokines and enhancing inflammation synergistically with TNF-α, and IL-1β.[71] IFN-γ is secreted by invading T cells and macrophages and together with IL-17 synergistically increases the expression of inflammatory mediators in the disc.[72,73] Lastly, IL-8 has been shown to play an important role in the pain generation pathway, as it has been shown that its co-inhibition with TNF-α decreases symptoms of mechanical hyperalgesia in disc autograft models.[74] In summary, these cytokines increase in response to the degenerative changes in the disc, upregulate inflammation, increase catabolic activity, induce neoinnervation and angiogenesis, and likely play a role in nociceptor sensitization (▶ Fig. 2.5). Many of these cytokines directly or indirectly lead to the upregulation of NF-κB, which induces the increased expression of aggrecanases and proteases that result in the direct breakdown of ECM in the IVD.[64] Overall, immune and inflammatory processes have been demonstrated to be key mediators of the degenerative process.

2.2.3 Proteases and Aggrecanases

Disc degeneration is associated with the upregulation of multiple aggrecanases and MMPs, which include disintegrin-like and metalloprotease with thrombospondin motifs ADAMTS-4, ADAMTS-5, ADAMTS-7, ADAMTS-12, MMP-1, MMP-2, MMP-3, MMP-9, MMP-13, and MMP-14.[75] The increased cytokine levels in the degenerative disc induce this protease upregulation. For example, NP cells from degenerated discs treated with TNF-α, IL-6, sIL-6 R, and IL-1β show a significant upregulation of MMP-13.[69] Furthermore, the NF-κB mediated pathways discussed in the previous section upregulate multiple MMPs and aggrecanases. A recent in vitro study on human NP cells demonstrated that inhibition of NF-κB decreased IL-1β–induced upregulation of MMP-3, MMP-9, MMP-13, ADAMTS-4, and ADAMTS-5.[76] This

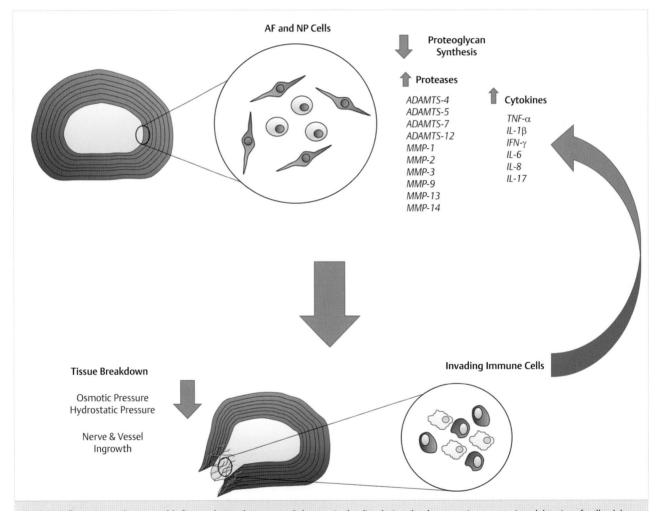

Fig. 2.5 Cells are primarily responsible for regulating the structural changes in the disc during the degenerative process in a deleterious feedback loop. Cells upregulate the expression of cytokines and proteases in the disc in addition to downregulating expression of critical proteoglycans that are involved with the maintenance of disc height and general mechanical function of the intervertebral disc. The upregulation of proteases results in further tissue breakdown and alterations to the disc environment that promotes inflammation and catabolism. This process results in the recruitment of immune cells that induce further upregulation of inflammatory cytokines along with angiogenesis and nociceptive nerve ingrowth. Once this cycle is entered, it is difficult to reverse the changes observed. Abbreviations: ADAMTS, disintegrin-like and metalloprotease with thrombospondin motifs; IL, interleukin; MMP, matrix metalloproteinase; TNF, tumor necrosis factor; IFN, interferon.

result can also be observed after TNF-α–induced NF-κB activity, which increases ADAMTS-4 and ADAMTS-5 expression and subsequently results in the degradation of collagen type II and aggrecan.[77] This link between cytokine and protease expression illustrates the cycle of disc degeneration, where inflammation induced by the initiating events induces further breakdown of the tissue.

2.2.4 Disc Nutrition

The nutrient supply of the IVD is provided via diffusion from blood vessels in vertebral bodies, through the cartilaginous end plates, and into the IVD. During the process of normal aging, the IVD nutrient supply is reduced by decreased vertebral body capillary density, integrity, and end plate calcification.[78] End plate calcification is hypothesized to drive disc degeneration by reducing nutrient transport between the disc and vertebral bodies; however, recent studies showing increased end plate and trabecular porosity in degenerative IVDs suggest capillary transport phenomena rather than end plate calcification cause decreased nutrient levels in degenerative IVDs.[79,80]

Transport of glucose, oxygen, and lactic acid is believed to be a driver of disc degeneration. IVD cells predominately produce energy via glycolysis even when oxygen is present.[81] Inadequate oxygen transport into IVDs, or removal of lactic acid from IVDs, may cause a noxious environment for the IVD cells. Severe drops in pH have been shown to cause cell death,[51] whereas less severe pH drops impact cell metabolism.[82] Similar drops in pH and nutrient levels observed in the degenerative IVD suggest that decreased IVD nutrient levels slows cell metabolism leading to the characteristic imbalance of catabolic and anabolic events in the degenerative IVD. Furthermore, finite element models have demonstrated that limited nutrient supply affects disc cell viability and metabolic activity, suggesting that glucose limitation and a decrease in pH are primary mediators of cell metabolism in degeneration.[83,84] Whereas disc cells can survive for at least 2 weeks without oxygen, disc cells exhibit cellular inactivity[51] and a loss of matrix synthesis[81] under hypoxic conditions, indicating that low pH, low glucose, and low oxygen provide an environment conducive to disc degeneration.

2.3 Conclusion

A delicate balance of biological processes maintains the healthy function of the IVD. In disc degeneration, altered mechanical loading, breakdown of disc tissue, inflammation, and altered nutrient supply in the disc interact to create a deleterious positive feedback loop that disrupts this balance and perpetuates disc degeneration. Discogenic pain is hypothesized to result from the interactions between the altered mechanics, inflammation, and neoinnervation of the degenerative disc.

2.4 References

[1] Murray CJ, Vos T, Lozano R, et al. Disability-adjusted life years (DALYs) for 291 diseases and injuries in 21 regions, 1990–2010: a systematic analysis for the Global Burden of Disease Study 2010. Lancet. 2012; 380(9859):2197–2223

[2] U.S. Department of Health and Human Services. Low back pain. 2015. http://www.ninds.nih.gov/disorders/backpain/low-back-pain-brochure.pdf. Accessed July 21, 2015

[3] Hoy D, Bain C, Williams G, et al. A systematic review of the global prevalence of low back pain. Arthritis Rheum. 2012; 64(6):2028–2037

[4] Katz, JN. Lumbar disc disorders and low-back pain: socioeconomic factors and consequences. J Bone Joint Surg Am. 2006; 88 Suppl 2:21–24

[5] Mayer JE, Iatridis JC, Chan D, Qureshi SA, Gottesman O, Hecht AC. Genetic polymorphisms associated with intervertebral disc degeneration. Spine J. 2013; 13(3):299–317

[6] Williams FMK, Bansal AT, van Meurs JB, et al. Novel genetic variants associated with lumbar disc degeneration in northern Europeans: a meta-analysis of 4600 subjects. Ann Rheum Dis. 2013; 72(7):1141–1148

[7] Shirazi-Adl A, Taheri M, Urban JPG. Analysis of cell viability in intervertebral disc: effect of endplate permeability on cell population. J Biomech. 2010; 43 (7):1330–1336

[8] Wang Y, Videman T, Battié MC. ISSLS prize winner: lumbar vertebral endplate lesions: associations with disc degeneration and back pain history. Spine. 2012; 37(17):1490–1496

[9] Adams MA, Roughley PJ. What is intervertebral disc degeneration, and what causes it? Spine. 2006; 31(18):2151–2161

[10] Adams M. Anatomy and physiology of the lumbar intervertebral disc and endplates. In: The Lumbar Intervertebral Disc. New York: Thieme Medical Publishers; 2010:14

[11] Pfirrmann CW, Metzdorf A, Zanetti M, Hodler J, Boos N. Magnetic resonance classification of lumbar intervertebral disc degeneration. Spine. 2001; 26 (17):1873–1878

[12] Thompson JP, Pearce RH, Schechter MT, Adams ME, Tsang IK, Bishop PB. Preliminary evaluation of a scheme for grading the gross morphology of the human intervertebral disc. Spine. 1990; 15(5):411–415

[13] Takaishi H, Nemoto O, Shiota M, et al. Type-II collagen gene expression is transiently upregulated in experimentally induced degeneration of rabbit intervertebral disc. J Orthop Res. 1997; 15(4):528–538

[14] Schollmeier G, Lahr-Eigen R, Lewandrowski KU. Observations on fiber-forming collagens in the anulus fibrosus. Spine. 2000; 25(21):2736–2741

[15] Le Maitre CL, Pockert A, Buttle DJ, Freemont AJ, Hoyland JA. Matrix synthesis and degradation in human intervertebral disc degeneration. BiochemSoc Trans. 2007; 35(Pt 4):652–655

[16] Cs-Szabo G, Ragasa-San Juan D, Turumella V, Masuda K, Thonar EJ-MA, An HS. Changes in mRNA and protein levels of proteoglycans of the anulus fibrosus and nucleus pulposus during intervertebral disc degeneration. Spine. 2002; 27(20):2212–2219

[17] Sztrolovics R, Grover J, Cs-Szabo G, et al. The characterization of versican and its message in human articular cartilage and intervertebral disc. J Orthop Res. 2002; 20(2):257–266

[18] Sztrolovics R, Alini M, Roughley PJ, Mort JS. Aggrecan degradation in human intervertebral disc and articular cartilage. Biochem J. 1997; 326(Pt 1):235–241

[19] Lyons G, Eisenstein SM, Sweet MB. Biochemical changes in intervertebral disc degeneration. Biochim Biophys Acta. 1981; 673(4):443–453

[20] Peng B, Hao J, Hou S, et al. Possible pathogenesis of painful intervertebral disc degeneration. Spine. 2006; 31(5):560–566

[21] Freemont AJ, Watkins A, Le Maitre C, et al. Nerve growth factor expression and innervation of the painful intervertebral disc. J Pathol. 2002; 197 (3):286–292

[22] Freemont AJ, Peacock TE, Goupille P, Hoyland JA, O'Brien J, Jayson MI. Nerve ingrowth into diseased intervertebral disc in chronic back pain. Lancet. 1997; 350(9072):178–181

[23] Buckwalter, JA. Aging and degeneration of the human intervertebral disc. Spine. 1995; 20(11):1307–1314

[24] Roberts S, Evans H, Trivedi J, Menage J. Histology and pathology of the human intervertebral disc. J Bone Joint Surg Am. 2006; 88 Suppl 2:10–14

[25] Adams P, Muir H. Qualitative changes with age of proteoglycans of human lumbar discs. Ann Rheum Dis. 1976; 35(4):289–296

[26] Melrose J, Ghosh P, Taylor TK. A comparative analysis of the differential spatial and temporal distributions of the large (aggrecan, versican) and small (decorin, biglycan, fibromodulin) proteoglycans of the intervertebral disc. J Anat. 2001; 198(Pt 1):3–15

[27] Kiani C, Chen L, Wu YJ, Yee AJ, Yang BB. Structure and function of aggrecan. Cell Res. 2002; 12(1):19–32

[28] Perie DS, Maclean JJ, Owen JP, Iatridis JC. Correlating material properties with tissue composition in enzymatically digested bovine annulus fibrosus and nucleus pulposus tissue. Ann Biomed Eng. 2006; 34(5):769–777

[29] Ebara S, Iatridis JC, Setton LA, Foster RJ, Mow VC, Weidenbaum M. Tensile properties of nondegenerate human lumbar anulus fibrosus. Spine. 1996; 21 (4):452–461

[30] Roughley PJ. Biology of intervertebral disc aging and degeneration: involvement of the extracellular matrix. Spine. 2004; 29(23):2691–2699

[31] O'Connell GD, Vresilovic EJ, Elliott DM. Human intervertebral disc internal strain in compression: the effect of disc region, loading position, and degeneration. J Orthop Res. 2011; 29(4):547–555

[32] O'Connell GD, Johannessen W, Vresilovic EJ, Elliott DM. Human internal disc strains in axial compression measured noninvasively using magnetic resonance imaging. Spine. 2007; 32(25):2860–2868

[33] Eyre DR, Muir H. Types I and II collagens in intervertebral disc. Interchanging radial distributions in annulus fibrosus. Biochem J. 1976; 157(1):267–270

[34] Guerin HAL, Elliott DM. Degeneration affects the fiber reorientation of human annulus fibrosus under tensile load. J Biomech. 2006; 39(8):1410–1418

[35] Hickey DS, Hukins DW. Relation between the structure of the annulus fibrosus and the function and failure of the intervertebral disc. Spine. 1980; 5(2):106–116

[36] García-Cosamalón J, del Valle ME, Calavia MG, et al. Intervertebral disc, sensory nerves and neurotrophins: who is who in discogenic pain? J Anat. 2010; 217(1):1–15

[37] Kokubo Y, Uchida K, Kobayashi S, et al. Herniated and spondylotic intervertebral discs of the human cervical spine: histological and immunohistological findings in 500 en bloc surgical samples. Laboratory investigation. J Neurosurg Spine. 2008; 9(3):285–295

[38] Risbud MV, Shapiro IM. Role of cytokines in intervertebral disc degeneration: pain and disc content. Nat Rev Rheumatol. 2014; 10(1):44–56

[39] Johnson WEB, Caterson B, Eisenstein SM, Hynds DL, Snow DM, Roberts S. Human intervertebral disc aggrecan inhibits nerve growth in vitro. Arthritis Rheum. 2002; 46(10):2658–2664

[40] Oprée A, Kress M. Involvement of the proinflammatory cytokines tumor necrosis factor-alpha, IL-1 beta, and IL-6 but not IL-8 in the development of heat hyperalgesia: effects on heat-evoked calcitonin gene-related peptide release from rat skin. J Neurosci. 2000; 20(16):6289–6293

[41] Brenn D, Richter F, Schaible H-G. Sensitization of unmyelinated sensory fibers of the joint nerve to mechanical stimuli by interleukin-6 in the rat: an inflammatory mechanism of joint pain. Arthritis Rheum. 2007; 56(1):351–359

[42] Stover JD, Bah I, Kotelsky A, Buckley MR, Bowles RD. Conditioned media from degenerative intervertebral discs sensitize dorsal root ganglion neurons to heat stimuli. Proc Summer Biomech Bioeng Biotransport Conf 2015: Abstract 1040

[43] Colombier P, Clouet J, Hamel O, Lescaudron L, Guicheux J. The lumbar intervertebral disc: from embryonic development to degeneration. Joint Bone Spine. 2014; 81(2):125–129

[44] Boos N, Weissbach S, Rohrbach H, Weiler C, Spratt KF, Nerlich AG. Classification of age-related changes in lumbar intervertebral discs: 2002 Volvo Award in basic science. Spine. 2002; 27(23):2631–2644

[45] Erwin WM, Ashman K, O'Donnel P, Inman RD. Nucleus pulposus notochord cells secrete connective tissue growth factor and up-regulate proteoglycan expression by intervertebral disc chondrocytes. Arthritis Rheum. 2006; 54(12):3859–3867

[46] de Vries SAH, Potier E, van Doeselaar M, Meij BP, Tryfonidou MA, Ito K. Conditioned medium derived from notochordal cell-rich nucleus pulposus tissue stimulates matrix production by canine nucleus pulposus cells and bone marrow-derived stromal cells. Tissue Eng Part A. 2015; 21(5–6):1077–1084

[47] Erwin WM, Islam D, Inman RD, Fehlings MG, Tsui FWL. Notochordal cells protect nucleus pulposus cells from degradation and apoptosis: implications for the mechanisms of intervertebral disc degeneration. Arthritis Res Ther. 2011; 13(6):R215

[48] Handa, T, Ishihara, H, Ohshima, H, Osada, R, Tsuji, H, Obata, K. Effects of hydrostatic pressure on matrix synthesis and matrix metalloproteinase production in the human lumbar intervertebral disc. Spine. 1997; 22(10):1085–1091

[49] Ishihara H, Warensjo K, Roberts S, Urban JP. Proteoglycan synthesis in the intervertebral disk nucleus: the role of extracellular osmolality. Am J Physiol. 1997; 272(5 Pt 1):C1499–C1506

[50] Nerlich AG, Schleicher ED, Boos N. 1997 Volvo Award winner in basic science studies. Immunohistologic markers for age-related changes of human lumbar intervertebral discs. Spine. 1997; 22(24):2781–2795

[51] Horner HA, Urban JP. 2001 Volvo Award Winner in Basic Science Studies: effect of nutrient supply on the viability of cells from the nucleus pulposus of the intervertebral disc. Spine. 2001; 26(23):2543–2549

[52] Gruber HE, Ingram JA, Norton HJ, Hanley EN , Jr. Senescence in cells of the aging and degenerating intervertebral disc: immunolocalization of senescence-associated beta-galactosidase in human and sand rat discs. Spine. 2007; 32(3):321–327

[53] Campisi J, d'Adda di Fagagna F. Cellular senescence: when bad things happen to good cells. Nat Rev Mol Cell Biol. 2007; 8(9):729–740

[54] Purmessur D, Walter BA, Roughley PJ, Laudier DM, Hecht AC, Iatridis J. A role for TNF in intervertebral disc degeneration: a non-recoverable catabolic shift. Biochem Biophys Res Commun. 2013; 433(1):151–156

[55] Zhao C-Q, Liu D, Li H, Jiang L-S, Dai L-Y. Interleukin-1beta enhances the effect of serum deprivation on rat annular cell apoptosis. Apoptosis. 2007; 12(12):2155–2161

[56] Risbud MV, Shapiro IM. Role of cytokines in intervertebral disc degeneration: pain and disc content. Nat Rev Rheumatol. 201 4; 10(1):44–56

[57] Kepler CK, Markova DZ, Dibra F, et al. Expression and relationship of proinflammatory chemokine RANTES/CCL5 and cytokine IL-1 in painful human intervertebral discs. Spine. 2013; 38(11):873–880

[58] Shamji MF, Setton LA, Jarvis W, et al. Proinflammatory cytokine expression profile in degenerated and herniated human intervertebral disc tissues. Arthritis Rheum. 2010; 62(7):1974–1982

[59] Vernon-Roberts B, Moore RJ, Fraser RD. The natural history of age-related disc degeneration: the pathology and sequelae of tears. Spine. 2007; 32(25):2797–2804

[60] Abe Y, Akeda K, An HS, et al. Proinflammatory cytokines stimulate the expression of nerve growth factor by human intervertebral disc cells. Spine. 2007; 32(6):635–642

[61] Ohtori S, Inoue G, Koshi T, et al. Up-regulation of acid-sensing ion channel 3 in dorsal root ganglion neurons following application of nucleus pulposus on nerve root in rats. Spine. 2006; 31(18):2048–2052

[62] Zhang X, Huang J, McNaughton PA. NGF rapidly increases membrane expression of TRPV1 heat-gated ion channels. EMBO J. 2005; 24(24):4211–4223

[63] Pelzer C, Thome M. IKK takes control of canonical NF-B activation. Nat Immunol. 2011; 12(9):815–816

[64] Wuertz K, Vo N, Kletsas D, Boos N. Inflammatory and catabolic signalling in intervertebral discs: the roles of NF-B and MAP kinases. Eur Cell Mater. 2012; 23:103–119, discussion 119–120

[65] Le Maitre CL, Hoyland JA, Freemont AJ. Catabolic cytokine expression in degenerate and herniated human intervertebral discs: IL-1beta and TNFalpha expression profile. Arthritis Res Ther. 2007; 9(4):R77

[66] Andrade P, Visser-Vandewalle V, Philippens M, et al. Tumor necrosis factor-levels correlate with postoperative pain severity in lumbar disc hernia patients: opposite clinical effects between tumor necrosis factor receptor 1 and 2. Pain. 2011; 152(11):2645–2652

[67] Nasto LA, Seo H-Y, Robinson AR, et al. ISSLS prize winner: inhibition of NF-B activity ameliorates age-associated disc degeneration in a mouse model of accelerated aging. Spine. 2012; 37(21):1819–1825

[68] Wang J, Tian Y, Phillips KLE, et al. Tumor necrosis factor - and interleukin-1-dependent induction of CCL3 expression by nucleus pulposus cells promotes macrophage migration through CCR1. Arthritis Rheum. 2013; 65(3):832–842

[69] Studer RK, Vo N, Sowa G, Ondeck C, Kang J. Human nucleus pulposus cells react to IL-6: independent actions and amplification of response to IL-1 and TNF-. Spine. 2011; 36(8):593–599

[70] Bowles RD, Karikari IO, VanDerwerken DN, et al. In vivo luminescent imaging of NF-B activity and NF-B-related serum cytokine levels predict pain sensitivities in a rodent model of peripheral neuropathy. Eur J Pain. 2016; 20(3):365–376

[71] Gaffen SL. Recent advances in the IL-17 cytokine family. Curr Opin Immunol. 2011; 23(5):613–619

[72] Schroder K, Hertzog PJ, Ravasi T, Hume DA. Interferon-gamma: an overview of signals, mechanisms and functions. J Leukoc Biol. 2004; 75(2):163–189

[73] Gabr MA, Jing L, Helbling AR, et al. Interleukin-17 synergizes with IFN or TNF to promote inflammatory mediator release and intercellular adhesion molecule-1 (ICAM-1) expression in human intervertebral disc cells. J Orthop Res. 2011; 29(1):1–7

[74] Takada T, Nishida K, Maeno K, et al. Intervertebral disc and macrophage interaction induces mechanical hyperalgesia and cytokine production in a herniated disc model in rats. Arthritis Rheum. 2012; 64(8):2601–2610

[75] Wang W-J, Yu X-H, Wang C, et al. MMPs and ADAMTSs in intervertebral disc degeneration. Clin Chim Acta. 2015; 448:238–246

[76] Zhongyi S, Sai Z, Chao L, Jiwei T. Effects of nuclear factor kappa B signaling pathway in human intervertebral disc degeneration. Spine. 2015; 40(4):224–232

[77] Wang Z, Hutton WC, Yoon ST. Bone morphogenetic protein-7 antagonizes tumor necrosis factor–induced activation of nuclear factor B and up-regulation of the ADAMTS, leading to decreased degradation of disc matrix macromolecules aggrecan and collagen II. Spine J. 2014; 14(3):505–512

[78] Bernick S, Cailliet R. Vertebral end-plate changes with aging of human vertebrae. Spine. 1982; 7(2):97–102

[79] Rodriguez AG, Slichter CK, Acosta FL, et al. Human disc nucleus properties and vertebral endplate permeability. Spine. 2011; 36(7):512–520

[80] Rodriguez AG, Rodriguez-Soto AE, Burghardt AJ, Berven S, Majumdar S, Lotz JC. Morphology of the human vertebral endplate. J Orthop Res. 2012; 30 (2):280–287

[81] Ishihara H, Urban JP. Effects of low oxygen concentrations and metabolic inhibitors on proteoglycan and protein synthesis rates in the intervertebral disc. J Orthop Res. 1999; 17(6):829–835

[82] Ohshima H, Urban JP. The effect of lactate and pH on proteoglycan and protein synthesis rates in the intervertebral disc. Spine. 1992; 17(9):1079–1082

[83] Malandrino A, Noailly J, Lacroix D. The effect of sustained compression on oxygen metabolic transport in the intervertebral disc decreases with degenerative changes. PLOS Comput Biol. 2011; 7(8):e1002112

[84] Jackson AR, Huang C-Y, Gu WY. Effect of endplate calcification and mechanical deformation on the distribution of glucose in intervertebral disc: a 3D finite element study. Comput Methods Biomech Biomed Engin. 2011; 14 (2):195–204

3 Imaging of the Healthy and Diseased Spinal Disc

Darryl B. Sneag and Hollis G. Potter

Abstract

Magnetic resonance imaging (MRI) plays a critical role in evaluating degenerative disc disease (DDD) and detecting other potential pain generators. As disc degeneration is prevalent in asymptomatic individuals, it is important for the managing physician to carefully correlate MRI findings with patient symptomatology.

Effective MRI evaluation of the spine, and specifically the intervertebral disc (IVD), requires an understanding of image acquisition and the normal appearance of both the disc and its adjacent endplates. This chapter provides a basic protocol, and its underlying rationale, for a spine MRI. It briefly summarizes quantitative MRI techniques to assess disc degeneration that are still largely research tools but may in the future play important roles in early disease detection and management. It also explains widely accepted classification schemes for grading disc and endplate degeneration.

A discussion of disc herniation nomenclature and appropriate descriptors is accompanied by relevant imaging examples and schematics, where appropriate, to help highlight important concepts. Finally, the chapter provides a description and imaging examples of more unusual disc pathology, which are sometimes encountered during routine MRI exams of the lumbar spine.

Keywords: disc degeneration, herniation, Modic classification, MRI, Pfirrmann classification, quantitative MRI, T1-rho, T2 mapping

3.1 Historical Perspective

Back pain is extremely prevalent in the general population, affecting up to 85% of individuals at some point in their lives.[1] Degenerative disc disease (DDD) is a common cause of both back pain and radicular symptoms and is a leading culprit of chronic disability in the working population.[2] DDD refers to biochemical and structural alterations of the disc under physiological and pathological stresses that result in collagen degradation and proteoglycan (PG) and water matrix depletion.

Historically, imaging of discogenic pain involved the combination of radiography and myelography and more recently, discography and computed tomography (CT) myelography. Although such studies are still ordered to evaluate back pain, these modalities fail to detect many types of disc pathology that magnetic resonance imaging (MRI) can demonstrate.[3] MRI is uniquely suited to evaluate disc degeneration and its associated pathology given its high contrast resolution, direct multiplanar capabilities, and lack of ionizing radiation. A large retrospective study evaluating 111 MR examination cases from the Spine Patient Outcomes Research Trial (SPORT) found MRI to be reliable in assessing nondisc contour degenerative findings of the lumbar spine.[4] The relationships between abnormalities detected by MRI and symptomatology, however, are controversial and incompletely understood,[4,5] and multiple studies have documented extensive imaging pathology in asymptomatic individuals.[6,7,8]

Quantitative, parametric MRI mapping sequences such as T1-rho[9] and T2* mapping,[10] ultrashort time-to-echo (UTE),[11] and diffusion weighted imaging (DWI),[12] including diffusion tensor imaging (DTI), may be able to bridge this knowledge gap by providing information about the microstructure of the intervertebral disc (IVD) and cartilaginous endplate and identify early biomarkers of DDD not detectable with conventional techniques (▶ Fig. 3.1). As these advanced imaging techniques are mainly used for research purposes and not for routine clinical practice, they lie beyond this chapter's scope. This chapter's goal is to describe and illustrate the role of conventional MRI in evaluating disc pathology, focusing on the lumbar motion segments.

3.2 MR Imaging Acquisition

At the authors' institution, all spine MRI exams are obtained on high field strength 1.5 or 3.0 T systems using dedicated surface coil arrays. For the lumbar spine, this typically involves sagittal

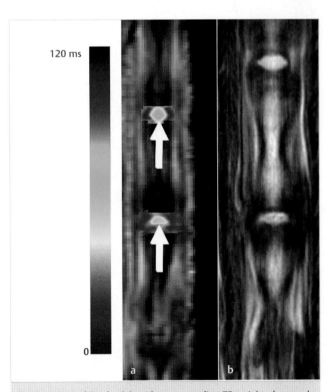

Fig. 3.1 Coronal T1-rho (a), with corresponding T2-weighted coronal fast spin echo (b), magnetic resonance imaging of the intervertebral discs of a tail of a healthy rat demonstrates higher T1-rho relaxation times of the central nucleus pulposus (*arrows*) compared with the peripheral annulus fibrosus, reflecting higher proteoglycan content of the nucleus and greater restriction of water and extracellular matrix molecules in the fibrocartilaginous annulus.

short tau inversion recovery (STIR) and T1-weighted fast spin echo (FSE) sequences, as well as axial, coronal, and sagittal T2-weighted techniques. The STIR sequence is used to detect bone marrow edema patterns, indicating stress reaction or fracture, as well as soft tissue abnormalities such as spinal cord and nerve root edema, annular fissures, facet joint cysts, and fascial/intramuscular edema. The coronal sequence is helpful to confirm transitional lumbosacral anatomy, assess coronal balance, and detect extraforaminal disc herniations. At our institution, axial sequences are obtained in multiple overlapped slices without gaps and parallel to the disc space, to best evaluate the degree of central stenosis and disc contour, and in the cervical spine to also assess the degree of neural foraminal stenosis. Protocols in which axial sequences are prescribed only through the disc space, with gaps between disc spaces, may fail to include a disc sequestration or extrusion extending cephalocaudal to the disc space (▶ Fig. 3.2). In the cervical spine, the coronal sequence is replaced with a 2D gradient recalled echo sequence to help differentiate between posterior endplate osseous remodeling and ridges, which are low signal intensity, and disc herniations, which are typically of higher signal intensity. Gadolinium T1-weighted sequences have a role both in the pre- and postoperative setting, but for disc pathology they are typically used to differentiate between postoperative epidural fibrosis, which will enhance, and residual or recurrent disc herniation, which will not enhance.[13] In the presence of metallic hardware, imaging parameters of conventional sequences are optimized to reduce susceptibility effects. Dedicated metal artifact reduction sequences developed mainly for arthroplasty imaging, such as MAVRIC (multiacquisition variable resonance image combination) and SEMAC (slice-encoding metal artifact correction), with proton-density weighting or inversion recovery, can also be employed to further reduce susceptibility effects (▶ Fig. 3.3).[14]

3.3 Disc Degeneration Pathoanatomy

The discovertebral complex is formed by the intervertebral disc (IVD) and its adjacent cartilaginous endplate. The disc comprises an inner nucleus pulposus (NP), eccentrically located toward the posterior disc margin, and peripheral annulus fibrosus (AF), which is attached to the cartilaginous endplates. The NP contains mostly water and proteoglycans in a loose network

of type II collagen, whereas the AF is a dense, fibrocartilaginous structure comprised mostly of type I collagen. The term *degeneration*, as defined by Modic et al., refers to various disc pathology including desiccation, fibrosis, disc space narrowing, annular fissuring, endplate changes, and osteophytes at the vertebral apophyses.[2]

3.4 Disc Degeneration Classification

Pfirrmann et al. developed a five-level grading scheme to describe lumbar disc degeneration using midsagittal T2-weighted FSE imaging and demonstrated adequate intra- and interobserver reliability to discriminate between the different grades (▶ Fig. 3.4).[15] The normal disc (Grade I) maintains its height and appears as homogeneous high signal intensity with clear distinction between the high signal intensity central NP and lower signal intensity AF. Grade II maintains a clear distinction between NP and AF but signal arising from the NP is more inhomogeneous. Grade III involves inhomogeneous, intermediate signal intensity of the NP, unclear distinction between the NP and AF, and normal to slightly decreased height. The distinction between NP and AF is lost in Grade IV and disc height can be normal to moderately decreased. In Grade V, the disc space is collapsed and the disc is diffusely hypointense.

One caveat of interpreting the Pfirrmann grading scheme is that to date, no studies have convincingly correlated disc abnormalities on MRI with patients' symptoms.[2] It is also important to understand that T2 signal intensity changes do not directly reflect decreased water content of the disc. A study of cadaveric spines of various ages demonstrated that absolute T2 measurements correlated more with glycosaminoglycan (GAG) concentration rather than absolute water content.[16] Thus, signal intensity likely reflects the state of water rather than total water content and as such, the term *disc desiccation* should be avoided when interpreting disc T2 signal changes. As disc degeneration progresses, the disc may undergo calcification that typically appears as internal regions of low signal intensity. However, the type and concentration of calcification impact signal intensity; concentrations of particulate calcium of up to 30% by weight may in fact shorten T1 relaxation times and result in T1 signal hyperintensity of the disc.[17]

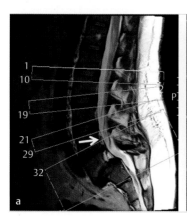
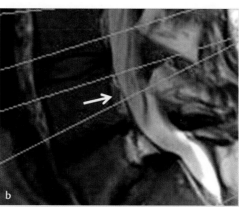

Fig. 3.2 Localizer lines delineate cephalad (e.g., parallel line 1) and caudal (parallel line 10) slices of each axial batch through the lumbar spine on this sagittal T2-weighted sequence (a). Note that as plotted, axial imaging would not include the sequestered disc fragment (*arrows*) posterior to the L4 vertebral body (magnified in sagittal image) (b).

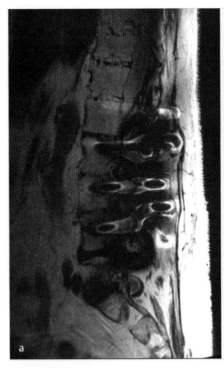
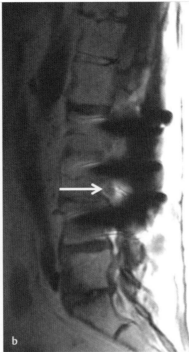

Fig. 3.3 Sagittal T2-weighted magnetic resonance image of the instrumented lumbar spine (a) demonstrates complete obscuration of the neural foramina by susceptibility effect. Corresponding multiacquisition variable resonance image combination (MAVRIC) proton-density sequence (b) during the same exam demonstrates markedly reduced susceptibility and clear visualization of the left L3 nerve root (*arrow*) within the L3–4 neural foramen.

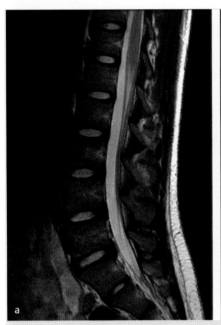
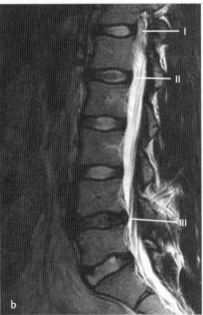
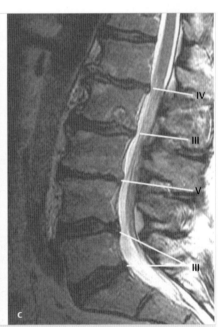

Fig. 3.4 Pfirrmann grades on sagittal T2-weighted magnetic resonance imaging. (a) Image demonstrates normal discs in an 11-year-old girl. (b,c) Images in an 18-year-old woman and a 51-year-old man, respectively, demonstrate varying degrees of disc degeneration, classified by the Pfirrmann grading scheme (Roman numerals).

3.5 Quantification of Disc Degeneration Based on MRI

Quantitative methods to analyze and characterize disc degeneration are not currently used in routine clinical practice and have been mainly explored for research purposes. If properly developed, however, these techniques might be used to identify individuals or individual IVDs at risk for symptomatic degeneration that could benefit from future therapeutic interventions such as cell-based and growth factor therapies. The IVD has three major constituents: water, collagen, and aggregan—proteoglycan (PG) core and GAG chains. With DDD, there is loss of PG and water, fibrocartilage formation, and disorganization of annular architecture. Several MRI techniques for biochemical evaluation of the IVD currently exist. T1-rho is a spin-lock sequence that employs a lower Larmor frequency to permit the detection of low-frequency physiochemical interactions between water and extracellular matrix (ECM) molecules.[18] A positive linear relationship between T1-rho relaxation times and GAG content has been observed in a cadaveric spine series,[18] and T1-rho values also appear to correlate with Pfirrmann grades in both human and animal species.[9] T2* mapping involves interrogation of T2 relaxation times of the disc that correlate strongly with water content and weakly with PG content[19] and also correlate with Pfirrmann grades of disc degeneration and patient age (▶ Fig. 3.1).[20] DWI apparent diffusion coefficient values of normal and degenerated discs show considerable overlap and subsequently may be less useful.[21] No prior studies to date have investigated the relationship between biochemical assessment of the IVD with DTI, which may reflect collagen fiber orientation of the disc, and patient symptoms.

3.6 Annulus Fibrosus

Annulus disruption, by conventional wisdom, is the initial mechanism leading to disc degeneration as annular fissures are present in almost all degenerated discs.[22,23] The AF is innervated by the recurrent meningeal nerve and thus can be a source of low back pain. Annulus disruption as the causative event of the degenerative disc cascade, however, has not been proven.[2] Ye et al. demonstrated that in early stages of disc degeneration, AF disruption was associated with faster subsequent degeneration of the NP,[2,24] but a recent longitudinal study found that discs with a Pfirrmann Grade > 2 and an annular fissure were not prone to accelerated degeneration when compared with matched control discs.[25]

The terms *annular fissure* and *annular tear* have been used to describe a localized high intensity zone (HIZ) within the annulus (▶ Fig. 3.5). HIZs reflect granulation tissue and will enhance following contrast administration.[26] Most spine societies recommend the term *annular fissure* be used rather than *annular tear* due to concern about misconstruing the abnormality as traumatic in etiology. Discography may play an additive role in detecting annular fissures as this modality may reveal fissures not visualized with MRI (▶ Fig. 3.6).[26]

3.7 Disc Herniation

Disc herniation, as defined in a recent multisociety consensus paper, refers to localized displacement involving less than 25% of the circumference of disc material (including NP, cartilage

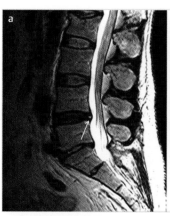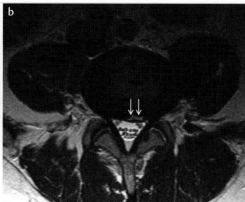

Fig. 3.5 Lumbar spine magnetic resonance sagittal **(a)** and axial **(b)** T2-weighted images in a 47-year-old man demonstrate a broad-based posterior left paracentral annular fissure (*arrows*).

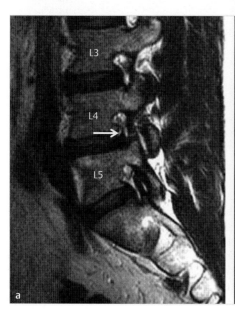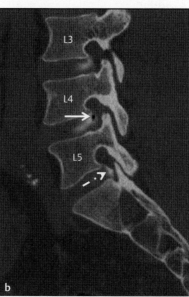

Fig. 3.6 **(a)** Sagittal T2-weighted magnetic resonance imaging (MRI) demonstrates a small annular fissure (*arrow*) at the level of the neural foramen at L4–5. Sagittal computed tomography discography image **(b)** demonstrates contrast material and a small focus of gas (possibly from the injection) extending into the annular fissure at L4–5 (*solid arrow*) but also reveals an additional fissure at L5–S1 (*dashed arrow*), not seen on MRI.

fragmented apophyseal bone, or fragmented annular tissue) beyond the IVD space.[26] The disc space is defined cephalad and caudal by the end plates and peripherally by the outer edges of the vertebral ring apophyses.[2] A *disc bulge* instead involves greater than 25% of the disc circumference and typically extends a short distance (< 3 mm) beyond the edges of the disc space. The same consensus group defines a *disc protrusion* if the transverse dimension of the base of the disc herniation is greater than the distance between the edges of the disc material extending beyond the disc space.

The group defines a *disc extrusion*, conversely, as a herniation whose base dimensions are less than the dimensions of the distance between the edges of the disc material extending beyond the disc space in any plane.[26] A *sequestered disc* is a subtype of disc extrusion in which disc material has lost continuity with its parent disc (▶ Fig. 3.2, ▶ Fig. 3.7). At the authors' institution, the distinction between a protrusion and extrusion is made by whether the herniation is contained by the posterior longitudinal ligament (PLL), visualized as a low signal intensity line posterior to the herniation on axial and/or sagittal sequences. The outer fibers of the annulus and the PLL blend with one another and thus their interface is indistinguishable. If the herniation is contained by the PLL, this is defined as a disc protrusion or *subligamentous herniation* (▶ Fig. 3.8), with or without cephalocaudal migration, and if there is extension beyond the PLL, this is considered a disc extrusion or *supraligamentous herniation* (▶ Fig. 3.9, ▶ Fig. 3.10).[27] Although the true clinical significance of distinguishing protrusion from extrusion has yet to be elucidated,[28] integrity of the PLL is a determining factor of whether minimally invasive treatment methods, such as percutaneous disc decompression and endoscopic discectomy, can be performed.[29] When this distinction cannot be confidently made by MRI,[30] we refrain from using the terms *protrusion* or *extrusion* and label the disc material as a disc herniation.

Disc herniations are also characterized by their location. The location of the herniation can be divided in the axial plane moving from central to left lateral as central, left central, left subarticular, left foraminal, or left extraforaminal, as defined by Fardon et al (▶ Fig. 3.11).[26] When reporting, disc herniations are also characterized by their cephalocaudal position with respect to the disc space and whether they have migrated into the lateral recess. The sagittal T1-weighted sequence, in the authors' opinion, is most valuable in detecting very small disc extrusions, including sequestered disc fragments that have migrated cephalad or caudal to the disc space.

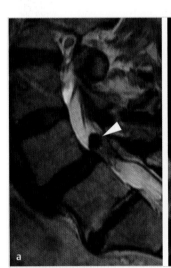
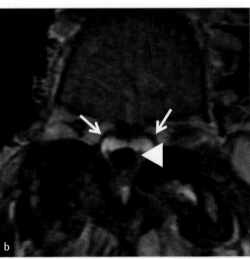

Fig. 3.7 Sagittal (a) and axial (b) magnetic resonance images demonstrate an intrathecal sequestration (*arrowheads*) impinging the cauda equina. Note the dura anteriorly (*arrows*), confirming its intrathecal location.

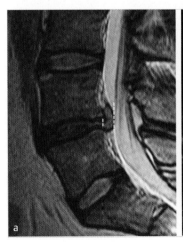
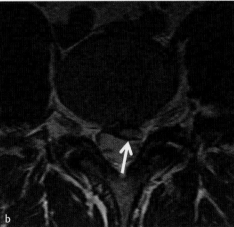

Fig. 3.8 Sagittal (a) and axial (b) T2-weighted magnetic resonance images demonstrate a left paracentral disc herniation at the L4–5 motion segment that extends cephalad to the disc space and causes mild thecal sac compression (b). Note in (a), that its base dimension (*short line*) is less than the dimension between the edges of the herniated disc material (*tall line*), but it appears to be contained by the (b) posterior longitudinal ligament (*arrow*). At the authors' institution, this would be designated a disc protrusion. Compare with ▶ Fig. 3.9.

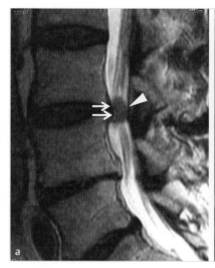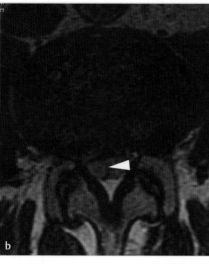

Fig. 3.9 Sagittal **(a)** and axial **(b)** T2-weighted lumbar spine magnetic resonance images in a 66-year-old man demonstrates a disc extrusion (*arrowheads*) that has extended beyond the posterior longitudinal ligament (*arrows*).

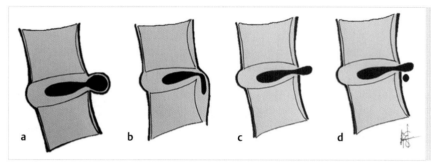

Fig. 3.10 A schematic drawing depicting the possible types of disc herniations in the sagittal plane, with respect to the posterior longitudinal ligament. **(a)** Disc protrusion without cephalocaudal migration. **(b)** Disc protrusion with caudal migration. **(c)** Disc extrusion. **(d)** Disc sequestration.

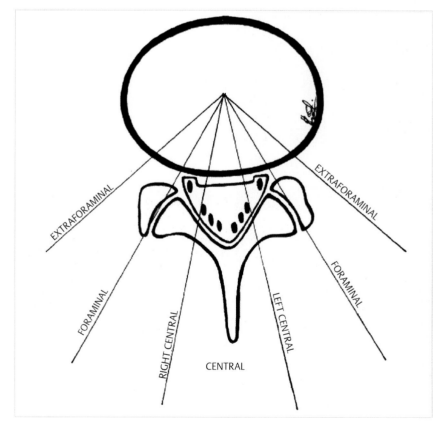

Fig. 3.11 A schematic drawing depicts the possible locations of disc herniations in the axial plane.

Most importantly, a disc herniation should be evaluated with respect to its relationship to the spinal cord and nerve roots, and whether the nerve root is being impinged (contacted) or compressed (between two osseous structures) and/or displaced. The extraforaminal root should be carefully assessed on water-sensitive T2-weighted, Dixon fat/water separation or STIR sequences for the presence of edema and/or enlargement as presumed indicators of nerve inflammation.

3.8 Unusual Disc Pathology

Lumbar *intradural disc herniations* are rare and thought to be caused by dural adhesions to the PLL and attenuation of the ventral dura.[31] Occasionally, this entity may be identified on MRI as an intradural mass, which can then be confirmed surgically by opening the dura and inspecting the thecal sac (► Fig. 3.7).

Atypical extradural masses, other than hematoma and neoplasms,[32] that are occasionally encountered include gas-containing disc herniations and discal cysts. The etiology of an epidural *gas-containing disc herniation* is uncertain but is thought to be associated with degenerative vacuum phenomenon. Gas-containing disc herniations tend to be located posterolaterally, possibly as a result of focal weakening of the outer annulus/PLL. A *discal cyst* (► Fig. 3.12) may present as an extradural mass in contiguity with the IVD and cause lumbar radiculopathy, typically in younger patients with lumbar DDD and most commonly at the L4–5 motion segment.[33] The discal cyst is theorized to either develop from an incompletely resorbed epidural hematoma, initially caused by a disc herniation,[34] or alternatively, a disc degeneration with leakage of "fluid content" that then becomes encapsulated.[35] The hallmark of a discal cyst is its communication with the IVD, demonstrated by discography.[33] Both gas-containing disc herniations and discal cysts[33] can be managed with CT-guided aspiration.

3.9 Endplate Changes

Signal intensity changes of the subchondral bone underlying degenerated discs were initially classified by Modic et al. into three different types. In Modic type 1 changes, the endplates demonstrate T1 hypointensity and T2 hyperintensity, reflecting edema related to more acute disc degeneration. Modic type 2 changes are defined by increased T1- and T2-weighted signal, reflecting fatty deposition. Modic type 3 changes are defined by decreased T1- and T2-weighted signal reflecting the presence of dense woven bone and corresponding to sclerotic changes on radiographs (► Fig. 3.13).[36] Modic changes are invariably only identified adjacent to degenerative discs and have been shown to be highly specific, but lacking sensitivity, for indicating the level of a painful IVD.[37] Other endplate changes include Schmorl's nodes, or intravertebral herniations, that are precipitated by disorders that weaken the endplate (► Fig. 3.14). These include DDD and trauma, Scheuermann's disease (juvenile kyphosis), metabolic disease (e.g., osteoporosis, hyperparathyroidism), and neoplasm.

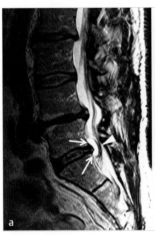
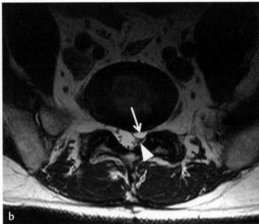

Fig. 3.12 Sagittal (**a**) and axial (**b**) T2-weighted lumbar spine magnetic resonance images in a 61-year-old man demonstrate a moderate-size discal cyst (*arrows*) along the posterior left L5–S1 disc margin that impinges the left S1 axillary sleeve (*arrowheads*).

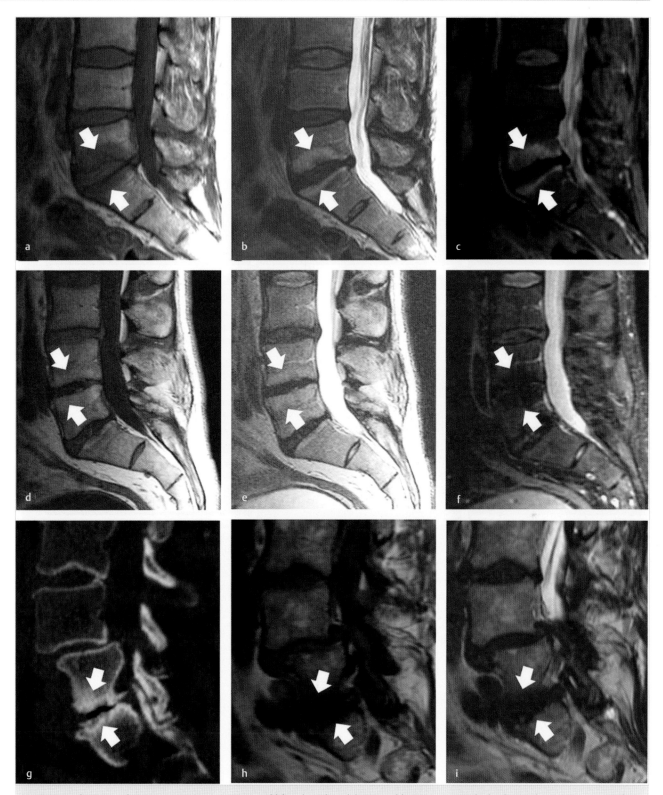

Fig. 3.13 Modic type 1 changes are present in a 49-year-old female with endplate signal hypointensity at the lumbosacral segment on sagittal T1-weighted imaging **(a)** and endplate hyperintensity on T2-weighted **(b)** and short tau inversion recovery (STIR) **(c)** sequences. Modic type 2 changes are present in a 44-year-old man with endplate signal hyperintensity at the L4–5 segment on sagittal T1- **(d)** and T2-weighted **(e)** images and hypointensity on the corresponding STIR image **(f)**. Modic type 3 changes are present in a 65-year-old woman with endplate sclerosis at the lumbosacral segment on sagittal computed tomography **(g)** and corresponding hypointensity on T1- **(h)** and T2-weighted **(i)** sequences on magnetic resonance imaging.

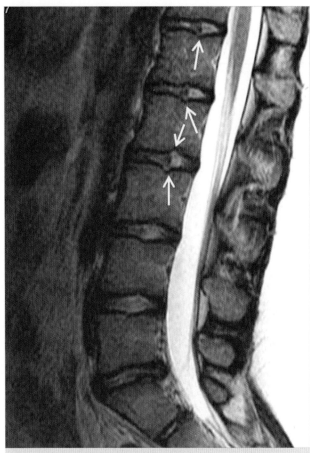

Fig. 3.14 Sagittal T2-weighted image of the lumbar spine in a 13-year-old girl demonstrates multisegmental Schmorl's nodes (*arrows*).

3.10 Conclusion

The etiology of symptoms in patients with DDD is likely multi-factorial but can be ambiguous. MRI is the most reliable imaging modality in evaluating DDD and detecting potential pain generators. Given the prevalence of disc degeneration in asymptomatic individuals, however, it is incumbent on both the referring clinician and interpreting radiologist to correlate MRI findings with patient symptomatology. Quantitative techniques such as T1-rho and T2 mapping, to detect early disc degeneration, and diffusion tensor imaging, mainly used to detect myelomalacia and nerve root integrity, are promising research tools, but further work is necessary to elucidate their roles in spine imaging and integrate them into routine clinical practice.

3.11 References

[1] Andersson GB. Epidemiological features of chronic low-back pain. Lancet. 1999; 354(9178):581–585

[2] Modic MTRJ, Ross JS. Lumbar degenerative disk disease. Radiology. 2007; 245(1):43–61

[3] Saboeiro GR. Lumbar discography. Radiol Clin North Am. 2009; 47(3):421–433

[4] Carrino JA, Lurie JD, Tosteson AN, et al. Lumbar spine: reliability of MR imaging findings. Radiology . 2009; 250(1):161–170

[5] Farshad-Amacker NA, Farshad M, Winklehner A, Andreisek G. MR imaging of degenerative disc disease. Eur J Radiol. 2015; 84(9):1768–1776

[6] Rajeswaran G, Turner M, Gissane C, Healy JC. MRI findings in the lumbar spines of asymptomatic elite junior tennis players. Skeletal Radiol. 2014; 43 (7):925–932

[7] Weishaupt D, Zanetti M, Hodler J, Boos N. MR imaging of the lumbar spine: prevalence of intervertebral disk extrusion and sequestration, nerve root compression, end plate abnormalities, and osteoarthritis of the facet joints in asymptomatic volunteers. Radiology. 1998; 209(3):661–666

[8] Stadnik TW, Lee RR, Coen HL, Neirynck EC, Buisseret TS, Osteaux MJ. Annular tears and disk herniation: prevalence and contrast enhancement on MR images in the absence of low back pain or sciatica. Radiology. 1998; 206 (1):49–55

[9] Zhou Z, Jiang B, Zhou Z, et al. Intervertebral disk degeneration: T1ρ MR imaging of human and animal models. Radiology. 2013; 268(2):492–500

[10] Welsch GH, Trattnig S, Paternostro-Sluga T, et al. Parametric T2 and T2* mapping techniques to visualize intervertebral disc degeneration in patients with low back pain: initial results on the clinical use of 3.0 Tesla MRI. Skeletal Radiol . 2011; 40(5):543–551

[11] Law T, Anthony MP, Chan Q, et al. Ultrashort time-to-echo MRI of the cartilaginous endplate: technique and association with intervertebral disc degeneration. J Med Imaging RadiatOncol . 2013; 57(4):427–434

[12] Zhang W, Ma X, Wang Y, et al. Assessment of apparent diffusion coefficient in lumbar intervertebral disc degeneration. Eur Spine J . 2014; 23(9):1830–1836

[13] Hueftle MG, Modic MT, Ross JS, et al. Lumbar spine: postoperative MR imaging with Gd-DTPA. Radiology . 1988; 167(3):817–824

[14] Koch, KM, Brau, AC, Chen, W, et al. Imaging near metal with a MAVRIC-SEMAC hybrid. Magn Reson Med . 2011; 65(1):71–82

[15] Pfirrmann CW, Metzdorf A, Zanetti M, Hodler J, Boos N. Magnetic resonance classification of lumbar intervertebral disc degeneration. Spine . 2001; 26(17):1873–1878

[16] Majors AW, McDevitt CA, Silgalis I, Modic MT. A correlative analysis of T2, ADC and MT radio with water, hydroxyproline and GAG content in excised human intervertebral disk. New Orleans, La: Orthopedic Research Society; 1994:116–120

[17] Bangert BA, Modic MT, Ross JS, et al. Hyperintense disks on T1-weighted MR images: correlation with calcification. Radiology . 1995; 195(2):437–443

[18] Nguyen AM, Johannessen W, Yoder JH, et al. Noninvasive quantification of human nucleus pulposus pressure with use of T1rho-weighted magnetic resonance imaging. J Bone Joint Surg Am . 2008; 90(4):796–802

[19] Marinelli NL, Haughton VM, Muñoz A, Anderson PA. T2 relaxation times of intervertebral disc tissue correlated with water content and proteoglycan content. Spine . 2009; 34(5):520–524

[20] Marinelli NL, Haughton VM, Anderson PA. T2 relaxation times correlated with stage of lumbar intervertebral disk degeneration and patient age. AJNR Am J Neuroradiol . 2010; 31(7):1278–1282

[21] Niinimäki J, Korkiakoski A, Ojala O, et al. Association between visual degeneration of intervertebral discs and the apparent diffusion coefficient. Magn Reson Imaging . 2009; 27(5):641–647

[22] Yu SW, Haughton VM, Sether LA, Wagner M. Anulus fibrosus in bulging intervertebral disks. Radiology . 1988; 169(3):761–763

[23] Yasuma T, Makino E, Saito S, Inui M. Histological development of intervertebral disc herniation. J Bone Joint Surg Am. 1986; 68(7):1066–1072

[24] Sharma A, Pilgram T, Wippold FJ, II. Association between annular tears and disk degeneration: a longitudinal study. AJNR Am J Neuroradiol. 2009; 30 (3):500–506

[25] Farshad-Amacker NA, Hughes AP, Aichmair A, Herzog RJ, Farshad M. Is an annular tear a predictor for accelerated disc degeneration? Eur Spine J. 2014; 23(9):1825–1829

[26] Fardon DF, Williams AL, Dohring EJ, Murtagh FR, Gabriel Rothman SL, Sze GK. Lumbar disc nomenclature: version 2.0: recommendations of the combined task forces of the North American Spine Society, the American Society of Spine Radiology and the American Society of Neuroradiology. Spine J. 2014; 14(11):2525–2545

[27] Grenier N, Greselle J-F, Vital J-M, et al. Normal and disrupted lumbar longitudinal ligaments: correlative MR and anatomic study. Radiology. 1989; 171 (1):197–205

[28] Lurie JD, Doman, DM, Spratt, KF, Tosteson, ANA, Weinstein, JN. Magnetic resonance imaging interpretation in patients with symptomatic lumbar spine disc herniations: comparison of clinician and radiologist readings. Spine. 2009; 34(7):701–705

[29] Oh KJ, Lee JW, Yun BL, et al. Comparison of MR imaging findings between extraligamentous and subligamentous disk herniations in the lumbar spine. AJNR Am J Neuroradiol. 2013; 34(3):683–687

[30] Silverman CS, Lenchik L, Shimkin PM, Lipow KL. The value of MR in differentiating subligamentous from supraligamentous lumbar disk herniations. AJNR Am J Neuroradiol. 1995; 16(3):571–579

[31] Krajewski KLRJ, Regelsberger J. Intradural lumbar disc herniation associated with degenerative spine disease and rheumatoid arthritis. Spine. 2013; 38 (12):E763–E765

[32] Jeong GK, Bendo JA. Lumbar intervertebral disc cyst as a cause of radiculopathy. Spine J. 2003; 3(3):242–246

[33] Endo Y, Miller TT, Saboeiro GR, Cooke PM. Lumbar discal cyst: diagnostic discography followed by therapeutic computed tomography-guided aspiration and injection. J Radiol Case Rep. 2014; 8(12):35–40

[34] Toyama Y, Kamata N, Matsumoto M, Nishizawa T, Koyanagi T, Suzuki N. Pathogenesis and diagnostic title of intraspinal cyst communicating with intervertebral disk in the lumbar spine. RinshoSeikeiGeka.. 1997; 32:393:400

[35] Kono K, Nakamura H, Inoue Y, Okamura T, Shakudo M, Yamada R. Intraspinal extradural cysts communicating with adjacent herniated disks: imaging characteristics and possible pathogenesis. AJNR Am J Neuroradiol. 1999; 20(7):1373–1377

[36] Modic MT, Steinberg PM, Ross JS, Masaryk TJ, Carter JR. Degenerative disk disease: assessment of changes in vertebral body marrow with MR imaging. Radiology. 1988; 166(1 Pt 1):193–199

[37] Braithwaite I, White J, Saifuddin A, Renton P, Taylor BA. Vertebral end-plate (Modic) changes on lumbar spine MRI: correlation with pain reproduction at lumbar discography. Eur Spine J. 1998; 7(5):363–368

4 Biomechanics of the Healthy and Diseased Spine

Hans-Joachim Wilke and Fabio Galbusera

Abstract

The intervertebral disc (IVD) is a pad of soft tissue that uniformly distributes the stresses due to spinal loads while ensuring the mobility of the motion segment. The disc consists of an inner nucleus pulposus (NP) with high water and proteoglycan content, and an outer annulus fibrosus (AF) mostly consisting of oriented lamellae of collagen fibers. Due to its structure and composition, the disc has the capability to imbibe water, and therefore develops an intradiscal pressure (IDP) that gives it a high capacity to sustain compressive loads and to act as a shock absorber.

Degenerative disorders of the IVD feature morphological changes (decreased disc height, end plate defects and sclerosis, osteophytes, and size reduction of the NP) as well as changes in the tissue composition (loss of water content, which causes the black disc appearance seen in magnetic resonance imaging [MRI]). These degenerative alterations have a direct impact on the biomechanics of the motion segment. The loss of water content induces a decrease of the IDP and the possible presence of stress peaks in the AF, which may be responsible for pain episodes.

Spinal fusion is considered the golden standard for the surgical treatment of symptomatic degenerative disorders of the IVD. Several authors have hypothesized that moderately degenerated discs may lead to spinal instability, that is, an abnormal motion response to physiological loads, which has paved the way for novel surgical treatments not aimed at spinal fusion, but rather at restoring the physiological spine stiffness. However, because numerous studies have contradicted the instability hypothesis, the issue is still under debate.

Keywords: compressive load, disc height, intradiscal pressure, spinal instability, stress distribution, swelling

4.1 Historical Perspective

Knowledge about the intervertebral disc (IVD) and its biomechanical functions dates back to the beginning of the scientific era. In 1680, Giovanni Alfonso Borelli published the first known essay about biomechanics, *De Motu Animalium*, in which the time-dependent mechanical response of the IVD was described.[1] The first modern extensive investigation of the structure of the disc as well as its changes due to aging and pathological processes was carried out in 1926 by Georg Schmorl, a pathologist who analyzed disc specimens gathered from human cadavers using laboratory techniques. For the first time, disc height loss, end plate defects, and annular tears were described; disc degeneration started to have an influence on the clinical and surgical management of pathologies such as back pain and sciatica.[2]

Spine fusion with autologous grafts and, beginning in the 1960s, with instrumentation such as pedicle screws and internal fixators remained the gold standards for the treatment of many degenerative spinal disorders for decades,[3] until the concept of spinal instability emerged in the 1980s. Despite being first mentioned 30 years before,[4] instability acquired a practical relevance after Kirkaldy-Willis and Farfan presented their theory about the degenerative cascade in which instability constitutes a key stage.[5] Supported by the work by Pope and Panjabi,[6] who defined instability as a pathological loss of spinal stiffness, i.e., hypermobility, the paper paved the way for novel surgical treatments not aimed at spinal fusion, but rather at restoring the physiological spine stiffness. Following the principle that restraining abnormal spinal motion to physiological levels may be an effective treatment for back pain, several motion-preserving, dynamic stabilization devices were introduced to the market and are still widely used.[7] Success rates appear to be satisfactory in select patients, but whether these implants constitute an improvement with respect to instrumented fusion is not clear yet.[8] Meanwhile, papers that refined the definition of spinal instability[9] as well as biomechanical studies aimed at proving or disproving the validity of this concept have been published.[10,11,12]

This chapter presents the changes occurring to IVDs due to aging and pathological processes and their implications in biomechanical terms. Special attention is given to the concept of spinal instability and to its relation to the radiological, morphological, and tissue composition changes of the degenerative IVD.

4.2 Biomechanics of the Healthy Intervertebral Disc

The IVD is a pad of soft tissue located between two adjacent vertebrae, the function of which is to uniformly distribute the stresses due to spinal loads while ensuring the mobility of the motion segment.[13] The disc consists of an inner nucleus pulposus (NP) with high water and proteoglycan content,[14] and an outer annulus fibrosus (AF) mostly consisting of oriented lamellae of collagen fibers. Proteoglycans are highly negatively charged molecules synthesized by the NP cells, which tend to attract cations in the interstitial fluid to achieve electrical equilibrium.[15] Their presence gives the disc the capability to imbibe water, which creates an osmotic pressure gradient between the disc itself and the external environment, commonly named as intradiscal pressure (IDP). Due to its peculiar structure, the IVD has a high capacity for sustaining compressive loads and acting as a shock absorber.[16] Pressure transducers implanted in living subjects have been employed to measure the IDP in different postures and during various daily activities. The technique was introduced by Nachemson and coworkers[17,18] and used in several later studies.[19,20] Values ranging from 0.1 MPa during bed rest up to 2.3 MPa during weight lifting were recorded[19] (► Fig. 4.1, ► Fig. 4.2, ► Table 4.1), thus demonstrating the capability of the disc to sustain high mechanical loads.

The AF has a fundamental role in determining the strength of the IVD. Under loading, the NP is pressurized and creates a tensile stress in the collagen fibers of the AF, which bulges outward.[21,22] The optimized organization of the fibers allows them

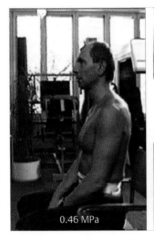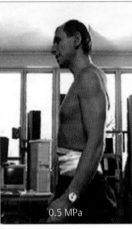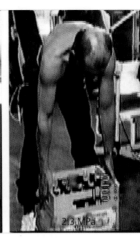

0.46 MPa   0.5 MPa   2.3 MPa

Fig. 4.1 Intradiscal pressure in a healthy L4–5 disc during relaxed sitting without backrest, relaxed standing, and lifting 20 kg, bent over with round back.[19]

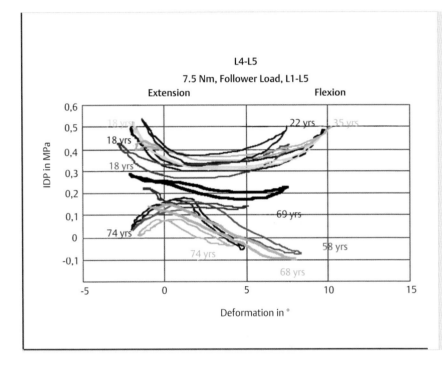

L4-L5
7.5 Nm, Follower Load, L1-L5

Fig. 4.2 Measurements from in vitro tests in flexion-extension applying ± 7.5 Nm plus a follower load of 280 N. Intradiscal pressure changes strongly with increasing age (degeneration).

to be loaded mostly in tension under loading conditions typical of daily life such as bending, thus acting similarly to the fiber reinforcement of a car tire. The IVD is connected to the vertebral bone through osseous and cartilaginous layers called end plates, which contribute in uniformly distributing the spinal stresses and in damping the response to fast loads.[23]

4.3 Radiological Changes with Potential Biomechanical Relevance

The assessment of the degenerative changes of the spine with biomedical imaging techniques has a fundamental importance in the clinical management of spinal disorders, because imaging constitutes a substantial part of the information available to the clinician in diagnostic and therapeutic decision making. Establishing a link between the degenerative changes that can be highlighted with imaging methods and their biomechanical relevance is therefore of critical importance to improving the clinical management of disc degeneration.

Planar radiography allows for an easy and direct visualization of some changes related to the degenerative disease. A degenerated motion segment commonly appears as having low intervertebral space due to disc height loss and reduced segmental lordosis, as well as increased bone density in the end plates and adjacent bony tissue (end plate sclerosis).[24] In frequent cases, osteophytes, that is, heterotopic bone formations commonly located near the anterior and posterior longitudinal ligaments, are also visible.[25] End plate anomalies and defects (Schmorl's nodes, notches, shape irregularities), either related to the degenerative processes or not, as well as foraminal stenosis can in some cases be detected. Subtle abnormalities and lesions of the IVD can be diagnosed by means of provocative discography, that is, injection of radiopaque contrast medium in the disc

Table 4.1 Absolute values of intradiscal pressure for different postures and exercises, normalized to relaxed standing (chosen arbitrarily as 100%) (after Wilke et al[19])

Position	Pressure (MPa)	%
Lying supine	0.1	20
Side-lying	0.12	24
Lying prone	0.11	22
Lying prone, extended back, supporting elbows	0.25	50
Laughing heartily, lying laterally	0.15	30
Sneezing, lying laterally	0.38	76
Peaks by turning around	0.7–0.8	140–160
Relaxed standing	0.5	100
Standing, performing Valsalva maneuver	0.92	184
Standing, bent forward	1.1	220
Sitting relaxed, without backrest	0.46	92
Sitting actively straightening the back	0.55	110
Sitting with maximum flexion	0.83	166
Sitting bent forward with thigh supporting the elbows	0.43	86
Sitting slouched into the chair	0.27	54
Standing up from the chair	1.1	220
Walking barefoot	0.53–0.65	106–130
Walking with tennis shoes	0.53–0.65	106–130
Jogging with hard street shoes	0.35–0.95	70–190
Jogging with tennis shoes	0.35–0.95	70–190
Climbing stairs, one at a time	0.5–0.7	100–140
Climbing stairs, two at a time	0.3–1.2	60–240
Walking down stairs, one at a time	0.38–0.6	76–120
Walking down stairs, two at a time	0.3–0.9	60–180
Lifting 20 kg, bent over with round back	2.3	460
Lifting 20 kg as taught in back school	1.7	340
Holding 20 kg close to the body	1.1	220
Holding 20 kg, 60 cm away from the chest	1.8	360
Carrying 20 kg (in the left or in the right hand)	1.0	200
Carrying 40 kg (20 kg left and 20 kg right)	0.9	180
Pressure increase during the night rest (over a period of 7 h)	0.1–0.24	20–48

aimed at highlighting small tears and provoking pain in symptomatic discs. This method is however currently under heated debate due to its high false-positive rate and the risk of degeneration in the long term due to the needle puncture.[26,27]

Sagittal radiographic projections in flexion-extension are commonly used to diagnose the so-called radiological instability of the lumbar spine, for which various definitions have been provided (e.g., sagittal translation > 3 mm,[28] 10–15% of the vertebral width,[29] or segmental range of motion > 20 degrees at L4–5[30]). However, the clinical relevance of radiological instability as well as its correlation with back pain remains unclear.

Magnetic resonance imaging (MRI) allows for a high contrast within soft tissues such as the IVD and ligaments.[31] As a matter of fact, the most commonly employed grading system for disc degeneration (the Pfirrmann scale) is based on MRI scans.[32] T2-weighted imaging of the NP shows a progressive reduction in the MRI signal with degeneration, which is related to a loss of water content and fibrotization of the tissue. A dehydrated, T2-hypointense disc is usually referred to as a *black disc* and is commonly considered one of the most important signs of disc degeneration. MRI also allows for an excellent characterization of the disc height and morphology; it is the method of choice for the detection of Schmorl's nodes and end plate defects, as well as for Modic changes.[31] Recent studies showed the potential of ultra high field MRI (> 7 T) for the detection of small disc tears that are currently not discernible with conventional clinical scanners, thus also highlighting the possible use of MRI as an alternative to provocative discography.[33]

Computed tomography (CT) is seldom used in cases of degenerative disc disease (DDD) for diagnostic purposes; nevertheless, it can be useful for assessing spinal stenosis and for planning decompression surgeries.[34] CT is also commonly employed in degenerative processes involving the facet joints, due to its capability to show reductions in the articular space and local calcifications.[35]

4.4 Morphological and Tissue Composition Changes in the Intervertebral Disc

The radiological signs mentioned above outline a degenerative disorder of the IVD featuring morphological changes (decreased disc height, end plate defects and sclerosis, osteophytes, and size reduction of the NP), as well as changes in the tissue composition (e.g., loss of water content, which results in the black disc appearance). Macroscopic analysis of cadaveric disc specimens with different degrees of degeneration showed that the radiographic signs correspond well, despite some exceptions, to the actual changes occurring in the motion segment[24] (▶ Fig. 4.3). Nevertheless, less apparent alterations in the tissue structure and composition not discernible by means of conventional biomedical imaging were also found to take place.[36]

Previous works conducted on cadaveric specimens showed that a clear relationship between symptoms and visible alterations in the discs due to the physiological aging process cannot

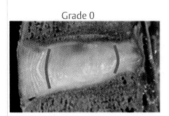 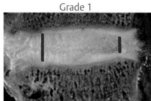 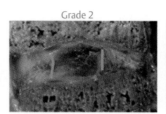 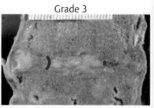

Grade 0   Grade 1   Grade 2   Grade 3

Fig. 4.3 Healthy and degenerated discs with increasing degrees of degeneration (after Wilke et al[24]). Macroscopic changes and inward and outward bulging of the nucleus.

be directly established. In other words, macroscopic and tissue composition changes usually occur with aging even in nonsymptomatic, nondegenerated discs.[36] Besides, back pain can only in a minority of cases be attributed to specific degenerative changes in the disc.[37,38] It appears that there is a "gray area" of aging discs, with possibly either subclinical or significant symptoms of difficult attribution, the classification of which as degenerated or nondegenerated could be somewhat arbitrary. It should also be noted that radiological examination is usually performed on patients seeking medical care, whereas little information about symptomatology can usually be gathered about donors of cadaveric specimens. Thus, translating information between symptomatology, radiological, and postmortem studies has necessarily some inherent limitations.

In accordance with radiographic observations, disc height loss is observed in most degenerated discs,[24,39,40] whereas aging nondegenerated discs show a slight tendency to a height increase.[41,42,43] Degenerated discs, and to a lesser extent aging nondegenerated discs, are subjected in many cases to a drop in fluid content, replaced by fibrotic tissue especially in the NP.[16,44] Indeed, as progressing degeneration induces a loss in the proteoglycan content, the capability of the disc to attract and imbibe water is decreased, thus leading to the decrease in the MRI signal and to the so-called black disc.[16] A thickening of the AF as well as a more disorganized appearance of the annulus itself and of the transition zone between it and the nucleus is also frequently visible.[45] Annular tears and clefts have been also reported in many specimens.[36,46] Indeed, the number of cases in which they could be observed (> 50% of adults, including asymptomatic subjects) may indicate that minor structural failure could be a part of the physiological aging process.[47] Among the different types of tears, radial and rim lesions seem to be more strongly related to a pathological degeneration process.[46] Sclerosis of the end plates and presence of osteophytes have been reported, in agreement with the radiological findings.[48,49,50]

These macroscopic changes are believed to originate by, or in combination with, cellular and biochemical alterations. In the physiological development, cell density in IVDs shows a continuous decrease from childhood onward, which explains the reduction of the proteoglycan content in the disc mentioned above as well as a decrease in matrix turnover.[51] Furthermore, cell senescence was reported to limit the per-cell proteoglycan synthesis rate. These phenomena lead to a weak self-repair capability of the IVD during adulthood, and thus to the persistence or progression of most mechanically initiated lesions.[52,53]

4.5 Biomechanical Implications of the Changes in the Intervertebral Disc

The degenerative alterations of the discal tissue have a direct impact on the biomechanics of the motion segment. Similarly to the alterations themselves, nondegenerated aging discs also exhibit changes in their biomechanical responses due to aging phenomena of the tissues,[16] and the distinction between aging and proper degenerated discs is somewhat arbitrary.

The decrease in proteoglycan synthesis and the consequent loss in water content induce a marked decrease of the IDP in the nucleus[15]—to negligible values in the case of severe degeneration[20]—and the possible presence of stress peaks in the AF as well as inward bulging of the annular fibers.[44] Having lost the capability of swelling and pressurization, the degenerated disc is not able to uniformly distribute the stresses of spine loading on the vertebral end plates. The consequent stress peaks and concentrations inside the disc as well as in the adjacent vertebrae may be responsible for pain episodes,[44] especially for specific postures and motions.[54] Based on these observations, a hypothesis colloquially referred to as the *stone-in-the-shoe theory*, in which discogenic pain is related to these stress peaks like a small stone in the shoe creates painful stress peaks on the foot sole, was proposed and is currently under heated debate.[55]

The concepts of radiological and clinical instability mentioned above are intimately related to the alteration of the composition of the disc matrix as well as structural failure of its components. Disc height loss is a direct consequence of the decrease in water content, and may have a critical impact on the stability of the motion segment. Parametric numerical studies showed that a decrease of the disc height alone results in a decrease of spinal flexibility.[56,57] Nevertheless, since the mechanical effects of disc collapse are linked to changes in tissue composition and therefore material properties, they cannot be predicted in an accurate manner. Using a computational model, Zhao et al[58] showed an increase in spinal flexibility with progressing dehydration of the discal tissue, thus counteracting the stabilizing effect of the height loss. However, due to the profound and complex interplay of the many factors that determine the mechanical properties of degenerated discs (i.e., water content, permeability, swelling), the relatively limited research conducted on this topic nowadays cannot provide any definitive answers regarding the biomechanical relevance of disc collapse and dehydration.

The presence of annular tears and clefts was hypothesized to be the key determinant of clinical instability.[5] However, only a few papers report investigation of this topic from a biomechanical point of view, and their conclusions are rather contradictive. Artificially created tears and lesions were found to determine only a minor destabilization of disc specimens.[59,60] Rim lesions induced more profound changes to the spine stiffness in comparison with concentric and radial tears, but their effect was still regarded as minor. However, the authors hypothesized that tears and lesions are able to alter the stress distribution inside the IVD, thus potentially supporting the degenerative process.[59]

On the contrary, vertebral osteophytes were found to increase spine stability and stiffness, especially in flexion-extension and lateral bending.[61,62,63] Therefore, current data support the concept that osteophytosis is a physiological adaptation process aimed to increase the stiffness of an unstable spine.

4.6 Clinical Instability: Myth or Reality?

Going beyond the original idea of hypermobility, White and Panjabi provided a rigorous definition of clinical instability as "the loss of the ability to maintain its patterns of displacement under physiologic loads so there is no initial or additional neurologic deficit, no major deformity, and no incapacitating pain."[13] The concept was further refined in two papers by Panjabi, in which the stabilizing system of the spine is described as being composed of three subsystems: a passive component (vertebrae, discs, ligaments), an active component (muscles), and a control subsystem (central and peripheral nervous systems), which monitors various transduced signals from the other two subsystems and activates the muscles to achieve the needed spine stability.[9,64] Alterations to the performance of the three subsystems may result in compensation strategies, long-term adaptation responses, and eventually back pain in some patients. The author also introduced the concept of a neutral zone, which is defined as the region around the neutral posture in which the passive component offers minimal resistance to motion, and which was hypothesized to be a better indicator of clinical instability than the overall range of motion.[9] This hypothesis was widely accepted, and the neutral zone is a fundamental parameter used in many current biomechanical studies.

The topic of spinal instability was investigated in several studies employing in vitro experimental tests on cadaver specimens. A hypothesis that has been reported on in many papers concerns the theory of the degenerative cascade described by Kirkaldy-Willis and Farfan,[5] in which hypermobility characterizes the early/mild stage of disc degeneration, and is followed by a spontaneous stabilization stage. Some researchers actually reported an increase of spine flexibility in the early stage of degeneration,[10,61,62] whereas other studies showed rather the opposite, with an increase of spinal stiffness even in mildly degenerated discs.[11,12,65] Other studies reported an erratic correlation between spinal flexibility and disc degeneration, with no discernible tendencies.[66] The trend recurring in several reports[11,12,61,62,65] can be summarized as modest flexibility alterations in flexion-extension and lateral bending, a tendency toward hypermobility in axial rotation, and an increase in spinal stiffness for severe disc degeneration.

The neutral zone was investigated and reported on in a smaller number of papers, which provided more interesting results. A consensus seemed to emerge that an increase of the size of the neutral zone correlated with disc degeneration,[9,11,67] despite contrasting results also being reported.[61] One study conducted on a large number of specimens (203 motion segments from 111 donors) generally reported small alterations of both stiffness and neutral zone, but a significant increment of the neutral zone in axial rotation with increasing degeneration.[12]

In summary, in vitro tests do not generally support the concept of clinical instability of the spine, with some exceptions. The theory that the degenerative cascade includes an unstable mild degeneration stage followed by spontaneous stabilization could not be proven by basic science studies. An increase in the size of the neutral zone may be a better indicator of an ongoing degenerative process; however, it should be noted that radiological instability as it could be diagnosed on living subjects may not correlate well with the neutral zone, as no scientific evidence exists. Due to these reasons, the translation of the concept of clinical instability from bench to bedside appears not to be straightforward.

4.7 References

[1] Borelli GA. De Motu Animalium. Rome: 1680
[2] Schmorl G, Junghanns H. The Human Spine in Health and Disease. Grune and Stratton; 1971
[3] Roy-Camille R, Saillant G, Mazel C. Internal fixation of the lumbar spine with pedicle screw plating. Clin OrthopRelat Res. 1986;(203):7–17
[4] Harris RI, Macnab I. Structural changes in the lumbar intervertebral discs; their relationship to low back pain and sciatica. J Bone Joint Surg Br. 1954; 36-B(2):304–322
[5] Kirkaldy-Willis WH, Farfan HF. Instability of the lumbar spine. Clin Orthop Relat Res. 1982;(165):110–123
[6] Pope MH, Panjabi M. Biomechanical definitions of spinal instability. Spine. 1985; 10(3):255–256
[7] Mulholland RC, Sengupta DK. Rationale, principles and experimental evaluation of the concept of soft stabilization. Eur Spine J. 2002; 11 Suppl 2:S198–S205
[8] Chou D, Lau D, Skelly A, Ecker E. Dynamic stabilization versus fusion for treatment of degenerative spine conditions. Evid Based Spine Care J. 2011; 2(3):33–42
[9] Panjabi MM. The stabilizing system of the spine. Part II. Neutral zone and instability hypothesis. J Spinal Disord. 1992; 5(4):390–396, discussion 397
[10] Krismer M, Haid C, Behensky H, Kapfinger P, Landauer F, Rachbauer F. Motion in lumbar functional spine units during side bending and axial rotation moments depending on the degree of degeneration. Spine. 2000; 25 (16):2020–2027
[11] Mimura M, Panjabi MM, Oxland TR, Crisco JJ, Yamamoto I, Vasavada A. Disc degeneration affects the multidirectional flexibility of the lumbar spine. Spine. 1994; 19(12):1371–1380
[12] Kettler A, Rohlmann F, Ring C, Mack C, Wilke HJ. Do early stages of lumbar intervertebral disc degeneration really cause instability? Evaluation of an in vitro database. Eur Spine J. 2011; 20(4):578–584
[13] White AA, Panjabi MM. Clinical Biomechanics of the Spine. 2nd ed. Lippincott Williams & Wilkins; 1990
[14] Iatridis JC, MacLean JJ, O'Brien M, Stokes IA. Measurements of proteoglycan and water content distribution in human lumbar intervertebral discs. Spine. 2007; 32(14):1493–1497
[15] Urban JP, McMullin JF. Swelling pressure of the inervertebral disc: influence of proteoglycan and collagen contents. Biorheology. 1985; 22(2):145–157
[16] Adams MA, Roughley PJ. What is intervertebral disc degeneration, and what causes it? Spine. 2006; 31(18):2151–2161
[17] Nachemson A. Measurement of intradiscal pressure. Acta Orthop Scand. 1959; 28:269–289

[18] Nachemson A, Morris JM. In vivo measurements of intradiscal pressure. Discometry, a method for the determination of pressure in the lower lumbar discs. J Bone Joint Surg Am. 1964; 46:1077–1092

[19] Wilke HJ, Neef P, Caimi M, Hoogland T, Claes LE. New in vivo measurements of pressures in the intervertebral disc in daily life. Spine. 1999; 24 (8):755–762

[20] Sato K, Kikuchi S, Yonezawa T. In vivo intradiscal pressure measurement in healthy individuals and in patients with ongoing back problems. Spine. 1999; 24(23):2468–2474

[21] Heuer, F, Schmitt, H, Schmidt, H, Claes, L, Wilke, HJ. Creep associated changes in intervertebral disc bulging obtained with a laser scanning device. Clin Biomech (Bristol, Avon). 2007; 22(7):737–744

[22] Brinckmann P, Porter RW. A laboratory model of lumbar disc protrusion. Fissure and fragment. Spine. 1994; 19(2):228–235

[23] Adams MA, McMillan DW, Green TP, Dolan P. Sustained loading generates stress concentrations in lumbar intervertebral discs. Spine. 1996; 21(4):434–438

[24] Wilke HJ, Rohlmann F, Neidlinger-Wilke C, Werner K, Claes L, Kettler A. Validity and interobserver agreement of a new radiographic grading system for intervertebral disc degeneration: Part I. Lumbar spine. Eur Spine J. 2006; 15(6):720–730

[25] Freund M, Sartor K. Degenerative spine disorders in the context of clinical findings. Eur J Radiol. 2006; 58(1):15–26

[26] Carragee EJ, Tanner CM, Khurana S, et al. The rates of false-positive lumbar discography in select patients without low back symptoms. Spine. 2000; 25 (11):1373–1380, discussion 1381

[27] Carragee EJ, Don AS, Hurwitz EL, Cuellar JM, Carrino JA, Herzog R. 2009 ISSLS Prize Winner: does discography cause accelerated progression of degeneration changes in the lumbar disc: a ten-year matched cohort study. Spine. 2009; 34(21):2338–2345

[28] Boden SD, Wiesel SW. Lumbosacral segmental motion in normal individuals. Have we been measuring instability properly? Spine. 1990; 15(6):571–576

[29] Hayes MA, Howard TC, Gruel CR, Kopta JA. Roentgenographic evaluation of lumbar spine flexion-extension in asymptomatic individuals. Spine. 1989; 14 (3):327–331

[30] Panjabi MM. Clinical spinal instability and low back pain. J Electromyogr Kinesiol. 2003; 13(4):371–379

[31] Adams A, Roche O, Mazumder A, Davagnanam I, Mankad K. Imaging of degenerative lumbar intervertebral discs; linking anatomy, pathology and imaging. Postgrad Med J. 2014; 90(1067):511–519

[32] Pfirrmann CW, Metzdorf A, Zanetti M, Hodler J, Boos N. Magnetic resonance classification of lumbar intervertebral disc degeneration. Spine. 2001; 26(17):1873–1878

[33] Berger-Roscher, N, Galbusera, F, Rasche, V, Wilke, HJ. Intervertebral disc lesions: visualisation with ultra-high field MRI at 11.7 T. Eur Spine J. 2015; 24 (11):2488–2495

[34] Schonstrom, NS, Bolender, NF, Spengler, DM. The pathomorphology of spinal stenosis as seen on CT scans of the lumbar spine. Spine. 1985; 10(9):806–811

[35] Goda Y, Sakai T, Harada T, et al. Degenerative changes of the facet joints in adults with lumbar spondylolysis. Clin Spine Surg. 2016

[36] Boos N, Weissbach S, Rohrbach H, Weiler C, Spratt KF, Nerlich AG. Classification of age-related changes in lumbar intervertebral discs: 2002 Volvo Award in basic science. Spine. 2002; 27(23):2631–2644

[37] Willems PC, Staal JB, Walenkamp GH, de Bie RA. Spinal fusion for chronic low back pain: systematic review on the accuracy of tests for patient selection. Spine J. 2013; 13(2):99–109

[38] Brayda-Bruno M, Tibiletti M, Ito K, et al. Advances in the diagnosis of degenerated lumbar discs and their possible clinical application. Eur Spine J. 2014; 23 Suppl 3:S315–S323

[39] Murata M, Morio Y, Kuranobu K. Lumbar disc degeneration and segmental instability: a comparison of magnetic resonance images and plain radiographs of patients with low back pain. Arch Orthop Trauma Surg. 1994; 113 (6):297–301

[40] Thompson JP, Pearce RH, Schechter MT, Adams ME, Tsang IK, Bishop PB. Preliminary evaluation of a scheme for grading the gross morphology of the human intervertebral disc. Spine. 1990; 15(5):411–415

[41] Frobin W, Brinckmann P, Biggemann M, Tillotson M, Burton K. Precision measurement of disc height, vertebral height and sagittal plane displacement from lateral radiographic views of the lumbar spine. Clin Biomech (Bristol, Avon). 1997; 12 Suppl 1:S1–S63

[42] Berlemann U, Gries NC, Moore RJ. The relationship between height, shape and histological changes in early degeneration of the lower lumbar discs. Eur Spine J. 1998; 7(3):212–217

[43] Amonoo-Kuofi HS. Morphometric changes in the heights and anteroposterior diameters of the lumbar intervertebral discs with age. J Anat. 1991; 175:159–168

[44] Adams MA, McNally DS, Dolan P. 'Stress' distributions inside intervertebral discs. The effects of age and degeneration. J Bone Joint Surg Br. 1996; 78 (6):965–972

[45] Schollum ML, Robertson PA, Broom ND. How age influences unravelling morphology of annular lamellae—a study of interfibrecohesivity in the lumbar disc. J Anat. 2010; 216(3):310–319

[46] Vernon-Roberts B, Moore RJ, Fraser RD. The natural history of age-related disc degeneration: the pathology and sequelae of tears. Spine. 2007; 32 (25):2797–2804

[47] Krismer M, Haid C, Ogon M, Behensky H, Wimmer C. [Biomechanics of lumbar instability]. Orthopade. 1997; 26(6):516–520

[48] Roberts, S, Menage, J, Eisenstein, SM. The cartilage end-plate and intervertebral disc in scoliosis: calcification and other sequelae. J Orthop Res. 1993; 11(5):747–757

[49] Roberts S, Urban JP, Evans H, Eisenstein SM. Transport properties of the human cartilage endplate in relation to its composition and calcification. Spine. 1996; 21(4):415–420

[50] Benneker LM, Heini PF, Alini M, Anderson SE, Ito K. 2004 Young Investigator Award Winner: vertebral endplate marrow contact channel occlusions and intervertebral disc degeneration. Spine. 2005; 30(2):167–173

[51] Urban JP, Smith S, Fairbank JC. Nutrition of the intervertebral disc. Spine. 2004; 29(23):2700–2709

[52] Roughley PJ. Biology of intervertebral disc aging and degeneration: involvement of the extracellular matrix. Spine. 2004; 29(23):2691–2699

[53] Maeda S, Kokubun S. Changes with age in proteoglycan synthesis in cells cultured in vitro from the inner and outer rabbit annulus fibrosus. Responses to interleukin-1 and interleukin-1 receptor antagonist protein. Spine. 2000; 25(2):166–169

[54] Karadimas EJ, Siddiqui M, Smith FW, Wardlaw D. Positional MRI changes in supine versus sitting postures in patients with degenerative lumbar spine. J Spinal Disord Tech. 2006; 19(7):495–500

[55] Mulholland RC. The myth of lumbar instability: the importance of abnormal loading as a cause of low back pain. Eur Spine J. 2008; 17(5):619–625

[56] Galbusera, F, Schmidt, H, Neidlinger-Wilke, C, Wilke, HJ. The effect of degenerative morphological changes of the intervertebral disc on the lumbar spine biomechanics: a poroelastic finite element investigation. Comput Methods Biomech Biomed Engin. 2011; 14(8):729–739

[57] Niemeyer F, Wilke HJ, Schmidt H. Geometry strongly influences the response of numerical models of the lumbar spine—a probabilistic finite element analysis. J Biomech. 2012; 45(8):1414–1423

[58] Zhao F, Pollintine P, Hole BD, Dolan P, Adams MA. Discogenic origins of spinal instability. Spine . 2005; 30(23):2621–2630

[59] Thompson RE, Pearcy MJ, Barker TM. The mechanical effects of intervertebral disc lesions. Clin Biomech (Bristol, Avon). 2004; 19(5):448–455

[60] Przybyla A, Pollintine P, Bedzinski R, Adams MA. Outer annulus tears have less effect than endplate fracture on stress distributions inside intervertebral discs: relevance to disc degeneration. Clin Biomech (Bristol, Avon). 2006; 21 (10):1013–1019

[61] Tanaka N, An HS, Lim TH, Fujiwara A, Jeon CH, Haughton VM. The relationship between disc degeneration and flexibility of the lumbar spine. Spine J. 2001; 1(1):47–56

[62] Fujiwara A, Lim TH, An HS, et al. The effect of disc degeneration and facet joint osteoarthritis on the segmental flexibility of the lumbar spine. Spine . 2000; 25(23):3036–3044

[63] Al-Rawahi M, Luo J, Pollintine P, Dolan P, Adams MA. Mechanical function of vertebral body osteophytes, as revealed by experiments on cadaveric spines. Spine. 2011; 36(10):770–777

[64] Panjabi MM. The stabilizing system of the spine.Part I. Function, dysfunction, adaptation, and enhancement. J Spinal Disord. 1992; 5(4):383–389, discussion 397

[65] Zirbel SA, Stolworthy DK, Howell LL, Bowden AE. Intervertebral disc degeneration alters lumbar spine segmental stiffness in all modes of loading under a compressive follower load. Spine J. 2013; 13(9):1134–1147

[66] Oxland TR, Lund T, Jost B, et al. The relative importance of vertebral bone density and disc degeneration in spinal flexibility and interbody implant performance. An in vitro study. Spine. 1996; 21(22):2558–2569

[67] Gay RE, Ilharreborde B, Zhao K, Boumediene E, An KN. The effect of loading rate and degeneration on neutral region motion in human cadaveric lumbar motion segments. Clin Biomech (Bristol, Avon). 2008; 23(1):1–7

Part II

Experimental Techniques

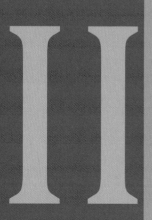

5 Differences between Human and Animal Discs: Pros and Cons of Current Animal Models for Preclinical Development of Biological Therapies for Low Back Pain

Jeffrey C. Lotz

Abstract

Animal models are an important component of preclinical therapy development for disc degeneration and discogenic pain. These models demonstrate the biological response and functional performance within context of in situ stressors that include load, host cells, and transport. Unfortunately, there is no consensus on the preferred model for preclinical purposes. Animal model factors that are commonly debated include disc size, cellular content, tissue composition, and in vivo loading. This review summarizes current literature regarding these factors and discusses how they should be integrated into the decision making for those developing biological therapies for the disc. Ultimately, the most significant barrier for identifying the ideal model is ambiguity regarding disc pain mechanisms in humans, and the lack of validated pain measures in animals that forecast clinical trial outcomes.

Keywords: animal models, low back pain, spinal disc degeneration

5.1 Introduction

Animal models allow investigators to collect data on physiological and pathological conditions that form the basis for developing clinical interventions. These models also provide a critical therapy development tool, and form a central component of preclinical evaluation of biological treatments for disc degeneration–related back pain. In situ factors such as physical stress, transport, immunity, and tissue spatial relationships will undoubtedly influence the retention and activity of regenerative products. Equally important, the consequences of therapy activity such as paracrine communication with host cells and new matrix formation will mature over time, and therefore the longitudinal assessment in vivo is required to judge the ultimate quality and safety of the desired clinical disease-modifying activity. These therapy aspects cannot be assessed purely with in vitro or computer models, and consequently, animal models are a necessary bridge to human clinical studies and provide the framework for submission, review, and regulatory approval.

A primary obstacle for disc regenerative therapies is whether the product (cells, matrices, and/or growth factors) can stimulate a desirable disease-modifying activity within the inhospitable niche of the degenerating human intervertebral disc (IVD).[1] This fact underscores the importance that the chosen animal model mimics the human situation relative to the salient technical and clinical features. The larger the discrepancy between the animal model and human, the greater the risk that the therapy will be ineffectual or even harmful.

Many animal models have been investigated in attempts to clarify disease mechanisms.[2,3,4,5] However, these are not necessarily appropriate for judging the quality of a regenerative response. Similarly, there is a diversity of animal models used for preclinical testing of bioactive disc therapies.[6] Yet, significant gaps between outcome measures in animals and pain mechanisms in humans muddle decision making when designing preclinical studies. The purpose of this review is to summarize factors that should be weighed when choosing an animal model for therapy development and validation.

5.2 Anatomy

Across the various species used for spine research, the IVD comprises the same basic subtissues: nucleus pulposus (NP), annulus fibrosus (AF), and cartilage end plate (▶ Fig. 5.1, ▶ Fig. 5.2, ▶ Fig. 5.3). This is not surprising given the similar developmental origins and functional requirements to facilitate spine flexibility while supporting load. However, species diversity, principally in size and bipedalism, leads to differences that can become significant in the context of disc tissue engineering.

5.2.1 Size

There is a tremendous range in disc size across species. For example, disc height can range between 0.25 mm for a mouse and up to 11 mm or more for a human (▶ Fig. 5.1; ▶ Table 5.1). However, when disc height is normalized by width as a measure of shape, the differences between animal and human are less extreme, and range between 12% for mouse and 31% for sheep.[7] Yet, these size differences have important biomechanical and biological consequences. Three centuries ago Galileo proposed the square-cube law, which states that as a structure's size increases, its volume (proportional to length cubed) grows faster than its surface area (proportional to length squared). For example, if an animal's disc size is doubled, then the surface area is increased by a factor of 4, whereas the volume is increased by a factor of 8. In this illustration, the square-cube law indicates that the larger disc may carry four times as much stress and nutritionally support 8 times as much tissue. Assuming that the same biomechanical and biological principles apply across species, then discs need to be redesigned and/or the animal behavior needs to be modified for tissue homeostasis as the animal becomes larger.

5.2.2 Biochemical Composition

Biomechanical properties of spinal discs can be linked to their biochemical composition and size.[8,9] Proteoglycans are a major constituent of the disc nucleus and, due to their fixed negative charge, provide the disc the capacity to osmotically swell to resist compressive mechanical forces.[10] Comparative tests indicate that nuclear proteoglycan and water contents are relatively similar between species (▶ Table 5.1), with the exception of

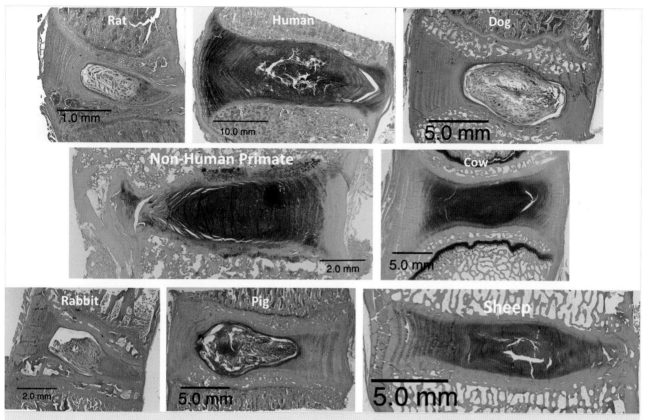

Fig. 5.1 Safranin-O stained mid-sagittal sections of various animal spinal discs. Scale bars indicate the range of disc sizes. In addition to size, images demonstrate diversity in several features, including nucleus/annulus distinction and presence of a vertebral growth plate.

rattail, which is significantly less, and baboon disc, which is significantly more.[11] Interestingly, despite the range of measured values, proteoglycan and water contents do not correlate with compressive properties across species.

The annulus is reinforced with collagen fibers that are oriented to support disc compression, bending, and axial torsion.[12,13] Disc collagen within the nucleus is similar between baboon, goat, and sheep disc, whereas that from pig is less than half and that from calf and cow is more than 3 times greater (▶ Table 5.1).[14] Similar variations are noted for the AF, where goat had 48% less and calf had 45% more than human. Yet, like proteoglycan and water composition, collagen content of annulus does not correlate strongly with disc torsional properties.

5.3 Biomechanics

Functionally, disc size, shape, and biochemical constituents affect biomechanical properties, which in turn, can influence how the regenerative effects of biological therapies observed in animals are scaled to judge an effect size for humans. Axial compressive stiffness varies between 13 N/mm in mouse and 2,491 N/mm in calf spines.[11] These differences can be narrowed by normalizing by a ratio of disc height to area, in which case disc stiffnesses from calf, cow, pig, baboon, sheep, rabbit, and rat are not statistically different from human.[11] Similar results have been reported for discs tested in axial torsion, where the normalized torsional stiffness (normalized by height divided by

the polar moment of inertia) of discs from goat and mouse (tail and lumbar) were within 10% of human, whereas calf and bovine discs were within 25%.[14] In this case, however, discs from pig and sheep were approximately 3 times stiffer, perhaps due to differences in annular material properties.[15] Taken together, these data indicate that the biomechanical effects of regenerative therapies as measured in animals may be scaled to human as an indicator of anticipated clinical effect size.

5.4 Transport

Because the disc is avascular, disc cells rely on transport to and from capillaries at the outer annulus and vertebral end plate.[16] This constraint creates opposing gradients of nutritional factors (e.g., glucose and oxygen) and products of cell metabolism (e.g., lactate[17]) from the disc periphery to the disc center. The square-cube law makes clear that the surface area for transport becomes disproportionately small compared with tissue volume as the disc size increases. Another consequence of size differences between species is the disc tolerance for metabolic demand. Computational studies demonstrate that the kinetics of solute transport into the disc significantly vary between species in relation to disc size (▶ Fig. 5.4).[18] By analogy, diffusion of disc metabolic products out of the disc will have a similar size dependency. These transport dynamics limit the extent of metabolic activity that can be supported within a disc of a particular size. This principle is beautifully depicted by experimental

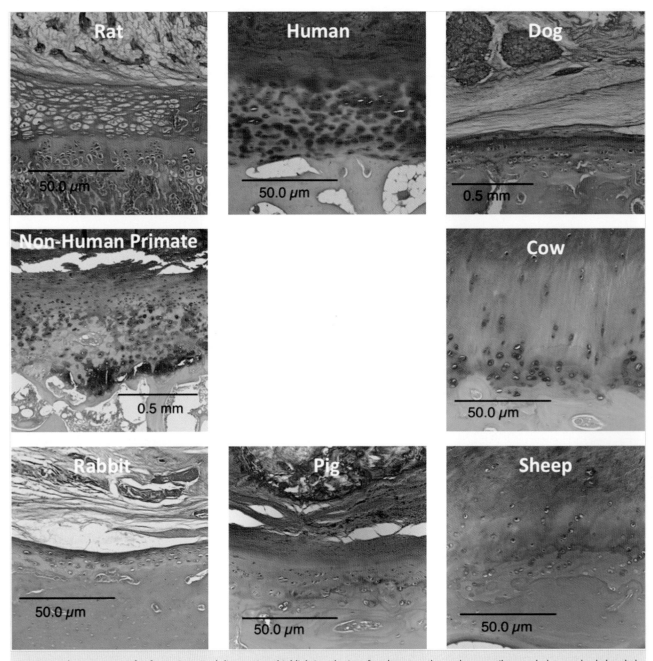

Fig. 5.2 High power view of Safranin-O–stained disc sections highlighting the interface between the nucleus, cartilage end plate, and subchondral bone. Species differences in end plate cartilage thickness are apparent.

data for nucleus cell density versus disc height across species (▶ Fig. 5.5).[19] Importantly, square-cube law scaling effects also explain why smaller discs have a greater healing capacity, as wound-site transport is better able to supply signals and a regenerative milieu, as seen in species-dependent healing of long bone fractures (▶ Fig. 5.6).[20]

5.5 Surgical Considerations

Variations of disc size across species have additional practical implications. A major disadvantage of small animals (mouse, rat, and to some extent rabbit) is that surgical techniques are limited, and it may not be meaningful or practical to study therapies that involve implants. It may also be difficult in small discs to reliably inject cells that may include viscous carriers (e.g., the mouse nucleus is approximately 0.13 μL[11]). Injecting through small-gage needles can damage cells due to high shear stress, as lower cell viability is associated with small needle diameter and long needle lengths.[21] Also, working with small volumes can lead to proportionately greater errors in the administered dose due to cell adherence within the syringe.

Size constraints are also a factor when attempting to implant tissues, scaffolds, and devices that are part of the regenerative therapy. Scaling to constructs appropriate for small animals

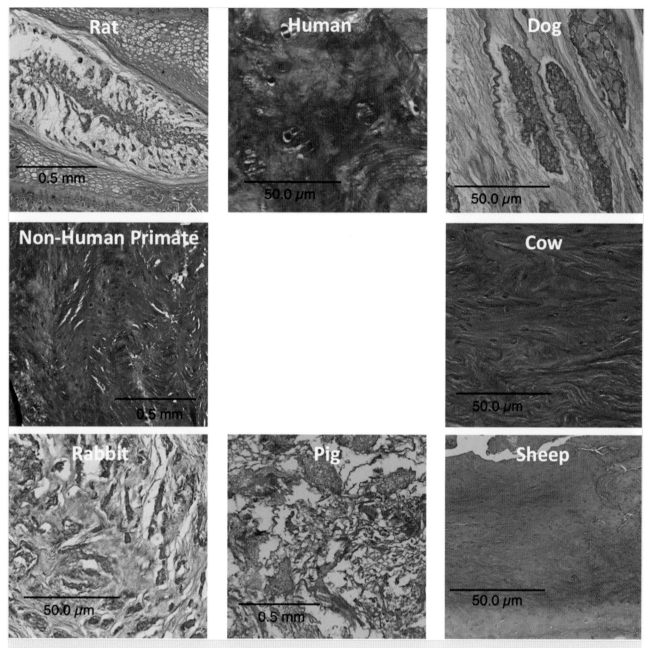

Fig. 5.3 High power view of Safranin-O–stained disc sections highlighting the cellularity of the nucleus pulposus. Species differences in cell type, density, and matrix homogeneity are notable.

may require significant deviation from the formulation and configuration of implants intended to be used in the clinical situation. For this reason, primates have been a model of choice for more traditional spinal implants and, more recently, disc arthroplasty devices.[22] Here, disc dimensions are more similar to human and hence more accommodating for implantation. Primates may also be valuable for refining the surgical approach and associated instrumentation.

Another factor is the availability of imaging to facilitate longitudinal studies. The use of magnetic resonance imaging (MRI) to assess disc healing longitudinally can help increase statistical power and reduce cost by using each animal as its own control. However, high field strength is needed to achieve a reasonable resolution in small animals (up to 7 T) and access to imaging resources may be limited for large animals.

5.6 Bipedalism

In addition to differences in metabolic stress between species, there may also be differences in physical loading. Although the common notion is that quadrupeds have lower spinal forces than humans due to their horizontal spine orientation, research in evolutionary biology indicates that in vivo biomechanical stresses are generally independent of animal size, and that tissues across species seem to be operating with a similar factor of

Table 5.1 Representative properties of animal model discs used for biological research, with human lumbar disc included for comparison

Animal	Disc height (mm)	Disc area (mm²)	Normalized compressive stiffness (MPa)	Normalized Torsional Stiffness (N-m/deg)	NP GAG per Dry Weight (ug/mg)	AF GAG per Dry Weight (ug/mg)	NP Water Content (%)	AF Water Content (%)	NP Collagen Content per Dry Weight (ug/mg)	AF Collagen Content per Dry Weight (ug/mg)
Human	10.91	1925	9.95	0.087	466	161	81	72	16	103
Calf	6.09	1100	12.72	0.108	384	66	80	69	60	149
Pig	5.46	872	15.77	0.403	379	72	83	59	6	122
Baboon	5.97	808	9.36	0.127	971	333	80	66	19	110
Goat	4.28	670	7.2	0.084	335	25	84	66	19	53
Sheep	3.4	511	9.78	0.356	547	133	75	57	20	107
Rabbit	2.4	90	10.44	0.152	579	160	82	62		78
Rat lumbar	0.77	11.85	5.09	0.04	384	47	82	65		
Mouse lumbar	0.31	1.61	2.93	0.083						
Cow tail	9.18	857	8.84	0.068	548	112	83	69	43	107
Rat tail	0.94	12.86	4.19	0.015	95	20.5	75	48		
Mouse tail				0.095						

Source: Adapted from[7,11,14]

Abbreviations: AF, annulus fibrosus; NP, nucleus pulposus.

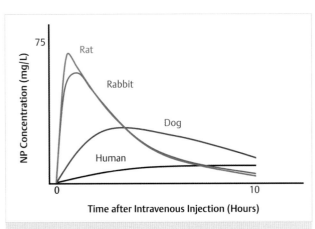

Fig. 5.4 Computational predictions of the time course of glucosamine uptake within the intervertebral disc after intravenous administration. Data indicate that disc size has a large effect on the postinjection concentration profiles. Adapted from Motaghinasab et al.[18]

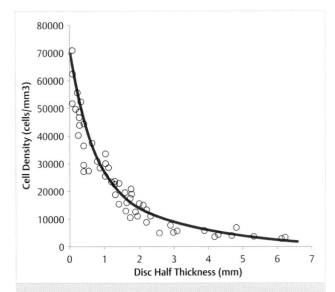

Fig. 5.5 Disc cell density as a function of disc size across several species. Red line indicates a curve fit proportional to disc height cubed, supporting that square-cube law scaling influences disc cell homeostasis. Adapted from Stairmand et al.[19]

safety (ratio of failure load to typical functional load)—of between 3 and 5.[23]

All animal spines are loaded by ligament and muscle forces developed during movement, and during maintenance of posture against gravitational loading. Even though the spines of quadrupeds are aligned parallel to gravitational forces, significant muscle forces are generated to support bending and torsional movements required for locomotion.[24] The observation that vertebral strength[24] and normalized disc stiffness (cited

above) in animals are comparable to, if not greater than human, also supports the notion that quadruped discs are subjected to significant in vivo force.

Some direct in vivo measurements have been made. Spine forces in baboon are generally proportionate (by body weight)

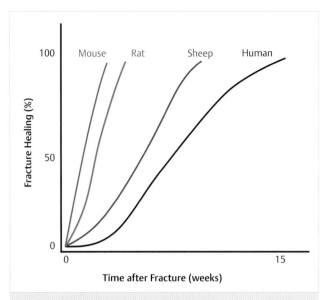

Fig. 5.6 Comparison of the time course of long bone fracture healing in mouse, rat, sheep, and human. Adapted from Garcia et al.[20]

Table 5.2 Important biological milestones of animals used in disc research

Animal	Age at skeletal maturity	Age at loss of notochordal cells	Age at onset of disc degeneration
Human	20 years	10 years	30–50 years
Chondrodystrophoid Dog	12 months	6 months	4 years
Nonchondrodystrophoid Dog	12 months	5 years	7 years
Sheep	20 months	>2 years	not reported
Rabbit	6 months	6 months	1 year
Cow	3 years	12 months	not reported
Rat	2 months	12 months	12 months
Horse	5 years	Birth	6 years

Source: Adapted from[28,86,87,88]

to human,[25] whereas those in sheep are approximately 50%.[26] Yet, the intradiscal pressures in sheep can be significantly higher than human depending on the activity.[26] Similar to baboon, bovine measurements show that loads and pressures are comparable to human during static postures, whereas dynamic pressures tend to be higher.[27]

These studies demonstrate that quadrupeds can generate significant spinal forces and pressures that are in the human range. Importantly, they indicate that animals with upright postures (e.g., primates) are not necessarily required to approximate human biomechanical conditions on tissue engineered constructs in vivo.

5.7 Cells

Cells are the heart of biological approaches for spinal disc repair. Although the therapeutic strategy may include delivery of donor cells, a bioactive agent that stimulates host cells, or a combination of both, the ultimate goal is to exploit a cellular disease-modifying activity. Several animal model features can impact the behavior of such strategies, potentially in ways that differ significantly from the human situation.

One main consideration is the fact that nucleus cells in animals may be notochordal, and have behaviors that differ from adult human NP cells. During embryonic development of the spinal column, the NP is formed by notochordal cells (NCs) that are sequestered from the developing vertebral bodies and AF.[28] Rodents, rabbits, and other nonchondrodystrophoid species[3] maintain a high NC number throughout their lifetime, whereas in other animals such as bovine, goat, and sheep, and in humans these cells disappear early in life[29,30,31] (▶ Table 5.2).

NCs are histologically and functionally distinct from human NP cells, appearing physaliferous or vacuolated. NCs express phenotypic markers such as CD44 s, galectin 3, vimentin, cytokeratins 8 and 19, chondroitin-sulfate proteoglycan (CSPG), and

collagen type IIA.[29] Molecular and immunologic studies show that NCs are more metabolically active than NP cells, and have been shown to produce significantly more lactate and proteoglycan than bovine NP cells.[32] Additionally, NCs have a number of beneficial activities: They can promote chondrogenesis of mesenchymal stem cells (MSCs),[33,34,35] protect NP cells from apoptosis,[36,37] increase glycosaminoglycan (GAG) production,[38] and secretion of regenerative factors.[39] Importantly, these therapeutic cell behaviors may vary by species, for example, porcine and canine NCs appear more potent than human.[40] By contrast, NP cells in degenerated human discs become senescent, display a catabolic phenotype,[41] and have diminished capacity to respond synthetically to mechanical load[42] and anabolic agents.[43]

A second important species difference that affects disc cell function is related to disc size, which influences transport and cell density. Therapies that aim to increase disc cell number and/or stimulate disc cell anabolic activity will, by definition, increase metabolic demand,[44] which can reduce nutrient concentrations to below critical levels.[45] Increased metabolic activity in the context of restricted glucose and oxygen can increase lactate production, which has known catabolic effects on disc cells.[46]

Consequently, given species differences in cell activity, transport, and cell density, the rate and magnitude of a biologically relevant response will likely be overestimated in studies performed on small animals and may overpredict clinical effects in humans. Therefore, treatments showing efficacy in smaller animals should have safety and efficacy profiles confirmed in larger animal models, where appropriate.[6]

5.8 The Degenerative Phenotype

As mentioned above, the unique microenvironment within the degenerated and painful disc presents an obstacle to biological manipulation for therapeutic purposes. It is becoming increasingly clear that symptomatic human discs have elevated levels of inflammatory cytokines, including tumor necrosis factor-α (TNF-α) and interleukins (ILs),[47,48,49,50] and other catabolic factors that can frustrate disc regeneration strategies. Inflammation is a normal response to tissue injury, but because the disc is avascular the response to inflammation is unique.[51] Within the disc, accumulation of metabolic waste products, matrix fragments, and cytokines inhibit matrix production and promote degeneration.[52,53,54] For example, IL-1 exposure increases expression of matrix-degrading enzymes,[55] and when combined with TNF-α, can stimulate nerve growth factor production in human IVD cells,[56] which can sensitize nociceptors and stimulate further cytokine production. Furthermore, IL-1β and TNF-α have been shown to inhibit chondrogenesis of human MSCs,[57] and prolonged exposure to an ischemic, nutrient-deprived microenvironment that resembles that of the degenerated IVD can lead to stem cell death[58,59] and potentiate inflammation.[60,61,62] Although cytokines secreted by the disc cells can stimulate wound healing, at the same time they can cause damage to transplanted cells. For example, TNF-α is a potent pro-death factor for MSCs.[63]

Many animal models of disc degeneration have been described in the literature.[3,4,64,65] These have been classified as either spontaneous or experimentally induced. Spontaneous degeneration models include certain rodents (sand rats and mice[66]), chondrodystrophoid breeds of dogs,[67] and primates.[68] Alternatively, degeneration can be produced by mechanical (in vivo compression, surgical instability), chemical (enzymatic treatment), or surgical (annular stab injury) means.[5] For the most part, these have been used to study degeneration mechanisms, and demonstrate many clinically relevant architectural, biochemical, and cellular changes—such as fibrous tissue formation in the nucleus, annular disorganization, loss of disc height, and decreases in nucleus cellularity.

Whether degeneration in animals mimics the inflammatory profile of painful human discs is less clear. Disc injury and herniation in animals can lead to a transient inflammation that lasts from days in mice and rats, to weeks in rabbits, and up to months in large animals.[5] However, the inflammation in surgically injured discs is primarily centered at the injury site and the granulation tissue that forms at the periphery of the wound tract.[69] Additionally, whether there is a clinically relevant inflammatory response to degeneration in spontaneous animal models has not been described. As a result, inflammation mechanisms, potential species differences, and their practical impact on regenerative therapies are yet to be disentangled.

5.9 Pain-Related Behavior

It may sound obvious, but low back patients seek clinical care because of pain and disability, not because of disc degeneration per se. Although in general, subjective self-ratings of back pain using questionnaires and scales are reliable,[70] the linkage between disc pathology and pain is variable.[71] This may be because chronic back pain in humans is commonly comorbid with a wide range of complex clinical conditions, all contributing to reductions in quality of life.[72] This fact is reinforced by the many studies that demonstrate disc degeneration in

asymptomatic volunteers,[73,74] and has significant implications for the preclinical development of back pain therapies and diagnostic tools that reliably identify discs appropriate for treatment. Specifically, if disc degeneration is necessary but not sufficient to cause back pain, then therapies targeting degeneration may not necessarily be clinically effective, particularly if it is difficult to distinguish degenerated/asymptomatic from degenerated/painful discs in the clinical setting.

Pain is a subjective experience associated with actual or impending tissue damage.[75] In humans, pain can have effects on behavior such as complaints of pain, reductions in activity, increased medication intake, or alterations in facial expression and body posture.[75] Although animals can't tell us about their pain, they may experience simple reflexive or innate pain behaviors such as withdrawal from a stimulus (hot, cold, or von Frey fibers) or other self-protective actions such as licking, biting, scratching, limited mobility, and vocalization. These behaviors may lack clinical face validity, but they can be reliably and objectively scored. Other proxy measures, such as gene expression, imaging, and neural activity have also been reported.[72]

Generally, the most used animals in pain research are mice and rats, and these have been most effective in backward validation—confirming activity of therapies already known to be effective in humans—rather than forward validation during therapy development.[72] Because an injured disc can chemically and mechanically irritate adjacent nerve roots, an early model for disc injury involved applying NP directly onto the nerve root in rats.[64] More recently, several groups have reported pain-related behaviors in rats secondary to surgical or chemical disc injury.[76,77,78,79] However, similar associations are not reliably reported for larger animals, such as rabbits, which make them less suitable to assess therapy efficacy for discogenic pain.[77]

5.10 Conclusion

In general, animal models are critical for evaluating the biological response and simulating the functional performance of new therapies. However, there is no consensus regarding the preferred animal model for regenerative therapies for spinal discs. Although there are often-debated species-specific considerations—size, tissue composition, and cellular content as described above—the primary barrier preventing progress is the uncertain pathogenesis for axial back pain in humans. If we don't know what causes the pain that brings patients to the clinic, then it is unreasonable to expect consensus on preclinical models to establish treatment efficacy.

Consequently, the logical first step toward animal model standardization is development and validation of diagnostic tools that localize spinal pathologies that associate with axial pain in human clinical studies.[80] Such studies will inform therapy development by providing evidence for biologically plausible disease-modifying activities. Without this, even promising therapies judged using standardized models may not be clinically effective. For example, there is an existing, generally accepted model for bioactive therapies for back pain—the rabbit model for intertransverse process spine fusion.[81,82] In this model, critical variables of disease-modifying activity are bony bridging and mechanical stability of the treated spinal level. Therapies tested in this model have been shown to be effective for many spinal indications, such as degenerative spondylolisthesis.[83] Yet, despite the availability of this standardized model and the generally agreed-upon mechanism of action (eliminating mechanical instability), the successful clinical application of spine fusion for axial back pain is not consistently demonstrated.[80,84] So, the lack of clinical success for new chronic low back pain therapies can't be blamed solely on the absence of an accepted animal model. The primary dilemma is our inability to reliably identify the origin of pain in this difficult patient population.

So, how should we proceed? Given the growing global burden of low back pain[85] we need to be aggressively advancing in parallel both improved diagnostic tools and therapies, given the circular reliance between proper diagnosis and efficacious treatment. First, it is critical that new therapies be grounded in current basic and clinical science, with mechanisms of action that are biologically plausible and clinically relevant. Scientists need to be working closely with diagnosticians and clinicians to understand how the proposed therapy would fit within the current diagnostic and patient management paradigms. How would patients and affected spinal levels for treatment be identified, and how would the outcomes be monitored? Second, biological plausibility of the desired disease-modifying activity should be established in models of increasing complexity, starting with cells in vitro and moving to small, and perhaps large animals. Given the absence of validated pain models, it will be important to push toward well-designed Phase I clinical studies once safety has been appropriately established. Incremental progress toward adoption of new low back pain therapies will come from an iterative and integrated development of both improved diagnostic algorithms plus promising therapeutics with clinically relevant mechanisms of action.

Still, animal models will continue to have a central role in preclinical development of biologics for low back pain—even in the absence of consensus on pain mechanisms. Investigators will need to select the model that best balances the therapy-specific constraints on how the treatment is delivered and what it is intended to accomplish. In this selection, the most critical variables to justify are size (relative to transport and surgical considerations) and host cell activity (e.g., notochordal versus adult disc cells). Other important model factors are reproducibility, and standardization of spinal level, therapy dose, choice of control, postoperative survival period, and postmortem evaluation metrics. Although some could contend that primates best approximate the human situation, there are significant ethical concerns, costs, and logistical constraints that limit their applicability. Moral considerations have appropriately led to significant oversight on primate studies,[86] and justification that this species is required is difficult to reconcile given the ambiguities inherent in the disc regeneration field summarized here. Arguably, perhaps the best current model from these perspectives is the rabbit, in which the disc stab injury has been shown to reliably create a degenerative phenotype and reproducibly simulate a therapeutic response.[87] Models of spontaneous degeneration may be argued to be more clinically relevant,[67] but come with practical challenges for conducting comprehensive studies with consistent starting points. Large animals with non-notochordal disc cells are similarly problematic due to cost, which creates difficulties in designing and justifying studies with sufficient statistical power, particularly given the lack of

relevant pain outcomes. Consequently, the combination of factors that include (1) good reproducibility and low cost of rabbits and (2) the push to Phase I human clinical studies to address pain outcomes once safety has been established, indicate that governing bodies, such as the US Food and Drug Administration (FDA), may accept smaller animals for therapies that aren't primarily structural, such as injectable biologics as contrasted with tissue engineered constructs for total disc replacement or annular repair in postdiscectomy patients. This clearly requires discussion with FDA to confirm that the chosen model meets the agency's qualification criteria.

This review highlights the pressing need for large animal models of discogenic pain that reliably forecast clinical trial outcomes. The ideal animal model for preclinical development of biological therapies for discogenic pain would (1) be of similar size to human so as to match in situ stressors such as load, transport, and cytokines; (2) include cells with similar activity to adult human; and (3) have a validated degenerative phenotype with relevant pain-related behavior.

Given the current ambiguity regarding disc degeneration and back pain mechanisms in humans, validated large animal models won't likely be available anytime soon. [88,89,90]

5.11 References

[1] Sakai D, Andersson GB. Stem cell therapy for intervertebral disc regeneration: obstacles and solutions. Nat Rev Rheumatol. 2015; 11(4):243–256

[2] Masuda K, Lotz JC. New challenges for intervertebral disc treatment using regenerative medicine. Tissue Eng Part B Rev. 2010; 16(1):147–158

[3] Alini M, Eisenstein SM, Ito K, et al. Are animal models useful for studying human disc disorders/degeneration? Eur Spine J. 2008; 17(1):2–19

[4] Lotz JC. Animal models of intervertebral disc degeneration: lessons learned. Spine. 2004; 29(23):2742–2750

[5] Lotz JC, Ulrich JA. Innervation, inflammation, and hypermobility may characterize pathologic disc degeneration: review of animal model data. J Bone Joint Surg Am. 2006; 88 Suppl 2:76–82

[6] Oehme D, Goldschlager T, Ghosh P, Rosenfeld JV, Jenkin G. Cell-based therapies used to treat lumbar degenerative disc disease: a systematic review of animal studies and human clinical trials. Stem Cells Int. 2015; 2015:946031

[7] O'Connell GD, Vresilovic EJ, Elliott DM. Comparison of animals used in disc research to human lumbar disc geometry. Spine. 2007; 32(3):328–333

[8] Lundon K, Bolton K. Structure and function of the lumbar intervertebral disk in health, aging, and pathologic conditions. J Orthop Sports Phys Ther. 2001; 31(6):291–303, discussion 304–306

[9] Akeson WH, Woo SL, Taylor TK, Ghosh P, Bushell GR. Biomechanics and biochemistry of the intervertebral disks: the need for correlation studies. Clin OrthopRelat Res. 1977(129):133–140

[10] Urban JP, Maroudas A, Bayliss MT, Dillon J. Swelling pressures of proteoglycans at the concentrations found in cartilaginous tissues. Biorheology. 1979; 16(6):447–464

[11] Beckstein JC, Sen S, Schaer TP, Vresilovic EJ, Elliott DM. Comparison of animal discs used in disc research to human lumbar disc: axial compression mechanics and glycosaminoglycan content. Spine. 2008; 33(6): E166–E173

[12] Hickey DS, Hukins DW. Collagen fibril diameters and elastic fibres in the annulus fibrosus of human fetal intervertebral disc. J Anat. 1981; 133(Pt 3):351–357

[13] Meakin JR, Hukins DW. Effect of removing the nucleus pulposus on the deformation of the annulus fibrosus during compression of the intervertebral disc. J Biomech. 2000; 33(5):575–580

[14] Showalter BL, Beckstein JC, Martin JT, et al. Comparison of animal discs used in disc research to human lumbar disc: torsion mechanics and collagen content. Spine. 2012; 37(15):E900–E907

[15] Monaco LA, DeWitte-Orr SJ, Gregory DE. A comparison between porcine, ovine, and bovine intervertebral disc anatomy and single lamella annulus fibrosus tensile properties. J Morphol. 2016; 277(2):244–251

[16] Urban JP, Smith S, Fairbank JC. Nutrition of the intervertebral disc. Spine. 2004; 29(23):2700–2709

[17] Holm S, Maroudas A, Urban JP, Selstam G, Nachemson A. Nutrition of the intervertebral disc: solute transport and metabolism. Connect Tissue Res. 1981; 8(2):101–119

[18] Motaghinasab S, Shirazi-Adl A, Parnianpour M, Urban JP. Disc size markedly influences concentration profiles of intravenously administered solutes in the intervertebral disc: a computational study on glucosamine as a model solute. Eur Spine J. 2014; 23(4):715–723

[19] Stairmand JW, Holm S, Urban JPG. Factors influencing oxygen concentration gradients in the intervertebral disc.A theoretical analysis. Spine. 1991; 16 (4):444–449

[20] Garcia P, Histing T, Holstein JH, et al. Rodent animal models of delayed bone healing and non-union formation: a comprehensive review. Eur Cell Mater. 2013; 26:1–12, discussion 12–14

[21] Amer MH, White LJ, Shakesheff KM. The effect of injection using narrow-bore needles on mammalian cells: administration and formulation considerations for cell therapies. J Pharm Pharmacol. 2015; 67(5):640–650

[22] Cunningham BW, Lowery GL, Serhan HA, et al. Total disc replacement arthroplasty using the AcroFlex lumbar disc: a non-human primate model. Eur Spine J. 2002; 11 Suppl 2:S115–S123

[23] Biewener AA. Safety factors in bone strength. Calcif Tissue Int. 1993; 53 Suppl 1:S68–S74

[24] Smit TH. The use of a quadruped as an in vivo model for the study of the spine - biomechanical considerations. Eur Spine J. 2002; 11(2):137–144

[25] Ledet EH, Tymeson MP, DiRisio DJ, Cohen B, Uhl RL. Direct real-time measurement of in vivo forces in the lumbar spine. Spine J. 2005; 5(1):85–94

[26] Reitmaier, S, Schmidt, H, Ihler, R, et al. Preliminary investigations on intradiscal pressures during daily activities: an in vivo study using the merino sheep. PLoS One. 2013; 8(7):e69610

[27] Buttermann GR, Beaubien BP, Saeger LC. Mature runt cow lumbar intradiscal pressures and motion segment biomechanics. Spine J. 2009; 9(2):105–114

[28] Urban JP, Roberts S, Ralphs JR. The nucleus of the intervertebral disc from development to degeneration. Am Zool. 2000; 40:53–61

[29] Hunter CJ, Matyas JR, Duncan NA. The notochordal cell in the nucleus pulposus: a review in the context of tissue engineering. Tissue Eng. 2003; 9 (4):667–677

[30] Weiler C, Nerlich AG, Schaaf R, Bachmeier BE, Wuertz K, Boos N. Immunohistochemical identification of notochordal markers in cells in the aging human lumbar intervertebral disc. Eur Spine J. 2010; 19(10):1761–1770

[31] Trout, JJ, Buckwalter, JA, Moore, KC, Landas, SK. Ultrastructure of the human intervertebral disc. I. Changes in notochordal cells with age. Tissue Cell. 1982; 14(2):359–369

[32] Miyazaki T, Kobayashi S, Takeno K, Meir A, Urban J, Baba H. A phenotypic comparison of proteoglycan production of intervertebral disc cells isolated from rats, rabbits, and bovine tails; which animal model is most suitable to study tissue engineering and biological repair of human disc disorders? Tissue Eng Part A. 2009; 15(12):3835–3846

[33] Korecki CL, Taboas JM, Tuan RS, Iatridis JC. Notochordal cell conditioned medium stimulates mesenchymal stem cell differentiation toward a young nucleus pulposus phenotype. Stem Cell Res Ther. 2010; 1(2):18

[34] Risbud MV, Schaer TP, Shapiro IM. Toward an understanding of the role of notochordal cells in the adult intervertebral disc: from discord to accord. Dev Dyn. 2010; 239(8):2141–2148

[35] Potier E, de Vries S, van Doeselaar M, Ito K. Potential application of notochordal cells for intervertebral disc regeneration: an in vitro assessment. Eur Cell Mater. 2014; 28:68–80, discussion 80–81

[36] Erwin WM, Islam D, Inman RD, Fehlings MG, Tsui FW. Notochordal cells protect nucleus pulposus cells from degradation and apoptosis: implications for the mechanisms of intervertebral disc degeneration. Arthritis Res Ther. 2011; 13(6):R215

[37] Mehrkens A, Karim MZ, Kim S, Hilario R, Fehlings MG, Erwin WM. Canine notochordal cell-secreted factors protect murine and human nucleus pulposus cells from apoptosis by inhibition of activated caspase-9 and caspase-3/7. Evid Based Spine Care J. 2013; 4(2):154–156

[38] Abbott RD, Purmessur D, Monsey RD, Iatridis JC. Regenerative potential of TGFβ3 + Dex and notochordal cell conditioned media on degenerated human intervertebral disc cells. J Orthop Res. 2012; 30(3):482–488

[39] Cornejo MC, Cho SK, Giannarelli C, Iatridis JC, Purmessur D. Soluble factors from the notochordal-rich intervertebral disc inhibit endothelial cell invasion and vessel formation in the presence and absence of pro-inflammatory cytokines. Osteoarthritis Cartilage. 2015; 23(3):487–496

[40] Bach FC, de Vries SA, Krouwels A, et al. The species-specific regenerative effects of notochordal cell-conditioned medium on chondrocyte-like cells derived from degenerated human intervertebral discs. Eur Cell Mater. 2015; 30:132–146, discussion 146–147

[41] Gruber HE, Ingram JA, Norton HJ, Hanley EN , Jr. Senescence in cells of the aging and degenerating intervertebral disc: immunolocalization of senescence-associated beta-galactosidase in human and sand rat discs. Spine. 2007; 32(3):321–327

[42] Le Maitre CL, Frain J, Millward-Sadler J, Fotheringham AP, Freemont AJ, Hoyland JA. Altered integrin mechanotransduction in human nucleus pulposus cells derived from degenerated discs. Arthritis Rheum. 2009; 60(2):460–469

[43] Abbott RD, Purmessur D, Monsey RD, Brigstock DR, Laudier DM, Iatridis JC. Degenerative grade affects the responses of human nucleus pulposus cells to link-N, CTGF, and TGFβ3. J Spinal Disord Tech. 2013; 26(3):E86–E94

[44] Huang YC, Urban JP, Luk KD. Intervertebral disc regeneration: do nutrients lead the way? Nat Rev Rheumatol. 2014; 10(9):561–566

[45] Shirazi-Adl A, Taheri M, Urban JP. Analysis of cell viability in intervertebral disc: effect of endplate permeability on cell population. J Biomech. 2010; 43 (7):1330–1336

[46] Grunhagen, T, Wilde, G, Soukane, DM, Shirazi-Adl, SA, Urban, JP. Nutrient supply and intervertebral disc metabolism. J Bone Joint Surg Am. 2006; 88 Suppl 2:30–35

[47] Weiler C, Nerlich AG, Bachmeier BE, Boos N. Expression and distribution of tumor necrosis factor alpha in human lumbar intervertebral discs: a study in surgical specimen and autopsy controls. Spine. 2005; 30(1):44–53, discussion 54

[48] Olmarker K, Larsson K. Tumor necrosis factor alpha and nucleus-pulposus-induced nerve root injury. Spine. 1998; 23(23):2538–2544

[49] Miyamoto H, Saura R, Harada T, Doita M, Mizuno K. The role of cyclooxygenase-2 and inflammatory cytokines in pain induction of herniated lumbar intervertebral disc. Kobe J Med Sci. 2000; 46(1–2):13–28

[50] Ahn SH, Cho YW, Ahn MW, Jang SH, Sohn YK, Kim HS. mRNA expression of cytokines and chemokines in herniated lumbar intervertebral discs. Spine. 2002; 27(9):911–917

[51] Molinos M, Almeida CR, Caldeira J, Cunha C, Gonçalves RM, Barbosa MA. Inflammation in intervertebral disc degeneration and regeneration. J R Soc Interface. 2015; 12(108):20150429

[52] Takegami K, Thonar EJ, An HS, Kamada H, Masuda K. Osteogenic protein-1 enhances matrix replenishment by intervertebral disc cells previously exposed to interleukin-1. Spine. 2002; 27(12):1318–1325

[53] Shen B, Melrose J, Ghosh P, Taylor F. Induction of matrix metalloproteinase-2 and -3 activity in ovine nucleus pulposus cells grown in three-dimensional agarose gel culture by interleukin-1beta: a potential pathway of disc degeneration. Eur Spine J. 2003; 12(1):66–75

[54] Séguin CA, Pilliar RM, Roughley PJ, Kandel RA. Tumor necrosis factor-alpha modulates matrix production and catabolism in nucleus pulposus tissue. Spine. 2005; 30(17):1940–1948

[55] Le Maitre CL, Freemont AJ, Hoyland JA. The role of interleukin-1 in the pathogenesis of human intervertebral disc degeneration. Arthritis Res Ther. 2005; 7(4):R732–R745

[56] Abe Y, Akeda K, An HS, et al. Proinflammatory cytokines stimulate the expression of nerve growth factor by human intervertebral disc cells. Spine. 2007; 32(6):635–642

[57] Wehling N, Palmer GD, Pilapil C, et al. Interleukin-1beta and tumor necrosis factor alpha inhibit chondrogenesis by human mesenchymal stem cells through NF-kappaB-dependent pathways. Arthritis Rheum. 2009; 60 (3):801–812

[58] Potier E, Ferreira E, Meunier A, Sedel L, Logeart-Avramoglou D, Petite H. Prolonged hypoxia concomitant with serum deprivation induces massive human mesenchymal stem cell death. Tissue Eng. 2007; 13(6):1325–1331

[59] Wuertz K, Godburn K, Neidlinger-Wilke C, Urban J, Iatridis JC. Behavior of mesenchymal stem cells in the chemical microenvironment of the intervertebral disc. Spine. 2008; 33(17):1843–1849

[60] Early SB, Hise K, Han JK, Borish L, Steinke JW. Hypoxia stimulates inflammatory and fibrotic responses from nasal-polyp derived fibroblasts. Laryngoscope. 2007; 117(3):511–515

[61] Westra J, Brouwer E, Bos R, et al. Regulation of cytokine-induced HIF-1alpha expression in rheumatoid synovial fibroblasts. Ann N Y AcadSci. 2007; 1108:340–348

[62] Ahn JK, Koh EM, Cha HS, et al. Role of hypoxia-inducible factor-1alpha in hypoxia-induced expressions of IL-8, MMP-1 and MMP-3 in rheumatoid fibroblast-like synoviocytes. Rheumatology (Oxford). 2008; 47(6):834–839

[63] Fan VH, Tamama K, Au A, et al. Tethered epidermal growth factor provides a survival advantage to mesenchymal stem cells. Stem Cells. 2007; 25 (5):1241–1251

[64] Strong JA, Xie W, Bataille FJ, Zhang JM. Preclinical studies of low back pain. Mol Pain. 2013; 9:17

[65] Singh K, Masuda K, An HS. Animal models for human disc degeneration. Spine J. 2005; 5(6) Suppl:267S–279S

[66] Gruber HE, Johnson T, Norton HJ, Hanley EN , Jr. The sand rat model for disc degeneration: radiologic characterization of age-related changes: cross-sectional and prospective analyses. Spine. 2002; 27(3):230–234

[67] Bergknut, N, Rutges, JP, Kranenburg, HJ, et al. The dog as an animal model for intervertebral disc degeneration? Spine. 2012; 37(5):351–358

[68] Bailey JF, Fields AJ, Liebenberg E, Mattison JA, Lotz JC, Kramer PA. Comparison of vertebral and intervertebral disc lesions in aging humans and rhesus monkeys. Osteoarthritis Cartilage. 2014; 22(7):980–985

[69] O'Neill CW, Liu JJ, Leibenberg E, et al. Percutaneous plasma decompression alters cytokine expression in injured porcine intervertebral discs. Spine J. 2004; 4(1):88–98

[70] Price DD, McGrath PA, Rafii A, Buckingham B. The validation of visual analogue scales as ratio scale measures for chronic and experimental pain. Pain. 1983; 17(1):45–56

[71] Cheung KM. The relationship between disc degeneration, low back pain, and human pain genetics. Spine J. 2010; 10(11):958–960

[72] Mogil JS. Animal models of pain: progress and challenges. Nat Rev Neurosci. 2009; 10(4):283–294

[73] Borenstein DG, et al. The value of magnetic resonance imaging of the lumbar spine to predict low-back pain in asymptomatic subjects: a seven-year follow up study. J Bone Joint Surg Am. 2001; 83-A:1306–1311

[74] Boden SD, Davis DO, Dina TS, Patronas NJ, Wiesel SW. Abnormal magnetic-resonance scans of the lumbar spine in asymptomatic subjects. A prospective investigation. J Bone Joint Surg Am. 1990; 72(3):403–408

[75] Keefe FJ, Fillingim RB, Williams DA. Behavioral assessment of pain: nonverbal measures in animals and humans. Ilar News. 1991; 33(1–2):3–13

[76] Olmarker K. Puncture of a lumbar intervertebral disc induces changes in spontaneous pain behavior: an experimental study in rats. Spine. 2008; 33 (8):850–855

[77] Kim JS, Kroin JS, Li X, et al. The rat intervertebral disk degeneration pain model: relationships between biological and structural alterations and pain. Arthritis Res Ther. 2011; 13(5):R165

[78] Lee M, Kim BJ, Lim EJ, et al. Complete Freund's adjuvant-induced intervertebral discitis as an animal model for discogenic low back pain. Anesth Analg. 2009; 109(4):1287–1296

[79] Rousseau MA, Ulrich JA, Bass EC, Rodriguez AG, Liu JJ, Lotz JC. Stab incision for inducing intervertebral disc degeneration in the rat. Spine. 2007; 32 (1):17–24

[80] Eck JC, Sharan A, Ghogawala Z, et al. Guideline update for the performance of fusion procedures for degenerative disease of the lumbar spine. Part 7: lumbar fusion for intractable low-back pain without stenosis or spondylolisthesis. J Neurosurg Spine. 2014; 21(1):42–47

[81] Ghodasra JH, Daley EL, Hsu EL, Hsu WK. Factors influencing arthrodesis rates in a rabbit posterolateral spine model with iliac crest autograft. Eur Spine J. 2014; 23(2):426–434

[82] Boden, SD, Schimandle, JH, Hutton, WC. An experimental lumbar inter-transverse process spinal fusion model.Radiographic, histologic, and biomechanical healing characteristics. Spine. 1995; 20(4):412–420

[83] Weinstein, JN, Lurie, JD, Tosteson, TD, et al. Surgical versus nonsurgical treatment for lumbar degenerative spondylolisthesis. N Engl J Med. 2007; 356(22):2257–2270

[84] Deyo RA, Mirza SK, Turner JA, Martin BI. Overtreating chronic back pain: time to back off? J Am Board Fam Med. 2009; 22(1):62–68

[85] Hoy D, March L, Brooks P, et al. Measuring the global burden of low back pain. Best Pract Res Clin Rheumatol. 2010; 24(2):155–165

[86] Phillips KA, Bales KL, Capitanio JP, et al. Why primate models matter. Am J Primatol. 2014; 76(9):801–827

[87] Masuda K, Aota Y, Muehleman C, et al. A novel rabbit model of mild, reproducible disc degeneration by an anulus needle puncture: correlation between the degree of disc injury and radiological and histological appearances of disc degeneration. Spine. 2005; 30(1):5–14

[88] Townsend HG, Leach DH, Doige CE, Kirkaldy-Willis WH. Relationship between spinal biomechanics and pathological changes in the equine thoracolumbar spine. Equine Vet J. 1986; 18(2):107–112

[89] Leung VY, Hung SC, Li L C, et al. Age-related degeneration of lumbar intervertebral discs in rabbits revealed by deuterium oxide-assisted MRI. Osteoarthritis Cartilage. 2008; 16(11):1312–1318

[90] Corlett SC, Couch M, Care AD, Sykes AR. Measurement of plasma osteocalcin in sheep: assessment of circadian variation, the effects of age and nutritional status and the response to perturbation of the adrenocortical axis. Exp Physiol. 1990; 75(4):515–527

6 Grading Scales for Disc Degeneration and Regeneration: Clinical and Experimental

Peter Grunert

Abstract

Several grading scales have been developed to quantify disc degeneration and regeneration. They are either based on macroscopic anatomy, histology or X-ray and magnetic resonance imaging (MRI). Macroscopic changes are evaluated ex vivo on mid-sagittal sections of explanted spinal segments. The most common grading system was developed by Thompson et al. It takes nucleus pulposus morphology, annulus fibrosus and end plate intactness as well as osteophyte formation into account. The Thompson grade is commonly used to validate degenerative changes assessed by novel imaging techniques or biochemical markers. Various histology based classifications have been developed for the human and animal spine. Boos et al established a grading scale for the human spine which takes matrix staining properties, cell quantity and as well as endplate morphology into account. Histological animal spine classifications are often used for in vivo disc regeneration experiments. Han et al developed a grading system in the rat spine which based on cell composition and morphology as well as staining properties of the extracellular matrix. X-Ray and MRI techniques allow for in vivo assessment of disc degeneration which makes it the most relevant assessment for clinical outcome studies. Pfirrmann developed an MR imaging grading system predominantly based on nucleus pulposus T2 signal intensity as well as loss of disc height. Recently quantitative MRI techniques have been introduced which allow for indirect assessments of the biochemical tissue composition of intervertebral discs. This facilitates to detect early degenerative changes in vivo.

Keywords: degeneration, grading system, histology, intervertebral disc, regeneration, MR imaging

6.1 Introduction

Grading scales for intervertebral disc (IVD) degeneration are important to evaluate degenerative processes and success of regenerative efforts. Scales allow researchers to present and compare study outcomes more objectively given that results on disc health are presented with a numeric value in contrast to nonquantitative assessments, which most commonly rely on an objective morphological description of disc pathology.

There are three different diagnostic assessments for which grading scales have been established to quantify degenerative changes of IVDs: (1) macroscopic anatomy, (2) histology, and (3) radiology.

6.2 Macroscopic Anatomy

Macroscopic anatomy is studied on gross sections of IVDs either by a mid-sagittal cut through a spinal segment or an axial cut through the middle of the disc. It allows ex vivo evaluation of native unstained tissue.

6.2.1 Grading Scales

Nachemson was the first to establish a grading scale for mid-axial (transverse) IVD sections in 1960.[1] This four-scale grading system takes into account nucleus pulposus (NP) morphology (gelatinous or fibrotic), the intactness of the annulus fibrosus (AF), and whether both structures maintain a visible border. The disadvantage of a mid-axial cut is that it does not allow for evaluation of changes in end plate cartilage and the vertebral body. In 1990, Thompson et al developed a grading system for mid-sagittal sections that included those structures and therefore allowed for a more complete evaluation of spinal segments.[2] It is the most commonly used macroscopic scale and became the standard system for quantifying degenerative changes in humans and animals.[3,4] The Thompson system involves five scales that are graded according to the progression of NP, AF, end plate, and vertebral body alterations. Nuclear changes involve formation of fibrous tissue and clefts throughout the NP; annular changes include disruption of the lamellar tissue and loss of demarcation to the nucleus. End plate alterations range from focal defects to diffuse sclerotic changes. Vertebral bodies are evaluated for osteophyte formation (▸ Table 6.1). The excess of these degenerative alterations have been shown to correlate with specimen age.[2]

6.2.2 Experimental Value

The Thompson grade has proven to be of high experimental value and is therefore broadly used for research purposes.[4] It has demonstrated a low intra- and interobserver variability[2,4] resulting in reproducible and comparable scores. It has shown a correlation to cellular and biochemical degenerative parameters as evidenced by Iatridis et al, who demonstrated an inverse correlation of decreasing proteoglycan and water content.[5] The same was found for the proteolytic enzyme aggrecanase.[6] Antoniou et al demonstrated a positive correlation to the amount of denatured type II collagen.[7] Additionally, the amount of senescent cells (without ability to proliferate) in the AF of degenerated discs has also shown a positive correlation.[8]

The Thompson grade also reflects degenerative changes on magnetic resonance imaging (MRI) in humans as well as in animals.[3,9] Loss of NP T2 signal intensity as well as loss of disc height has been shown to correlates to increasing Thompson grades.[3]

6.2.3 Clinical Value

In contrast to its experimental value, the Thompson grade is of low clinical relevance given that it is based on gross sections from human cadavers. However, it is often used to validate clinical diagnostic tests such as MRI or X-ray imaging.[10]

Table 6.1 Macroscopic grading introduced by Thompson et al[2] of lumbar disc degeneration on sagittal sections

Grade	Nucleus	Annulus	End plate	Vertebral body
I	Bulging gel	Discrete fibrous lamellae	Hyaline, uniformly thick	Margins rounded
II	White fibrous tissue peripherally	Mucinous material between lamellae	Thickness irregular	Margins pointed
III	Consolidated fibrous tissue	Extensive mucinous infiltration; loss of annular–nuclear demarcation	Focal defects in cartilage	Early chondrophytes or osteophytes at margins
IV	Horizontal clefts parallel to end plate	Focal disruptions	Fibrocartilage extending from subchondral bone; irregularity and focal sclerosis in subchondral bone	Osteophytes less than 2 mm
V	Clefts extended through nucleus and annulus		Diffuse sclerosis	Osteophytes greater than 2 mm

6.3 Histology

Histology is used to study IVD tissue samples microscopically most commonly using mid-sagittal cuts through the segment. Histology analysis is used for ex vivo and in vivo[11] evaluation of stained tissue in humans and animals. Compared with macroscopic anatomy it allows for evaluation of changes of cell density and composition as well as evaluation of matrix components via different staining methods. Besides hematoxylin and eosin (H&E), various stains are used for specific IVD structures. Alcian blue and Safranin-O are used to stain for proteoglycans[12] and picrosirius red for collagen.[13]Recently, a combination of both has been proposed.[14]

6.3.1 Grading Scales

Boos et al first introduced a histological grading system for human spinal segments using H&E and alcian blue stains.[15] Degenerative changes were subdivided into changes of the IVD, cartilage end plate, and end plate bone. The disc is graded based on chondrocyte cell decay and density, mucus degeneration (accumulation of eosinophilic tissue), tear or cleft formation, and granular changes (basophilic tissue on alcian blue stains).

End plate changes are graded according to intactness of cartilage tissue and bony sclerosis (▶ Table 6.2). These histological alterations showed a significant positive correlation with specimen age.[15] Due to its complex design and large number of grading parameters, the Boos classification often had to be modified for research purposes.[16,17] Another disadvantage is that the IVD is evaluated as a whole and not by its NP and AF component individually.

Rutges et al designed a simpler grading system that evaluates the AF and NP separately.[18] This classification system is similar to the macroscopic Thompson grading. The AF is described as organized or ruptured with a sharp or not distinguishable border to the NP. Nuclear alterations are classified with NP chondrocyte cellularity (cluster or no cluster formation) and nuclear matrix organization and staining with Safranin-O and alcian blue (▶ Table 6.3).

Different histological grading systems had to be developed for the animal spine. This is due to spinal segments of animals showing a varying degree of anatomical differences compared with humans. Animal IVDs are also often studied using specimen at a relatively young age with an NP predominantly composed of notochordal cells[3] in contrast to adult human discs which have a predominant chondrocyte cell composition.[19] In addition, animal spines are often used as disc degeneration models with an artificially induced degenerative process[20] that has an altered histological presentation[21] compared with naturally occurring degeneration.

Bergknut et al introduced a classification specifically for the canine spine. The NP and AF are graded according to their approximate percentage of notochordal cells or fibroblast cells, respectively, and by the amount of chondrocyte metaplasia or proliferation in those structures.[22] As in the Boos and Rutges grading systems it also includes staining characteristics of the NP (picosirius red and alcian blue) as well as morphological changes of the end plate (thickness and intactness).[22]

Han et al established a classification for needle-punctured rattail IVDs, a common degeneration model.[23] The NP is categorized according to the reduction of stellar-shaped notochordal cells and changes of cellular shape. The AF is categorized according to cell composition and the ratio of fibroblastic cells to chondrocytes (▶ Table 6.4) as well as fiber intactness.

6.3.2 Experimental Value

All the above mentioned grading systems are of experimental value. They have shown a high inter- and intraobserver agreement according to Cohen's weighted kappa analysis.[24] Except the Han system, they all have shown a significant positive correlation to the macroscopic Thompson grading and a negative correlation to the nuclear glycosaminoglycan (GAG) content.[3,18] Further, the Boos classification has also been shown to correlate with studied biochemical degenerative processes such as an increase in matrix metalloproteinases as well as matrix aggrecanases.[25,26] Due to its applicability for animal degeneration models, the Han grading system has been widely used to study success for biological disc regeneration approaches.[27]

Table 6.2 Histology grading by Boos et al[15] of intervertebral disc degeneration. Grading is based on sagittal paraffin sections stained with H&E, Masson-Goldner, and alcian blue–PAS.

Intervertebral disc	End plate
Cells (chondrocyte proliferation) 0 = No proliferation 1 = Increased cell density 2 = Connection of two chondrocytes 3 = Small size clones (i.e., several chondrocytes group together, i.e., 2–7 cells) 4 = Moderate-size clones (i.e., > 8 cells) 5 = Huge clones (i.e., 15 cells) 6 = Scar/tissue defects	**Cells** 0 = Normal cellularity 1 = Localized cell proliferation 2 = Diffuse cell proliferation 3 = Extensive cell proliferation 4 = Scar/tissue defects
Mucous degeneration 0 = Absent 1 = Rarely present 2 = Present in intermediate amounts 3 = Abundantly present 4 = Scar/tissue defects	**Cartilage disorganization** 0 = Well-structured hyaline cartilage 1 = Cartilage irregularities (obliterated vessels?) 2 = Disorganized matrix with thinning 3 = Complete cartilage disorganization with defects 4 = Scar/tissue defects
Cell death 0 = Absent 1 = Rarely present 2 = Present in intermediate amounts 3 = Abundantly present 4 = Scar/tissue defects	**Cartilage cracks** 0 = Absent 1 = Rarely present 2 = Present in intermediate amounts 3 = Abundantly present 4 = Scar/tissue defects
Tear and cleft formation 0 = Absent 1 = Rarely present 2 = Present in intermediate amounts 3 = Abundantly present 4 = Scar/tissue defects	**Microfracture** 0 = Absent 1 = Present 2 = Scar/tissue defects
Granular changes 0 = Absent 1 = Rarely present 2 = Present in intermediate amounts 3 = Abundantly present 4 = Scar/tissue defects	**New bone formation** 0 = Absent 1 = Present 2 = Scar/tissue defects **Bony sclerosis** 0 = Absent 1 = Present 2 = Scar/tissue defects

Abbreviations: H&E, hematoxylin and eosin; PAS, periodic acid–Schiff.

Similar to macroscopic sections, histology grading is not used clinically.

6.4 Radiology

X-ray as well as MR imaging has been used to evaluate and classify disc degeneration. In contrast to histology or anatomical cross sections they allow assessment of structural changes in vivo. X-rays, which have a high bone contrast, allow assessment of bone morphology, disc height, and spinal alignment. MR imaging with high tissue contrast allows for the evaluation of disc morphology and hydration as well as spinal neural structures. Computed tomography has not been used to establish a grading system for IVDs.

6.4.1 Grading Scales

Kellgren and Lawrence[28] were the first to introduce a grading system for spine degeneration on X-rays using lateral views.

This classification described the fundamental signs of radiographic alterations of spinal segments such as end plate sclerosis, "lipping" (osteophytes) of the vertebral body, disc height loss, and increased or decreased segmental mobility. In 1994, Mimura et al established a system based on lateral and anterior-posterior views that are more specific for IVD degeneration and that also quantify the amount of degenerative changes in contrast to the Kellgren system.[29] In this four-grade system loss of disc height ranges from mild (75% of adjacent healthy) to severe (25% of adjacent healthy). Osteophyte formation is scored according to the size (< 3 mm or > 3 mm) and the amount of bone spurs on each segment. End plate sclerosis is scored according to the involvement of a single or both end plates (► Table 6.5). Madan et al introduced a similar scoring system that also involves the vacuum sign of IVDs (gas accumulation within the disc tissue as an indicator of degeneration).[30]

In 1987, Schneiderman et al first introduced an MRI-based scale for disc degeneration using only T2 signal intensity as a radiological parameter. T2 signal intensity has been shown to

Table 6.3 Histology scoring items and grades according to Rutges[18] classification.

End plate H&E	0 Homogeneous structure; regular thickness 1 Slight irregularity with limited number of microfractures and locally decreased thickness 2 Severe irregularity with multiple microfractures of the EP and generalized decreased thickness
Morphology AF H&E/Saf O	0 Well-organized, half ring–shaped structure, collagen lamellae 1 Partly ruptured AF; loss of half ring–shaped structure 2 Completely ruptured AF; no intact half ring–shaped collagen lamellae
Boundary AF and NP H&E/Saf O	0 Clear boundary between AF and NP tissue 1 Boundary less clear; loss of annular–nuclear demarcation 2 No distinguishable boundary between AF and NP tissue
Cellularity NP H&E	0 Normal cellularity; no cell clusters 1 Mixed cellularity; normal pattern with some cell clusters 2 Mainly clustered cellularity, chondroid nests present
Matrix NP H&E	0 Well-organized structure of nucleus matrix 1 Partly disorganized structure of nucleus matrix 2 Complete disorganization and loss of nucleus matrix
NP matrix staining Saf O	0 Intense staining; red stain dominates 1 Reduced staining; mixture of red and slight green staining 2 Faint staining; increased green staining
NP matrix staining ABPR	0 Intense staining; blue staining dominates 1 Reduced staining; mixture of blue and slight red staining 2 Faint staining; increased red staining

Abbreviations: ABPR, alcian blue–picrosirius red; AF, annulus fibrosus; H&E, hematoxylin and eosin; NP, nucleus pulposus; Saf O, Safranin-O.

Table 6.4 Disc degeneration histology classification by Han et al[23] for needle punctured rattail intervertebral discs

I. Cellularity of the annulus fibrosus
Grade:
1 Fibroblasts comprise more than 75% of the cells
2 Neither fibroblasts nor chondrocytes comprise more than 75% of the cells
3 Chondrocytes comprise more than 75% of the cells

II. Morphology of the annulus fibrosus
Grade:
1 Well-organized collagen lamellae without ruptured or serpentine fibers
2 Inward bulging, ruptured, or serpentine fibers in less than one third of the annulus
3 Inward bulging, ruptured, or serpentine fibers in more than one third of the annulus

III. Border between the annulus fibrosus and nucleus pulposus
Grade:
1 Normal, without any interruption
2 Minimal interruption
3 Moderate or severe interruption

IV. Cellularity of the nucleus pulposus
Grade:
1. Normal cellularity with stellar-shaped nuclear cells evenly distributed throughout the nucleus
2 Slight decrease in the number of cells with some clustering
3 Moderate or severe decrease (50%) in the number of cells with all the remaining cells clustered and separated by dense areas of proteoglycans

V. Morphology of the nucleus pulposus
Grade:
1 Round, comprising at least half of the disc area in mid-sagittal sections
2 Rounded or irregularly shaped, comprising one quarter to half of the disc area in mid-sagittal sections
3 Irregularly shaped, comprising less than one quarter of the disc area in mid-sagittal sections

correlate with the hydration of the disc.[31] Signal intensity was qualitatively evaluated as normal, intermediate loss, marked loss, and absent. In 2001 Pfirrmann introduced the most commonly used MRI grading system that besides T2 signal intensity also takes disc structure (homogeneous or inhomogeneous), disc height (ranging from normal to collapsed), and AF/NP distinction (clear or lost) into account (► Table 6.6).[9] This five-grade classification was later modified by quantifying the loss of disc height (<30%, 30–60% and >60%) into an eight-grade system with the intention to improve discrimination in the older population spine.[32] Riesenburger et al introduced a classification system that additionally included Modic changes (T2 hyperintense signal at the vertebral end plates representing edema formation), and high intensity zone (T2 hyperintense signal in the AF indicating annular fissures).[33]

6.4.2 Experimental Value

X-ray based grading systems are not commonly used for research purposes because MRIs offer much higher soft-tissue contrast and are available at most research institutes. However, plain X-rays are still often used for indirect disc height measurements in animal studies.[34,35]

The MRI Pfirrmann grading has been used for various disc degeneration and regeneration studies in the human as well as the animal spine.[27] It has shown a high inter- and intraobserver agreement.[9,36] Similar to histological or macroscopical classifi-

cations, the Pfirrmann grading correlates with biochemical degenerative parameters of IVDs such as matrix metalloproteinases and bone morphogenic protein expression in human and animal discs.[37,38]

Although correlations to biochemical changes can be identified, morphology based MRI assessments such as the Pfirrmann grading do not analyze tissue composition. Giving that biochemical alterations occur prior to morphological changes captured by MR imaging,[39] the ability to measure these alterations could be crucial to sensitively assess early disc degeneration processes and regeneration efforts.

Recently, quantitative MR imaging based on T1 or T2 relaxation time measurements were introduced for disc research proposes. Quantitative measurements allow for indirect assessment of biochemical tissue composition[40] and its mechanical behavior.[41] T2 relaxation time measurements have been shown to positively correlate with disc water content and inversely with disc degeneration.[42] T1-rho relaxation time has been shown to positively correlate with disc proteoglycan content[43] and inversely with degenerative changes.[39]

6.4.3 Clinical Value

Radiological grading systems have been used for various clinical studies.[44] However, radiological grading classifications, whether on MRI or X-rays, have so far not proven applicable to influence clinical decision making or predict clinical outcome.[45]

6.5 Conclusion

Anatomical, radiological, and histological grades have been demonstrated to be useful to quantify degenerative changes in IVDs. However, there is limited use for these grades to quantify regenerative efforts. Recently, several biological approaches such as growth factors and stem cell injections, as well as tissue-engineered disc implantation have been studied in animal models to reverse disc degeneration. The anatomical, histological, or radiological disc morphology after biological treatment can differ from established grades making it difficult to quantify the success of disc regeneration by simple reversion of

Table 6.5 X-ray radiographic classification by Kellgren[28] of disc degeneration

Grade 1	Minimal anterior osteophytosis
Grade 2	Definite anterior osteophytosis with possible narrowing of the disc space and some sclerosis of vertebral plates
Grade 3	Moderate narrowing of the disc space with definite sclerosis of vertebral plates and osteophytosis
Grade 4	Severe narrowing of the disc space with sclerosis of vertebral plates and multiple large osteophytes

Table 6.6 MRI-based Pfirrmann grading scale.[9]

Grade	Structure	Distinction of nucleus and annulus	Signal intensity	Height of intervertebral disc
I	Homogeneous, bright white	Clear	Hyperintense, isointense to cerebrospinal fluid	Normal
II	Inhomogeneous with or without horizontal bands	Clear	Hyperintense, isointense to cerebrospinal fluid	Normal
III	Inhomogeneous, gray	Unclear	Intermediate	Normal to slightly decreased
IV	Inhomogeneous, gray to black	Lost	Intermediate to hypointense	Normal to moderately decreased
V	Inhomogeneous, black	Lost	Hypointense	Collapsed disc space

Abbreviations: MRI, magnetic resonance imaging.

degeneration grades. As more study groups assess biological treatment options, it will be critical to establish specific regeneration grades to improve quantification of the success of regenerative efforts.

6.6 References

[1] Nachemson A. Lumbar intradiscal pressure. Experimental studies on post-mortem material. Acta OrthopScand Suppl. 1960; 43:1–104

[2] Thompson JP, Pearce RH, Schechter MT, Adams ME, Tsang IK, Bishop PB. Preliminary evaluation of a scheme for grading the gross morphology of the human intervertebral disc. Spine. 1990; 15(5):411–415

[3] Bergknut N, Grinwis G, Pickee E, et al. Reliability of macroscopic grading of intervertebral disk degeneration in dogs by use of the Thompson system and comparison with low-field magnetic resonance imaging findings. Am J Vet Res. 2011; 72(7):899–904

[4] Kettler A, Wilke HJ. Review of existing grading systems for cervical or lumbar disc and facet joint degeneration. Eur Spine J. 2006; 15(6):705–718

[5] Iatridis JC, MacLean JJ, O'Brien M, Stokes IA. Measurements of proteoglycan and water content distribution in human lumbar intervertebral discs. Spine. 2007; 32(14):1493–1497

[6] Patel KP, Sandy JD, Akeda K, et al. Aggrecanases and aggrecanase-generated fragments in the human intervertebral disc at early and advanced stages of disc degeneration. Spine. 2007; 32(23):2596–2603

[7] Antoniou J, Steffen T, Nelson F, et al. The human lumbar intervertebral disc: evidence for changes in the biosynthesis and denaturation of the extracellular matrix with growth, maturation, ageing, and degeneration. J Clin Invest. 1996; 98(4):996–1003

[8] Gruber HE, Ingram JA, Norton HJ, Hanley EN , Jr. Senescence in cells of the aging and degenerating intervertebral disc: immunolocalization of senescence-associated beta-galactosidase in human and sand rat discs. Spine. 2007; 32(3):321–327

[9] Pfirrmann CWA, Metzdorf A, Zanetti M, Hodler J, Boos N. Magnetic resonance classification of lumbar intervertebral disc degeneration. Spine. 2001; 26(17):1873–1878

[10] Benneker LM, Heini PF, Anderson SE, Alini M, Ito K. Correlation of radiographic and MRI parameters to morphological and biochemical assessment of intervertebral disc degeneration. Eur Spine J. 2005; 14(1):27–35

[11] Roberts S, Evans H, Trivedi J, Menage J. Histology and pathology of the human intervertebral disc. J Bone Joint Surg Am. 2006; 88 Suppl 2:10–14

[12] Butler WF, Heap PF. Correlation between Alcian Blue stainig of glycosaminoglycans of cat nucleus pulposus and TEM x-ray probe microanalysis. Histochem J. 1979; 11(2):137–143

[13] Issy AC, Castania V, Castania M, et al. Experimental model of intervertebral disc degeneration by needle puncture in Wistar rats. Braz J Med Biol Res. 2013; 46(3):235–244

[14] Gruber HE, Ingram J, Hanley EN , Jr. An improved staining method for intervertebral disc tissue. Biotech Histochem. 2002; 77(2):81–83

[15] Boos N, Weissbach S, Rohrbach H, Weiler C, Spratt KF, Nerlich AG. Classification of age-related changes in lumbar intervertebral discs: 2002 Volvo Award in basic science. Spine. 2002; 27(23):2631–2644

[16] Bachmeier BE, Nerlich A, Mittermaier N, et al. Matrix metalloproteinase expression levels suggest distinct enzyme roles during lumbar disc herniation and degeneration. Eur Spine J. 2009; 18(11):1573–1586

[17] Kroeber M, Unglaub F, Guehring T, et al. Effects of controlled dynamic disc distraction on degenerated intervertebral discs: an in vivo study on the rabbit lumbar spine model. Spine. 2005; 30(2):181–187

[18] Rutges JP, Duit RA, Kummer JA, et al. A validated new histological classification for intervertebral disc degeneration. Osteoarthritis Cartilage. 2013; 21 (12):2039–2047

[19] Risbud MV, Shapiro IM. Notochordal cells in the adult intervertebral disc: new perspective on an old question. Crit Rev Eukaryot Gene Expr. 2011; 21 (1):29–41

[20] Sobajima S, Kompel JF, Kim JS, et al. A slowly progressive and reproducible animal model of intervertebral disc degeneration characterized by MRI, X-ray, and histology. Spine. 2005; 30(1):15–24

[21] Grunert P, Hudson KD, Macielak MR, et al. Assessment of intervertebral disc degeneration based on quantitative magnetic resonance imaging analysis: an in vivo study. Spine. 2014; 39(6):E369–E378

[22] Bergknut N, Meij BP, Hagman R, et al. Intervertebral disc disease in dogs - part 1: a new histological grading scheme for classification of intervertebral disc degeneration in dogs. Vet J. 2013; 195(2):156–163

[23] Han B, Zhu K, Li F C, et al. A simple disc degeneration model induced by percutaneous needle puncture in the rat tail. Spine. 2008; 33(18):1925–1934

[24] Koch GG, Landis JR, Freeman JL, Freeman DH, Jr, Lehnen RC. A general methodology for the analysis of experiments with repeated measurement of categorical data. Biometrics. 1977; 33(1):133–158

[25] Zigouris A, Alexiou GA, Batistatou A, Voulgaris S, Kyritsis APJ. The role of matrix metalloproteinase 9 in intervertebral disc degeneration. J Clin Neurosci. 2011; 18(10):1424–1425

[26] Le Maitre CL, Freemont AJ, Hoyland JA. Human disc degeneration is associated with increased MMP 7 expression. Biotech Histochem. 2006; 81(4–6):125–131

[27] Grunert P, Borde BH, Hudson KD, Macielak MR, Bonassar LJ, Härtl R. Annular repair using high-density collagen gel: a rat-tail in vivo model. Spine. 2014; 39(3):198–206

[28] Kellgren JH, Lawrence JS. Rheumatism in miners.II. X-ray study. Br J Ind Med. 1952; 9(3):197–207

[29] Mimura M, Panjabi MM, Oxland TR, Crisco JJ, Yamamoto I, Vasavada A. Disc degeneration affects the multidirectional flexibility of the lumbar spine. Spine. 1994; 19(12):1371–1380

[30] Madan SS, Rai A, Harley JM. Interobserver error in interpretation of the radiographs for degeneration of the lumbar spine. Iowa Orthop J. 2003; 23:51–56

[31] Schneiderman G, Flannigan B, Kingston S, Thomas J, Dillin WH, Watkins RG. Magnetic resonance imaging in the diagnosis of disc degeneration: correlation with discography. Spine. 1987; 12(3):276–281

[32] Griffith JF, Wang YX, Antonio GE, et al. Modified Pfirrmann grading system for lumbar intervertebral disc degeneration. Spine. 2007; 32(24):E708–E712

[33] Riesenburger RI, Safain MG, Ogbuji R, Hayes J, Hwang SW. A novel classification system of lumbar disc degeneration. J Clin Neurosci. 2015; 22(2):346–351

[34] Imai Y, Okuma M, An HS, et al. Restoration of disc height loss by recombinant human osteogenic protein-1 injection into intervertebral discs undergoing degeneration induced by an intradiscal injection of chondroitinase ABC. Spine. 2007; 32(11):1197–1205

[35] Acosta FL , Jr, Metz L, Adkisson HD, et al. Porcine intervertebral disc repair using allogeneic juvenile articular chondrocytes or mesenchymal stem cells. Tissue Eng Part A. 2011; 17(23–24):3045–3055

[36] Kanna RM, Shetty AP, Rajasekaran S. Patterns of lumbar disc degeneration are different in degenerative disc disease and disc prolapse magnetic resonance imaging analysis of 224 patients. Spine J. 2014; 14(2):300–307

[37] Canbay S, Turhan N, Bozkurt M, Arda K, Caglar S. Correlation of matrix metalloproteinase-3 expression with patient age, magnetic resonance imaging and histopathological grade in lumbar disc degeneration. Turk Neurosurg. 2013; 23(4):427–433

[38] Clouet J, Pot-Vaucel M, Grimandi G, et al. Characterization of the age-dependent intervertebral disc changes in rabbit by correlation between MRI, histology and gene expression. BMC MusculoskeletDisord. 2011; 12:147

[39] Zobel BB, Vadalà G, Del Vescovo R, et al. T1ρ magnetic resonance imaging quantification of early lumbar intervertebral disc degeneration in healthy young adults. Spine. 2012; 37(14):1224–1230

[40] Chai JW, Kang HS, Lee JW, Kim S-J, Hong SH. Quantitative analysis of disc degeneration using axial T2 mapping in a percutaneous annular puncture model in rabbits. Korean J Radiol. 2016; 17(1):103–110

[41] Mariappan YK, Glaser KJ, Ehman RL. Magnetic resonance elastography: a review. Clin Anat. 2010; 23(5):497–511

[42] Marinelli NL, Haughton VM, Muñoz A, Anderson PA. T2 relaxation times of intervertebral disc tissue correlated with water content and proteoglycan content. Spine. 2009; 34(5):520–524

[43] Johannessen W, Auerbach JD, Wheaton AJ, et al. Assessment of human disc degeneration and proteoglycan content using T1rho-weighted magnetic resonance imaging. Spine. 2006; 31(11):1253–1257

[44] Teichtahl AJ, Urquhart DM, Wang Y, Wluka AE, Heritier S, Cicuttini FM. A dose-response relationship between severity of disc degeneration and intervertebral disc height in the lumbosacral spine. Arthritis Res Ther. 2015; 17:297

[45] Yu LP, Qian WW, Yin GY, Ren YX, Hu ZY. MRI assessment of lumbar intervertebral disc degeneration with lumbar degenerative disease using the Pfirrmann grading systems. PLoS One. 2012; 7(12):e48074

7 Disc Regeneration: In Vitro Approaches and Experimental Results

John T. Martin, Harvey E. Smith, Lachlan J. Smith, and Robert L. Mauck

Abstract

There has been substantial progress toward disc regeneration in the past years and an array of promising strategies have been developed. In vitro culture systems are fundamental to the development and validation of these regenerative therapies, and serve as a prerequisite for preclinical animal research and ultimately clinical translation. This chapter describes the in vitro methods used to evaluate disc regeneration strategies in terms of the cell sources (i.e., pluripotent, multipotent, fully differentiated), the platforms (i.e., monolayer culture, three-dimensional, organ culture), and the external variables for eliciting a cell response (i.e., oxygen tension, pH, glucose, inflammatory factors, mechanical loading, growth factors). Using these in vitro systems, we have learned much about disc cell biology and biomaterials, and have generated a foundation for future research that will inform the implementation of these strategies to rescue disc disease.

Keywords: growth factors, hydrogels, mechanical loading, organ culture, scaffolds, stem cells, tissue engineering

7.1 Historical Perspective

Restoring degenerated or injured intervertebral discs (IVDs) by rescuing or replacing damaged tissue, reestablishing mechanical function, and developing homeostasis in the challenging disc microenvironment is the fundamental goal of IVD regeneration. The last decade has demonstrated marked progress in this field, including the delivery of growth factors and cell-based therapeutics, improvements in bioactive and cell-laden materials for annulus fibrosus (AF) and nucleus pulposus (NP) replacement, and the rise of composite materials for total disc tissue engineering. In vitro evaluation of these strategies is required to address many of the fundamental questions regarding disc repair and regeneration. For example, early in vitro studies focusing on growth factor and cell therapies generated critical data that led to clinical trials, whereas tissue engineering strategies have been advanced from basic work on biomaterials and engineered tissue replacements to implementation in various translational animal models. Finally, new methods of whole disc organ culture and the advancement of bioreactor technologies allow for the evaluation of disc biology and degeneration therapies in the disc microenvironment ex situ. Although these techniques have demonstrated early success, a number of fundamental hurdles still exist before effective, long-term tissue regeneration for early- and late-stage disc disease can be realized. This chapter highlights current in vitro methods for developing and validating regenerative strategies, and outlines persisting challenges in the realization of this important goal.

The first section of this chapter discusses the current clinical state-of-the-art treatments for symptomatic disc disease and provides an overview of experimental regeneration strategies now under investigation. This provides a framework in which to review current in vitro tissue regeneration and replacement methods. Subsequent sections describe the in vitro model systems designed to evaluate regeneration techniques in terms of cell sources, biomaterials, growth factors, and culture methods, and discusses relevant findings generated from each of these techniques. Finally, the outstanding issues and limitations of current regeneration strategies are summarized to provide a foundation and outline for future research in this area.

7.2 Overview of Regeneration Strategies

Although spinal fusion and total disc arthroplasty have seen increasing use in recent years, these interventions do not restore normal spine function; in both cases, the disc is removed and the original structure and mechanical functions of the spine are not replicated. Consequently, while these interventions may initially relieve pain, they are subject to postoperative complications and may not constitute a long-term solution for disc disease. Disc degeneration presents clinically as a spectrum ranging from mild to severe, with the level of tissue degradation correlating to the age of the individual.[1] Emerging regenerative strategies are thus calibrated to these stages of disease, with the aim of rescuing the disc from either early- or late-stage degeneration. These methods promise to improve upon current techniques by returning the intervertebral joint to a healthy state. Two general strategies have emerged for treatment at different points along the spectrum of IVD disease.

1. Injectable therapeutics. For early-stage degeneration, where the intrinsic ability of the tissue to repair itself may still be intact but in need of supplementation, the injection of therapeutics into the native disc may slow or even reverse the degenerative cascade. These techniques are aimed at directly improving the quality of the NP, the disc region in which degenerative changes often first manifest. Research on injectable therapeutics is largely based either on the injection of cells to replenish the diseased tissue, or the injection of growth factors that can directly stimulate anabolic behavior of endogenous cells. Additionally, the delivery of anti-inflammatory agents has been proposed to attenuate local inflammation and provide a microenvironment more conducive to regeneration by endogenous or exogenous cells.

2. Total or partial disc replacement. For end-stage degeneration when the native tissue likely has little capacity for regeneration, the removal of the native diseased AF and/or NP tissues and their replacement with an engineered substitute may restore healthy joint structure and function. Efforts to replace the native disc structure through the development of

viable engineered tissues leverage the growing knowledge base on cells, biomaterials, and their interactions.

The basic science that underlies each of these approaches is discussed below.

7.2.1 In Vitro Culture Systems

To test if cells, growth factors, and biomaterials can function in a regenerative capacity, numerous in vitro model systems have been developed to mimic specific features of the IVD microenvironment. These in vitro model systems are useful for studying basic physiological processes, injectable therapies, and engineered tissue replacements. In vitro model systems generally include a *cell source* with regenerative potential, a *material substrate* on which the cells are cultured, and a set of *external variables* that can be controlled to replicate the disc microenvironment. The following section introduces these three topics and provides examples from ongoing research in the field to present the current state of the art in this area.

7.2.2 Cell Sources

In the field of regenerative medicine, there are a wide variety of cell sources available for therapeutic use. In general, these can be categorized by their differentiation potential, that is, by their ability to assume phenotypic features similar to cells from different tissue types when provided with the appropriate environmental cues.

Pluripotent Cell Sources

Pluripotent stem cells can differentiate into all cell types and form all tissues derived from the three germ layers. Embryonic stem cells (ESCs), for example, are considered pluripotent and there has been some effort to use these as an injectable therapeutic for disc regeneration.[2] ESCs require special handling given their phenotype is difficult to direct and maintain. In addition, clinical use of ESCs requires allogeneic cells which are prone to immune rejection and infection. Likewise, the supply of such cells is currently limited and there are well-known ethical issues related to obtaining fetal cells.

As an alternative to ESCs, fully differentiated cells, such as skin fibroblasts, can be induced into pluripotency by introducing a series of reprogramming genes through viral transduction and other mechanisms.[3] These are aptly named *induced pluripotent* stem cells or iPSCs. Similar to ESCs, iPSCs require a fibroblast feeder layer and a number of chemical factors to first maintain the cells in an undifferentiated state and then to induce differentiation. In contrast to ESCs, however, there is an unlimited supply of donor cells from adult skin tissue. This is a promising, although new, line of research for the regeneration of the IVD[4,5] as well as other musculoskeletal tissues.[6,7] One drawback of iPSCs is that their preparation is time-consuming, requiring months to generate, differentiate, expand, and direct toward skeletal lineages,[8] which may limit their use as an autogenous source. To overcome this, researchers in Japan, Europe, and the United States are developing iPSC banks with fully differentiated cell lines for on-demand access.

Multipotent Cell Sources

There are a number of *multipotent* stem cell sources under investigation for disc regeneration. Multipotent cells have limited differentiation potential compared with pluripotent cells, but have more clinical relevance given that they can be harvested from adults. For applications in orthopaedics, there are multipotent sources with the ability to adopt phenotypes of a number of musculoskeletal tissues,[9,10] including cartilage and fibrocartilage, such as the NP and AF. Mesenchymal stem cells (MSCs), for example, are a popular source because they can be isolated from a number of locations, most commonly bone marrow, adipose tissue, and synovium, and can generate tissues with compositional and functional properties similar to native cartilage.[11,12,13] There is a growing body of work on MSCs for disc regeneration that ranges from in vitro experiments to animal models to clinical trials.[14] A minor surgical procedure is required in most cases for retrieving MSCs from the donor, and so donor site morbidity remains an issue. Likewise, it is not clear that every MSC has the same potential, and so methods to sort and use optimized subpopulations of MSCs is an area of considerable interest.

Notochordal Cells, Nucleus Pulposus Progenitor Cells

Another source of cells relevant to regeneration are cells that reside within the disc at early development stages that are notochordal in origin. During development, the NP forms from the embryonic notochord,[15] and cells that retain a notochordal-like phenotype make up a portion of the NP cellular composition early in life. The disappearance of these cells, potentially due to either differentiation into less metabolically active chondrocyte-like cells or apoptosis, may be associated with the onset of degenerative change at older ages. Thus, it has been hypothesized that notochordal cells play an important role in disc homeostasis and may have regenerative properties. Currently, there is significant research interest in notochordal cells for disc regeneration,[16,17,18,19,20,21,22,23,24,25] either through direct injection into a degenerate disc, or for use in co-culture with another cell source such as MSCs or degenerate NP cells. Although studying the function of notochordal cells will likely elucidate mechanisms for regenerative therapies, a reliable source of notochordal cells, one that can be harvested and expanded for injection or tissue engineering, has yet to be identified.

Fully Differentiated Cell Sources

Fully differentiated cells also have the potential for regeneration, despite their terminally differentiated state. It has been well demonstrated that AF and NP cells can be isolated and cultured in vitro, and that these cells can produce tissue whose composition largely mirrors that of the native extracellular matrix (ECM); gene expression data suggest that AF cells maintain a fibrochondrogenic phenotype, with high levels of types I and II collagen messenger RNA (mRNA); the NP phenotype is more chondrogenic and, similar to articular chondrocytes, NP cells express mRNA-related type II collagen, the chondrogenic transcription factor SOX9, and aggrecan.[26,27] NP cells also express unique factors that likely reflect their notochordal origin and the unique microenvironmental niche in which they must survive and function.[28] Potential sources for therapeutic AF and NP cells are from discarded disc tissue, such as degenerate tissue removed prior to spinal fusion for spondylolisthesis/ disc disease. However, there exist technical hurdles related to this cell source given that degenerate tissue yields cells with an altered phenotype characterized by decreased proteoglycan production, senescence, catabolism, and a number of inflammatory markers.[29,30,31,32] However, these cells may be rescued from their degenerate state prior to their injection into the disc space, for example, by co-culture with a healthy cell population.[33,34]

Other terminally differentiated cells can be sourced from cartilage at various anatomical locations; these cells have demonstrated potential for musculoskeletal regeneration as well. Articular chondrocytes from non–load-bearing regions of the knee have been widely used for cartilage restoration procedures such as autologous chondrocyte implantation.[35,36] Whereas these cells have robust chondrogenic potential, their isolation is associated with local tissue damage. Nasal[37] and auricular[38] chondrocytes have demonstrated potential for in vitro chondrogenesis, and local donor site morbidity related to the isolation of these cells may be preferable when compared with articular chondrocytes because they are not in an environment that has potential for joint-level communication of inflammatory signals, as is the case for a synovial joint. Additionally, allogeneic articular chondrocytes have recently become commercially available. As these cells are prepared from juvenile (deceased) donors, this is a source of highly active chondrocytes that has shown some clinical success in treating articular cartilage defects[39]; these cells may likewise have potential for disc regeneration applications.

7.2.3 Culture Systems

The physical environment in which cells are cultured has a significant influence on experimental outcomes; cells read cues from material substrates to regulate phenotype and metabolic activity.[40,41] The standard material platforms for disc cell culture fit into one of three categories: cells cultured in a thin layer on plastic dishes (monolayer culture); cells aggregated as pellets, encapsulated in hydrogels, or seeded onto fibrous scaffolds (three-dimensional [3D] culture); live disc explants removed from animals or human cadavers and cultured in the lab (organ culture) (▶ Fig. 7.1).

Monolayer Culture

Due to ease of manipulation and experimental assays, simple monolayer culture conditions have been used to generate the majority of our knowledge regarding mammalian cell behavior, and IVD cells are no exception. The procedure for culturing disc cells or other cell types in monolayer involves first isolating cells from donor tissue, suspending these cells in a growth medium, and plating the cell suspension onto a sterile polystyrene culture dish. Cells attach directly to the dish and can be serially passaged to expand their number. A number of outcomes can be measured; cells can be retrieved and their RNA can be extracted for gene expression analysis; cultures can be directly

stained for protein and ECM components; cell appearance and morphology can be evaluated by microscopy; culture media can be extracted and its composition can be analyzed.

One or more cell types and their interactions can be evaluated by simple modifications to a monolayer culture system. For example, the influence of NP cells on AF cells can be evaluated through co-culture; NP and AF cells can be seeded in direct apposition to study the influence of direct cell–cell communication, or seeded in culture dishes that have two tiers (one of which is porous) to study the influence of paracrine signaling between these two cell types. These are popular techniques in disc regeneration to evaluate the influence of one cell type on another, for example, to generate an NP-like phenotype in MSCs, MSCs can be co-cultured with NP cells.[42]

Three-Dimensional Culture

In vivo, disc cells reside in a three-dimensional microenvironment that is not well represented by monolayer culture systems. Phenotypic differences are evident when comparing NP cells cultured in monolayer, where they develop a fibroblast-like phenotype, with NP cells cultured in a 3D environment.[43,44] Indeed, the "de-differentiation" that invariably occurs during monolayer cell expansion complicates interpretation of data acquired using monolayer culture methods.

A more realistic culture system would provide 3D spatial cues for cells to promote or preserve their phenotype, and although the types of experimental assays suitable for application to cells in 3D culture are more limited than for monolayer culture, advantages include the ability to more effectively assess matrix elaboration and mechanical function. In vitro NP and AF models can be scaffold-free (as in pellet culture) or can be generated from naturally occurring (agarose, alginate, collagen, fibrin, and hyaluronic acid [HA]) or synthetic (polyethylene glycol, polyvinyl alcohol, polylactic acid, and polycaprolactone) biomaterials (▶ Fig. 7.2a). Material topographies include homogeneous materials, composite networks of a bulk polymer and an additional interpenetrating polymer, and aligned and randomly oriented fibrous scaffolds. These materials are typically cross-linked to infer stability to the polymer network; this can be initiated through photo, thermal, and chemical stimuli, and depending on processing parameters, can lead to sparsely or densely cross-linked networks to enable tight control over the physical properties of the bulk material. Additionally, direct regulation of cellular phenotype and adhesion can be exerted by including growth factors and adhesion ligands that mimic natural ECM proteins (▶ Fig. 7.2b). As cell phenotype is driven by mechanical cues, biomaterial substrates selected for AF and NP cell studies often reflect the physical properties of the native NP and AF; soft hydrogels that induce an NP-like phenotype are used for NP cell studies, whereas fibrous scaffolds that instruct seeded AF cells to elongate and develop a fibrochondogenic phenotype are often used in AF cell studies.

Pellet Culture

Cells in a high density suspension can be centrifuged and concentrated in a pellet, forming a spheroid scaffold-free cell aggregate. Cell-generated ECM accumulates in the pellet over time, forming a physiological 3D microenvironment. Pellet

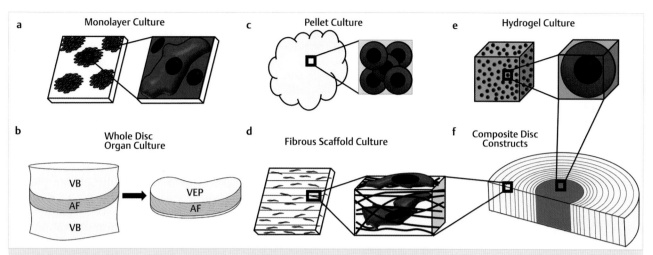

Fig. 7.1 In vitro model systems. **(a)** Monolayer culture allows for simple high-throughput studies of cell behavior. **(b)** Organ culture allows for studies of disc cells in their native environment. AF, annulus fibrosus; VB, vertebral body; VEP, vertebral end plate. **(c)** By removing the bulk of the vertebral body, the disc can remain viable in culture. This allows for the study of disc cells in their native environment. **(d)** To simulate the AF, cells can be cultured on scaffolds that mimic the organization of collagen fibers found in the AF region. **(e)** To simulate the nucleus pulposus (NP), cells can be cultured in hydrogels so as to reproduce a spherical cell morphology. **(f)** A combination of fibrous AF scaffolds and hydrogel NPs allows for co-culture of cells in a simulated disc environment.

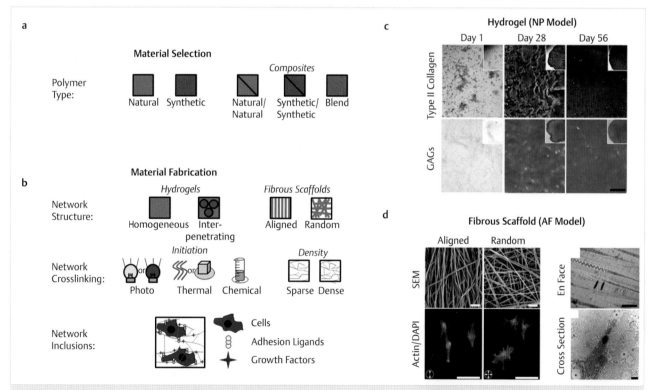

Fig. 7.2 Three-dimensional culture systems: material selection, fabrication, and examples. **(a)** A variety of naturally occurring and synthetic biomaterials, with specific physical and chemical properties, are available individually or as composite materials as a framework for cell culture. **(b)** Fabrication processes allow control over structural features and physical properties, and can incorporate bioactive components to better match the intervertebral niche or to elicit a desired cellular response. **(c)** In vitro nucleus pulposus (NP) model: NP cells cast in hyaluronic acid hydrogels develop a disc-like phenotype over 8 weeks of culture. This is evidenced by increasing levels of type II collagen and glycosaminoglycans (GAGs; scale = 100 μm).[54] **(d)** In vitro annulus fibrosus (AF) model: **(Top left)** scanning electron microscopy (SEM) images of electrospun scaffold with aligned and random orientations (scale = 10 μm). **(Bottom left)** Mesenchymal stem cells seeded on aligned scaffold demonstrate preferential alignment in the fiber direction (scale = 20 μm). **(Top right)** En face transmission electron microscopy (TEM) image of cell bodies aligned with the fiber direction (a cell nucleus is outlined with dotted white line; scale = 10 μm).[111] **(Bottom right)** Cross-sectional TEM image of a cell anchored at two electrospun fibers (starred). Collagen fibrils deposited by the cell (dark puncta) populate the space between the cell and the electrospun fibers (scale = 10 μm).[111,112]

culture is often used as a simple and more realistic alternative to monolayer culture to study basic cell functions, such as their response to inflammatory factors and hypoxia.[45] Additionally, scaffold-free aggregates are emerging for tissue engineering applications,[46] where multiple pellets can be combined into large structures, or aggregation geometry can be controlled to match a defect shape such as those common to the articulating surface of the tibia. One could envision exploiting this method for disc tissue engineering, though these studies have not yet been conducted. One drawback of the pellet culture approach is that, in most connective tissues, cell density is low and cell–cell contact is not common; thus, high density cell aggregates produce abnormal cell–cell contact that may influence experimental findings.

Hydrogels

For 3D culture systems specific to the IVD, hydrogels are often preferred for NP cell studies (▶ Fig. 7.2c); the physical cues provided by soft hydrogels tend to induce a spherical cell shape and promote an NP-like phenotype. In contrast to pellet monolayer culture, hydrogel encapsulation provides a 3D environment that better mimics the native NP environment and limits cell–cell contact.

There are a number of applications in NP regeneration in which hydrogels can be useful. Hydrogel culture systems allow for studying basic cell responses; for example, hydrogel systems are used to determine how NP cells respond to inflammatory challenge and anti-inflammatory interventions.[47] In a very active area of study, hydrogel vehicles are used to deliver cells for NP regeneration.[48,49,50,51,52] Hydrogel-mediated cell delivery serves as an alternative to delivery in a liquid carrier (such as saline or media), and physical parameters such as viscosity of the hydrogel can be tuned to both protect the cells during delivery as well as improve their retention at the delivery site. In addition, the chemistry of the hydrogel may be exploited to modulate cell activity; for example, a polyethylene glycol hydrogel can be modified to include cell adhesion ligands designed to influence cell phenotype.[53] Alternatively, the backbone of these hydrogels may be designed based on naturally occurring materials within the disc; another study demonstrated that the encapsulation of NP cells in HA, a ubiquitous ECM component, drives cells to express NP-specific markers.[54]

Due to their inherent physical properties, acellular hydrogels may allow for functional restoration by restoring native tissue mechanical properties in the disc space.[55,56] This restitution of disc mechanics may have a regenerative impact on endogenous cells by normalizing stresses and strains that they experience.

Whereas hydrogels are largely used for the study of NP cells, they have also been used for AF regeneration studies. To study basic cell functions, AF cells can be encapsulated in hydrogels; for example, AF cells in agarose respond to growth factor stimulation and osmotic loading.[57] Others have also taken advantage of cell-mediated remodeling of hydrogels to build engineered AF-like tissues; fiber alignment can be generated by depositing cell-laden collagen around a post and allowing the gel to contract, producing circumferential fiber architecture similar to the native AF[58]; adhesive gels are also in evaluation for the repair of AF fenestrations that remain after microdiscectomy.[59,60]

Fibrous Scaffolds

Given the ordered structure of the AF, scaffolds composed of aligned polymer fibers, of geometry ranging from nanoscale to microscale, are preferred for AF tissue engineering (▶ Fig. 7.2d). These scaffolds provide a topographical template; when cells are seeded on fibrous scaffolds, they will orient and elongate in the prevailing fiber direction. These topographical cues direct cells toward a phenotype similar to that of AF cells,[61,62,63] depositing ordered ECM that acts as a mechanical reinforcement in the fiber direction. The hierarchical fiber structure in the AF, with alternating angles ± 30 degrees in apposed layers, can be constructed from sheets of aligned fibers using a layering technique,[64] and this structure can be maintained after in vivo implantation.[65] This methodology has also been exploited to develop engineered fibrous tissues composed of MSCs with mechanical properties matching that of the native AF.[66]

Composite Disc Constructs

Beyond simple realization of the component parts of the disc, recent research efforts have expanded to include the ambitious goal of total disc replacement with an engineered, cellularized artificial disc, combining hydrogel NP regions with fibrous AF regions (▶ Fig. 7.3). This methodology allows for the evaluation of NP and AF cells in co-culture, and for the evaluation of other

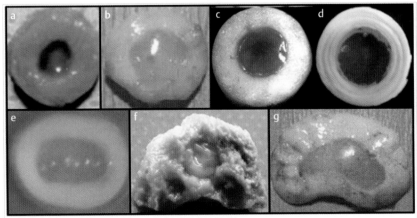

Fig. 7.3 Composite engineered discs. Engineered discs are fabricated from a variety of materials and cell types. **(a)** Silk annulus fibrosus (AF), fibrin and hyaluronic acid nucleus pulposus (NP), porcine disc cells and chondrocytes[113]; **(b)** poly(glycolic acid) AF, alginate NP, ovine disc cells[114]; **(c)** poly(e-caprolactone) foam AF, hyaluronic acid NP, bovine disc cells or mesenchymal stem cells (MSCs) (unpublished work from our lab); **(d)** electrospun poly(e-caprolactone) AF, alginate NP, bovine disc cells or MSCs[64]; **(e)** collagen AF, alginate NP, ovine disc cells[58]; **(f)** demineralized bone matrix gelatin AF, collagen, hyaluronic acid, chondroitin sulfate NP, lapine disc cells[115]; **(g)** poly(glycolic acid) AF, alginate NP, ovine disc cells.[116]

potential cell types like MSCs. It also allows for the interrogation of total disc mechanical properties, which are of particular importance for engineered total disc replacement. NP and AF regions that comprise the total disc constructs have taken a number of forms with varying levels of complexity, ranging from 3D-printed polymer discs,[67] to nanofibrous scaffold AFs wrapped around hydrogel NPs,[64] to collagen gels with circumferential fiber alignment about a central hydrogel NP region.[68] Even more recently, this work has been extended to include engineered end plates into total disc constructs to improve potential attachment at the vertebral junction.[69]

The last decade has witnessed significant advances in the development of engineered total disc replacements, with benchtop work now transitioning to in vivo total disc replacement in animal models. In some studies, these engineered discs proved to be biocompatible and match motion segment mechanical properties,[70] with early work in murine models now transitioning to large animal models.[71] These constructs have the potential to improve upon current clinical treatments for degenerative disc disease (DDD), such as spinal fusion and metal-on-plastic arthroplasty, by restoring native spinal mechanics with a self-sustaining, cell-based, viable, and continually remodeling engineered replacement.

Organ Culture

Whereas in vivo large animal models are an essential platform for preclinical evaluation of disc regeneration strategies, IVD organ culture allows for the investigation of therapeutic strategies in the native environment without the expense and logistical or ethical considerations involved in large animal trials.[72] Organ culture involves isolating discs from recently deceased subjects, ranging from murine to bovine to human, and culturing the disc in standard incubator and media conditions (▶ Fig. 7.4). Through use of live, cadaveric human disc explants, organ culture can explore unique research questions that cannot be answered with animal models, particularly in the absence of robust large animal models that accurately recapitulate the human degenerative disc phenotype.

Previous studies on large animal and human discs demonstrate that cells in the NP and AF in whole disc organ culture can remain viable and active for periods up to a month.[73,74,75] For long-term studies it is of particular importance to maintain

appropriate end plate conditions (removal of bony end plate, but maintenance of cartilage end plate) and dynamic mechanical loading conditions to maintain cell viability. Sophisticated bioreactors, machines that replicate select features of the physiological environment, have been developed to apply complex static,[76] dynamic,[77] and impact loading[78] to identify organ- and cell-level functions. These technical considerations have allowed whole disc organ culture studies to address a number of basic physiological mechanisms, such as cellular response to inflammatory factors and hypoxia,[79] and also to generate disc degeneration models through chemonucleolysis.[80]

Using organ culture systems, therapies for the treatment of DDD can be screened for efficacy prior to their use in an animal model or human clinical trial. The delivery of cells to the disc, through direct injection,[81] hydrogel vehicle injection,[82] and cell homing,[83] has demonstrated regenerative benefits in organ culture models. Growth factor treatment has also been successful in organ culture models of disc degeneration.[84] Currently, there is no clinical treatment to prevent reherniation following microdiscectomy. It may be possible to mend the AF with a fibrous patch or polymer plug, as has been demonstrated successfully in organ culture.[85] One of the most exciting possibilities associated with organ culture is the ability to culture, maintain, and perform experiments on live human discs for realistic studies of physiology and regeneration.[73,86] However, it is still not known how well the organ culture framework can generate translatable clinical therapies as this method can not reproduce all aspects of the physiological environment (e.g., the host immune response); so although the technique is very promising, in vivo validation is still required.

7.3 Controllable External Variables

The disc microenvironment comprises a complex interconnected set of precisely balanced external variables that are required to maintain disc homeostasis. These external variables are often controlled in vitro to mimic the native physiological environment and are often controlled in in vitro culture systems to mimic cell behavior. This section discusses these relevant variables and summarizes results related to their impact on disc culture.

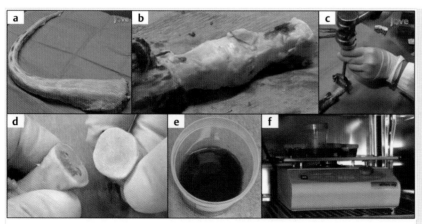

Fig. 7.4 Isolation of a bovine caudal disc for organ culture. The bovine caudal disc is one of the most common models used in organ culture. The procedure for isolating a bovine disc is pictured here as documented by Chan and Gantenbein-Ritter.[117] **(a)** A bovine tail is procured from a local stockyard and prepared for aseptic dissection. **(b)** The disc can be visualized after removal of the contiguous connective tissues and muscle. **(c)** A device similar to an osteotome is used to sharply dissect the disc from the tail proper, leaving a small amount of vertebral bone. **(d)** The vertebral end plate is visualized, **(e)** the disc is submerged in growth media, and **(f)** then placed on an orbital shaker plate inside an incubator for long-term culture.

7.3.1 Oxygen Tension, pH, and Glucose

As the IVD is primarily avascular, it acquires oxygen by diffusion through a network of vessels in the cartilaginous end plates. Consequently, there are steep oxygen gradients in the NP and areas of low oxygen tension. This can be replicated in vitro; specialized incubators designed for oxygen regulation are available to induce a hypoxic environment similar to the intervertebral niche. Hypoxia studies have been conducted in a number of formats including monolayer[87] and hydrogel culture[88] systems. These studies collectively show that NP cells are uniquely suited to survive in strenuous conditions, deprived of both oxygen and serum, with minimal changes in viability; an ability that is closely tied to the transcription factor hypoxia-inducible factor (HIF)-1α.[89] Consequently, one school of thought suggests that preconditioning engineered replacements in a hypoxic in vitro environment will induce an NP-like phenotype and improve transplantation results, affecting in vivo survival and phenotype retention. Other cell types with potential for disc regeneration, such as MSCs, which normally reside in an oxygen-rich environment, demonstrate muted functional ECM deposition when cultured under hypoxic conditions in vitro,[90] perhaps foretelling their poor performance when implanted into the disc space.

A number of factors contribute to an acidic pH in the IVD space. Due to disc avascularity and an insufficient oxygen supply, NP cells are powered primarily through anaerobic glycolysis. A byproduct of this metabolic process is lactic acid, which accumulates in the extracellular space due to impaired transport out of the disc space as a result of poor vascular supply, resulting in a low local pH.

As demonstrated by hydrogel NP cell culture experiments, pH set at a neutral level provides an anabolic boost in ECM metabolism, whereas pH set at lower levels (a state with physiological relevance to the disc) causes a profound disruption of ECM metabolism.[91] It may be necessary to examine and challenge potential therapeutic strategies, such as engineered tissue replacements, in a low pH environment prior to clinical use to ensure successful translation.

Glucose is transported into the disc through the limited vascular supply in the cartilage end plates. As a result, this important energy source for disc cells is in low supply in healthy discs and the supply is further compromised with degeneration due to changes in tissue permeability. The effects of low glucose are often simulated in vitro by formulating media with varying glucose concentrations. Low glucose was shown to have a significant effect on NP cells in hydrogel culture, causing decreases in many metabolic markers.[92] Similar effects of glucose deprivation have been demonstrated for MSCs as well.[90]

The implications of limited glucose on tissue regeneration are important to consider. The degenerate disc space may not be able to sustain injectables with highly concentrated cells or engineered tissue replacements with a high cell density, given the finite glucose reserves. Thus, high cell concentrates may be subjected to increased levels of apoptosis soon after injection. Appropriately tuning the cell source for the in vivo environment is of critical importance for cell therapies.[93]

7.3.2 Inflammatory Factors

For resident cells, conditions in the disc microenvironment adversely affect normal function in a healthy state and are exacerbated in a degenerate state; the physiological niche is characterized in normal conditions by low pH, low glucose, and low oxygen (as described above), and in degeneration by disc-wide inflammation, as pro-inflammatory factors are produced by cells of both the NP and AF.[32,94,95,96] These factors, which induce downstream production of collagen- and proteoglycan-degrading enzymes, create an environment of catabolism, contributing to fibrosis, compaction, and loss of structure in the NP, and are a significant hurdle for regeneration.

This pathological inflammatory milieu will influence both injectable therapies and engineered tissue replacements. In vitro studies have confirmed that powerful pro-inflammatory cytokines, such as tumor necrosis factor (TNF)-α and interleukin (IL)-1β, which are ubiquitous in disc degeneration, have a negative impact on ECM production by disc cells. Matrix synthesis can be rescued by including antagonists to these molecules, such as a soluble TNF receptor,[97] the IL-1 receptor antagonist (IL-1ra),[47,98] or an NF-κB inhibitor,[99] suggesting molecules like these have significant potential for regeneration. Codelivery of such anticatabolic agents at the time of cell injection or engineered construct implantation may improve long-term outcomes.

7.3.3 Mechanical Loading

The disc experiences multiaxial static and dynamic loading during routine daily activities. Loading directly affects behavior at the cell level through mechanotransduction events. In addition, loading has an effect on nutrient transport and waste removal, and in a nutrient-deficient homeostatic state, loading can have a profound impact on the precarious balance of the intervertebral niche. Depending on the load magnitude, frequency, and duration, physical forces can positively or negatively affect cell metabolism,[76,77,100,101,102] and consequently mechanical loading conditions are often replicated in in vitro studies to analyze these effects.

Mechanical loading events can be simulated in vitro on the organ and tissue scale to study the effects on ECM metabolism and regeneration. For tissue engineering purposes, dynamic loading is used to stimulate ECM production to generate more robust tissues for implantation. On the tissue subcomponent level, dynamic compressive loading has been evaluated in hydrogel culture for both NP cells[103] and MSCs,[104] and dynamic tensile loading has been evaluated for both AF cells on flexible membranes[105] and MSCs on fibrous scaffolds.[106] On the whole disc level, dynamic loading has been used for mechanical stimulation of engineered discs comprising AF and NP cells[107] and MSCs,[108] as well as in organ culture[74] (▶ Fig. 7.5). A general summary of findings from these studies is that low frequency, moderate magnitude physical forces allow for anabolic in vitro stimulation of engineered tissues and disc explants.

7.3.4 Growth Factors

Growth factors that regulate cell metabolism are present in the disc space, and can be applied in vitro at supraphysiological

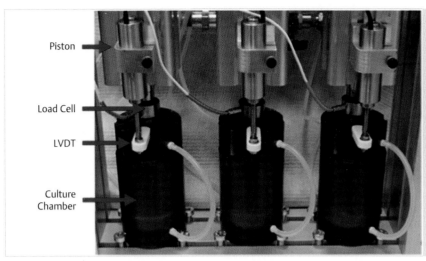

Fig. 7.5 A bioreactor for whole disc organ culture.[74] In this example of a bioreactor used for whole disc organ culture, a human or bovine disc is submerged in media and cultured under dynamic compressive loading in each of the three red culture chambers. A piston controlled by hydraulics is used to apply compressive forces, while force is recorded by the load cell and displacement is recorded by the displacement sensor (LVDT).

concentrations to achieve a specific cell phenotype or provide an anabolic stimulus to promote regeneration. A wealth of experiments on growth factor stimulation are available to support growth factor injections,[109] as well as to stimulate engineered tissues for disc repair or replacement.[70] The bone morphogenetic protein (BMP) family of growth factors is of specific interest, as two members of this family (osteogenic protein [OP-1]/BMP-7 and growth and differentiation [GDF]-5/BMP-14) have demonstrated sufficient in vitro success to motivate clinical trials.[110]

Growth factors have shown promising results in in vitro models, but significant hurdles must be overcome for growth factor injection to be translatable. In vitro studies allow for growth factors to be continuously supplemented by refreshing the culture media. The standard route for growth factor delivery in vivo, however, is by needle injection through the AF, and delivery through multiple injections for continuous supplementation is not feasible. One method for prolonged growth factor delivery with a single injection is through the sustained release of these factors from biomaterials. This can be achieved through a number of mechanisms including delivery from slow-releasing microspheres, hydrogels, and electrospun scaffolds. Release profiles can be tuned in vitro through polymer engineering to achieve continuous release that lasts on the order of weeks, obviating the need for multiple injections.

7.4 Outstanding Challenges

The IVD and its resident cells have a difficult assignment; the disc must meet substantial functional demands, resisting physical forces that are on the order of multiple body weights in compression, shear, torsion, and bending modes, and it must do so in an avascular environment, with minimal nutritional support for healthy ECM maintenance. These two aspects, high functional demands and limited nutrition, present a challenge not only for disc survival but also for the restoration of diseased discs to a healthy state. In the previous sections, we reviewed a number of potential cell sources, biomaterial frameworks, and culture systems that have advanced our knowledge of disc

biology and that can serve as experimental tools toward realizing disc regeneration. However, numerous challenges remain, many of which can be addressed using in vitro experimentation. The remaining challenges are summarized as follows for each mode of regenerative therapeutic under development:

- Injectable cell therapies:
  - Low O_2, glucose, and pH
  - Inflammatory signals present in diseased tissue
  - Mechanical stress
  - Maintenance of cell regenerative phenotype after injection
  - Delivery route is damaging to AF
- Injectable growth factor therapies:
  - Limited number of endogenous cells available for regeneration
  - Resident cells have a degenerate phenotype
  - Limited activity and/or half-life of growth factors
  - Growth factors may have limited activity in acidic environment
  - Delivery route is damaging to AF
- Biological NP replacements:
  - Low O_2, glucose, and pH
  - Mechanical stress
  - Maintenance of cell regenerative phenotype after implantation
- Biological AF replacements
  - Low O_2, glucose, and pH
  - Mechanical stress
  - Mechanical properties vary with fiber orientation
  - Method of fixation to native tissue
  - Maintenance of cell regenerative phenotype after implantation
- Biological total disc replacements:
  - Low O_2, glucose, and pH
  - Must match multiaxial mechanical properties of native tissue
  - Integration into vertebrae
  - Meeting nutritional demands through diffusion over long distances
  - Maintenance of cell regenerative phenotype after implantation

7.5 Conclusion

There has been substantial progress toward disc regeneration in the past years and an array of strategies have been developed that show promise in vitro and in early preclinical models. From these studies, we have learned much about disc cell biology and biomaterials, generating a foundation for future research that will inform the implementation of new strategies. Additional work is now required to systematically evaluate the second iterations of these earlier regeneration strategies, bearing in mind that the challenging environment present in the disc may counteract the regenerative potential of these approaches. These in vitro efforts, using many of the strategies documented in this chapter, are the critical experiments to define and optimize therapeutic approaches as they progress toward preclinical animal studies and ultimately to clinical trials in humans.

7.6 Evidence-based Results

1. Gantenbein B, Illien-Junger S, Chan SC, Walser J, Haglund L, Ferguson SJ, et al. Organ culture bioreactors–platforms to study human intervertebral disc degeneration and regenerative therapy. Curr Stem Cell Res Ther 2015;10:339–352
This recently published review of bioreactor technologies for whole disc organ culture was written by the leaders of the field and details the state-of-the-art techniques and current thoughts on using this methodology for disc research.

2. Walter BA, Illien-Junger S, Nasser PR, Hecht AC, Iatridis JC. Development and validation of a bioreactor system for dynamic loading and mechanical characterization of whole human intervertebral discs in organ culture. J Biomech 2014;47:2095–2101
This paper documents the development and thorough validation of a bioreactor for whole disc organ culture that applies dynamic mechanical loads to bovine caudal discs. The bioreactor is used to simulate diurnal loading, applying cyclic compressive loads during the day and allowing for recovery overnight. Discs cultured 21 days in the bioreactor maintain ~ 80% cell viability and show no changes in mechanical properties over time.

3. Alkhatib B, Rosenzweig DH, Krock E, Roughley PJ, Beckman L, Steffen T, et al. Acute mechanical injury of the human intervertebral disc: link to degeneration and pain. Eur Cell Mater 2014;28:98–110, discussion 110-1
In this paper, whole human discs were exposed to impact loads and subsequently cultured for 14 days. The loading protocol caused end plate fracture and fissure formation in the AF region. In comparison with controls, injured discs exhibited a loss of cell viability and glycosaminoglycan (GAG) content, and conditioned media from the injured group caused neurite sprouting in a neuronal cell line, highlighting a possible mechanism for discogenic pain.

4. Mwale F, Wang HT, Roughley P, Antoniou J, Haglund L. Link N and mesenchymal stem cells can induce regeneration of the early degenerate intervertebral disc. Tissue Eng Part A 2014;20:2942–2949
Bovine caudal discs were injected with trypsin to induce a degenerative-like condition and then, following 4 days of culture, MSCs, link N (a peptide with regenerative potential), or

both MSCs and link N were injected into the NP to evaluate their potential for regeneration. Within 14 days, discs in all treatment groups had restored GAG and normal type II collagen levels, indicating the potential of these therapeutic strategies.

7.7 References

[1] Miller JA, Schmatz C, Schultz AB. Lumbar disc degeneration: correlation with age, sex, and spine level in 600 autopsy specimens. Spine. 1988; 13 (2):173–178

[2] Sheikh H, Zakharian K, De La Torre RP, et al. In vivo intervertebral disc regeneration using stem cell-derived chondroprogenitors. J Neurosurg Spine. 2009; 10(3):265–272

[3] Takahashi K, Yamanaka S. Induction of pluripotent stem cells from mouse embryonic and adult fibroblast cultures by defined factors. Cell. 2006; 126 (4):663–676

[4] Liu Y, Fu S, Rahaman MN, Mao JJ, Bal BS. Native nucleus pulposus tissue matrix promotes notochordal differentiation of human induced pluripotent stem cells with potential for treating intervertebral disc degeneration. J Biomed Mater Res A. 2015; 103(3):1053–1059

[5] Chen J, Lee EJ, Jing L, Christoforou N, Leong KW, Setton LA. Differentiation of mouse induced pluripotent stem cells (iPSCs) into nucleus pulposus-like cells in vitro. PLoS One. 2013; 8(9):e75548

[6] Diekman BO, Christoforou N, Willard VP, et al. Cartilage tissue engineering using differentiated and purified induced pluripotent stem cells. Proc Natl AcadSci U S A. 2012; 109(47):19172–19177

[7] Zhang C, Yuan H, Liu H, et al. Well-aligned chitosan-based ultrafine fibers committed teno-lineage differentiation of human induced pluripotent stem cells for Achilles tendon regeneration. Biomaterials. 2015; 53:716–730

[8] Barruet E, Hsiao EC. Using human induced pluripotent stem cells to model skeletal diseases. Methods Mol Biol. 2016; 1353:101–118

[9] Johnstone B, Hering TM, Caplan AI, Goldberg VM, Yoo JU. In vitro chondrogenesis of bone marrow-derived mesenchymal progenitor cells. Exp Cell Res. 1998; 238(1):265–272

[10] Pittenger MF, Mackay AM, Beck SC, et al. Multilineage potential of adult human mesenchymal stem cells. Science. 1999; 284(5411):143–147

[11] Kim M, Erickson IE, Choudhury M, Pleshko N, Mauck RL. Transient exposure to TGF-β3 improves the functional chondrogenesis of MSC-laden hyaluronic acid hydrogels. J MechBehav Biomed Mater. 2012; 11:92–101

[12] Pei M, He F, Kish VL, Vunjak-Novakovic G. Engineering of functional cartilage tissue using stem cells from synovial lining: a preliminary study. Clin OrthopRelat Res. 2008; 466(8):1880–1889

[13] Awad HA, Wickham MQ, Leddy HA, Gimble JM, Guilak F. Chondrogenic differentiation of adipose-derived adult stem cells in agarose, alginate, and gelatin scaffolds. Biomaterials. 2004; 25(16):3211–3222

[14] Sakai D, Andersson GB. Stem cell therapy for intervertebral disc regeneration: obstacles and solutions. Nat Rev Rheumatol. 2015; 11(4):243–256

[15] Choi KS, Cohn MJ, Harfe BD. Identification of nucleus pulposus precursor cells and notochordal remnants in the mouse: implications for disk degeneration and chordoma formation. Dev Dyn. 2008; 237(12):3953–3958

[16] Bach FC, de Vries SA, Krouwels A, et al. The species-specific regenerative effects of notochordal cell-conditioned medium on chondrocyte-like cells derived from degenerated human intervertebral discs. Eur Cell Mater. 2015; 30:132–146, discussion 146–147

[17] Hwang PY, Jing L, Michael KW, Richardson WJ, Chen J, Setton LA. N-cadherin-mediated signaling regulates cell phenotype for nucleus pulposus cells of the intervertebral disc. Cell Mol Bioeng. 2015; 8(1):51–62

[18] Chen J, Yan W, Setton LA. Molecular phenotypes of notochordal cells purified from immature nucleus pulposus. Eur Spine J. 2006; 15 Suppl 3:S303–S311

[19] Cornejo MC, Cho SK, Giannarelli C, Iatridis JC, Purmessur D. Soluble factors from the notochordal-rich intervertebral disc inhibit endothelial cell invasion and vessel formation in the presence and absence of pro-inflammatory cytokines. Osteoarthritis Cartilage. 2015; 23(3):487–496

[20] Gantenbein B, Calandriello E, Wuertz-Kozak K, Benneker LM, Keel MJ, Chan SC. Activation of intervertebral disc cells by co-culture with notochordal cells, conditioned medium and hypoxia. BMC Musculoskelet Disord. 2014; 15:422

[21] Merceron C, Mangiavini L, Robling A, et al. Loss of HIF-1α in the notochord results in cell death and complete disappearance of the nucleus pulposus. PLoS One. 2014; 9(10):e110768

[22] Rodrigues-Pinto R, Richardson SM, Hoyland JA. An understanding of intervertebral disc development, maturation and cell phenotype provides clues to direct cell-based tissue regeneration therapies for disc degeneration. Eur Spine J. 2014; 23(9):1803–1814

[23] Guehring T, Wilde G, Sumner M, et al. Notochordal intervertebral disc cells: sensitivity to nutrient deprivation. Arthritis Rheum. 2009; 60 (4):1026–1034

[24] Purmessur D, Schek RM, Abbott RD, Ballif BA, Godburn KE, Iatridis JC. Notochordal conditioned media from tissue increases proteoglycan accumulation and promotes a healthy nucleus pulposus phenotype in human mesenchymal stem cells. Arthritis Res Ther. 2011; 13(3):R81

[25] de Vries SA, Potier E, van Doeselaar M, Meij BP, Tryfonidou MA, Ito K. Conditioned medium derived from notochordal cell-rich nucleus pulposus tissue stimulates matrix production by canine nucleus pulposus cells and bone marrow-derived stromal cells. Tissue Eng Part A. 2015; 21(5–6):1077–1084

[26] Minogue BM, Richardson SM, Zeef LA, Freemont AJ, Hoyland JA. Transcriptional profiling of bovine intervertebral disc cells: implications for identification of normal and degenerate human intervertebral disc cell phenotypes. Arthritis Res Ther. 2010; 12(1):R22

[27] Clouet J, Grimandi G, Pot-Vaucel M, et al. Identification of phenotypic discriminating markers for intervertebral disc cells and articular chondrocytes. Rheumatology (Oxford). 2009; 48(11):1447–1450

[28] Risbud MV, Schoepflin ZR, Mwale F, et al. Defining the phenotype of young healthy nucleus pulposus cells: recommendations of the Spine Research Interest Group at the 2014 annual ORS meeting. J Orthop Res. 2015; 33 (3):283–293

[29] Le Maitre CL, Freemont AJ, Hoyland JA. Accelerated cellular senescence in degenerate intervertebral discs: a possible role in the pathogenesis of intervertebral disc degeneration. Arthritis Res Ther. 2007; 9(3):R45

[30] Roberts S, Caterson B, Menage J, Evans EH, Jaffray DC, Eisenstein SM. Matrix metalloproteinases and aggrecanase: their role in disorders of the human intervertebral disc. Spine. 2000; 25(23):3005–3013

[31] Le Maitre CL, Freemont AJ, Hoyland JA. Localization of degradative enzymes and their inhibitors in the degenerate human intervertebral disc. J Pathol. 2004; 204(1):47–54

[32] Le Maitre CL, Hoyland JA, Freemont AJ. Catabolic cytokine expression in degenerate and herniated human intervertebral discs: IL-1beta and TNF alpha expression profile. Arthritis Res Ther. 2007; 9(4):R77

[33] Strassburg S, Richardson SM, Freemont AJ, Hoyland JA. Co-culture induces mesenchymal stem cell differentiation and modulation of the degenerate human nucleus pulposus cell phenotype. Regen Med. 2010; 5(5):701–711

[34] Mochida J, Sakai D, Nakamura Y, Watanabe T, Yamamoto Y, Kato S. Intervertebral disc repair with activated nucleus pulposus cell transplantation: a three-year, prospective clinical study of its safety. Eur Cell Mater. 2015; 29:202–212, discussion 212

[35] Peterson L, Vasiliadis HS, Brittberg M, Lindahl A. Autologous chondrocyte implantation: a long-term follow-up. Am J Sports Med. 2010; 38(6):1117–1124

[36] Nawaz SZ, Bentley G, Briggs TW, et al. Autologous chondrocyte implantation in the knee: mid-term to long-term results. J Bone Joint Surg Am. 2014; 96(10):824–830

[37] Fulco I, Miot S, Haug MD, et al. Engineered autologous cartilage tissue for nasal reconstruction after tumour resection: an observational first-in-human trial. Lancet. 2014; 384(9940):337–346

[38] Kang N, Liu X, Guan Y, et al. Effects of co-culturing BMSCs and auricular chondrocytes on the elastic modulus and hypertrophy of tissue engineered cartilage. Biomaterials. 2012; 33(18):4535–4544

[39] Farr J, Yao JQ. Chondral defect repair with particulated juvenile cartilage allograft. Cartilage. 2011; 2(4):346–353

[40] Engler AJ, Sen S, Sweeney HL, Discher DE. Matrix elasticity directs stem cell lineage specification. Cell. 2006; 126(4):677–689

[41] Khetan S, Guvendiren M, Legant WR, Cohen DM, Chen CS, Burdick JA. Degradation-mediated cellular traction directs stem cell fate in covalently crosslinked three-dimensional hydrogels. Nat Mater. 2013; 12(5):458–465

[42] Watanabe T, Sakai D, Yamamoto Y, et al. Human nucleus pulposus cells significantly enhanced biological properties in a coculture system with direct cell-to-cell contact with autologous mesenchymal stem cells. J Orthop Res. 2010; 28(5):623–630

[43] Kluba T, Niemeyer T, Gaissmaier C, Gründer T. Human anulus fibrosis and nucleus pulposus cells of the intervertebral disc: effect of degeneration and culture system on cell phenotype. Spine. 2005; 30(24):2743–2748

[44] Wang JY, Baer AE, Kraus VB, Setton LA. Intervertebral disc cells exhibit differences in gene expression in alginate and monolayer culture. Spine. 2001; 26(16):1747–1751, discussion 1752

[45] Allon AA, Butcher K, Schneider RA, Lotz JC. Structured bilaminar coculture outperforms stem cells and disc cells in a simulated degenerate disc environment. Spine. 2012; 37(10):813–818

[46] DuRaine GD, Brown WE, Hu JC, Athanasiou KA. Emergence of scaffold-free approaches for tissue engineering musculoskeletal cartilages. Ann Biomed Eng. 2015; 43(3):543–554

[47] Gorth DJ, Mauck RL, Chiaro JA, et al. IL-1ra delivered from poly(lactic-co-glycolic acid) microspheres attenuates IL-1β-mediated degradation of nucleus pulposus in vitro. Arthritis Res Ther. 2012; 14(4):R179

[48] Gupta MS, Nicoll SB. Duration of TGF-β3 exposure impacts the chondrogenic maturation of human MSCs in photocrosslinked carboxymethylcellulose hydrogels. Ann Biomed Eng. 2015; 43(5):1145–1157

[49] Frith JE, Cameron AR, Menzies DJ, et al. An injectable hydrogel incorporating mesenchymal precursor cells and pentosan polysulphate for intervertebral disc regeneration. Biomaterials. 2013; 34(37):9430–9440

[50] Naqvi SM, Buckley CT. Differential response of encapsulated nucleus pulposus and bone marrow stem cells in isolation and coculture in alginate and chitosan hydrogels. Tissue Eng Part A. 2015; 21(1–2):288–299

[51] Zeng Y, Chen C, Liu W, et al. Injectable microcryogels reinforced alginate encapsulation of mesenchymal stromal cells for leak-proof delivery and alleviation of canine disc degeneration. Biomaterials. 2015; 59:53–65

[52] Collin EC, Grad S, Zeugolis DI, et al. An injectable vehicle for nucleus pulposus cell-based therapy. Biomaterials. 2011; 32(11):2862–2870

[53] Francisco AT, Hwang PY, Jeong CG, Jing L, Chen J, Setton LA. Photocrosslinkable laminin-functionalized polyethylene glycol hydrogel for intervertebral disc regeneration. Acta Biomater. 2014; 10(3):1102–1111

[54] Kim DH, Martin JT, Elliott DM, Smith LJ, Mauck RL. Phenotypic stability, matrix elaboration and functional maturation of nucleus pulposus cells encapsulated in photocrosslinkable hyaluronic acid hydrogels. Acta Biomater. 2015; 12:21–29

[55] Smith LJ, Gorth DJ, Showalter BL, et al. In vitro characterization of a stem-cell-seeded triple-interpenetrating-network hydrogel for functional regeneration of the nucleus pulposus. Tissue Eng Part A. 2014; 20(13–14):1841–1849

[56] Showalter BL, Elliott DM, Chen W, Malhotra NR. Evaluation of an in situ gelable and injectable hydrogel treatment to preserve human disc mechanical function undergoing physiologic cyclic loading followed by hydrated recovery. J BiomechEng. 2015; 137(8):081008

[57] O'Connell GD, Carapezza MA, Newman IB. 2014

[58] Bowles RD, Williams RM, Zipfel WR, Bonassar LJ. Self-assembly of aligned tissue-engineered annulus fibrosus and intervertebral disc composite via collagen gel contraction. Tissue Eng Part A. 2010; 16(4):1339–1348

[59] Grunert P, Borde BH, Towne SB, et al. Riboflavin crosslinked high-density collagen gel for the repair of annular defects in intervertebral discs: An in vivo study. Acta Biomater. 2015; 26:215–224

[60] Schek RM, Michalek AJ, Iatridis JC. Genipin-crosslinked fibrin hydrogels as a potential adhesive to augment intervertebral disc annulus repair. Eur Cell Mater. 2011; 21:373–383

[61] Iu J, Santerre JP, Kandel RA. Inner and outer annulus fibrosus cells exhibit differentiated phenotypes and yield changes in extracellular matrix protein composition in vitro on a polycarbonate urethane scaffold. Tissue Eng Part A. 2014; 20(23–24):3261–3269

[62] Attia M, Santerre JP, Kandel RA. The response of annulus fibrosus cell to fibronectin-coated nanofibrous polyurethane-anionic dihydroxyligomer scaffolds. Biomaterials. 2011; 32(2):450–460

[63] Wismer N, Grad S, Fortunato G, Ferguson SJ, Alini M, Eglin D. Biodegradable electrospun scaffolds for annulus fibrosus tissue engineering: effect of scaffold structure and composition on annulus fibrosus cells in vitro. Tissue Eng Part A. 2014; 20(3–4):672–682

[64] Nerurkar NL, Sen S, Huang AH, Elliott DM, Mauck RL. Engineered disc-like angle-ply structures for intervertebral disc replacement. Spine. 2010; 35 (8):867–873

[65] Martin JT, Milby AH, Chiaro JA, et al. Translation of an engineered nanofibrous disc-like angle-ply structure for intervertebral disc replacement in a small animal model. Acta Biomater. 2014; 10(6):2473–2481

[66] Nerurkar NL, Baker BM, Sen S, Wible EE, Elliott DM, Mauck RL. Nanofibrous biologic laminates replicate the form and function of the annulus fibrosus. Nat Mater. 2009; 8(12):986–992

[67] van Uden S, Silva-Correia J, Correlo VM, Oliveira JM, Reis RL. Custom-tailored tissue engineered polycaprolactone scaffolds for total disc replacement. Biofabrication. 2015; 7(1):015008

[68] Bowles RD, Gebhard HH, Härtl R, Bonassar LJ. Tissue-engineered intervertebral discs produce new matrix, maintain disc height, and restore biomechanical function to the rodent spine. Proc Natl AcadSci U S A. 2011; 108 (32):13106–13111

[69] Chik TK, Chooi WH, Li YY, et al. Bioengineering a multicomponent spinal motion segment construct–a 3D model for complex tissue engineering. Adv Healthc Mater. 2015; 4(1):99–112

[70] Martin JT, Kim DH, Ikuta K. 2015

[71] Moriguchi Y, Navarro R, Grunert P. 2015

[72] Gantenbein B, Illien-Jünger S, Chan SC, et al. Organ culture bioreactors—platforms to study human intervertebral disc degeneration and regenerative therapy. Curr Stem Cell Res Ther. 2015; 10(4):339–352

[73] Gawri R, Mwale F, Ouellet J, et al. Development of an organ culture system for long-term survival of the intact human intervertebral disc. Spine. 2011; 36(22):1835–1842

[74] Walter BA, Illien-Jünger S, Nasser PR, Hecht AC, Iatridis JC. Development and validation of a bioreactor system for dynamic loading and mechanical characterization of whole human intervertebral discs in organ culture. J Biomech. 2014; 47(9):2095–2101

[75] Haglund L, Moir J, Beckman L, et al. Development of a bioreactor for axially loaded intervertebral disc organ culture. Tissue Eng Part C Methods. 2011; 17(10):1011–1019

[76] Walter BA, Korecki CL, Purmessur D, Roughley PJ, Michalek AJ, Iatridis JC. Complex loading affects intervertebral disc mechanics and biology. Osteoarthritis Cartilage. 2011; 19(8):1011–1018

[77] Chan SC, Walser J, Käppeli P, Shamsollahi MJ, Ferguson SJ, Gantenbein-Ritter B. Region specific response of intervertebral disc cells to complex dynamic loading: an organ culture study using a dynamic torsion-compression bioreactor. PLoS One. 2013; 8(8):e72489

[78] Dudli S, Haschtmann D, Ferguson SJ. Fracture of the vertebral endplates, but not equienergetic impact load, promotes disc degeneration in vitro. J Orthop Res. 2012; 30(5):809–816

[79] Ponnappan RK, Markova DZ, Antonio PJ, et al. An organ culture system to model early degenerative changes of the intervertebral disc. Arthritis Res Ther. 2011; 13(5):R171

[80] Chan SC, Bürki A, Bonél HM, Benneker LM, Gantenbein-Ritter B. Papain-induced in vitro disc degeneration model for the study of injectable nucleus pulposus therapy. Spine J. 2013; 13(3):273–283

[81] Mwale F, Wang HT, Roughley P, Antoniou J, Haglund L. Link N and mesenchymal stem cells can induce regeneration of the early degenerate intervertebral disc. Tissue Eng Part A. 2014; 20(21–22):2942–2949

[82] Peroglio M, Eglin D, Benneker LM, Alini M, Grad S. Thermoreversible hyaluronan-based hydrogel supports in vitro and ex vivo disc-like differentiation of human mesenchymal stem cells. Spine J. 2013; 13(11):1627–1639

[83] Illien-Jünger S, Pattappa G, Peroglio M, et al. Homing of mesenchymal stem cells in induced degenerative intervertebral discs in a whole organ culture system. Spine. 2012; 37(22):1865–1873

[84] Illien-Jünger S, Lu Y, Purmessur D, et al. Detrimental effects of discectomy on intervertebral disc biology can be decelerated by growth factor treatment during surgery: a large animal organ culture model. Spine J. 2014; 14 (11):2724–2732

[85] Likhitpanichkul M, Dreischarf M, Illien-Junger S, et al. Fibrin-genipin adhesive hydrogel for annulus fibrosus repair: performance evaluation with large animal organ culture, in situ biomechanics, and in vivo degradation tests. Eur Cell Mater. 2014; 28:25–37, discussion 37–38

[86] Alkhatib B, Rosenzweig DH, Krock E, et al. Acute mechanical injury of the human intervertebral disc: link to degeneration and pain. Eur Cell Mater. 2014; 28:98–110, discussion 110–111

[87] Risbud MV, Fertala J, Vresilovic EJ, Albert TJ, Shapiro IM. Nucleus pulposus cells upregulate PI3K/Akt and MEK/ERK signaling pathways under hypoxic conditions and resist apoptosis induced by serum withdrawal. Spine. 2005; 30(8):882–889

[88] Gorth DJ, Lothstein KE, Chiaro JA, et al. Hypoxic regulation of functional extracellular matrix elaboration by nucleus pulposus cells in long-term agarose culture. J Orthop Res. 2015; 33(5):747–754

[89] Risbud MV, Schipani E, Shapiro IM. Hypoxic regulation of nucleus pulposus cell survival: from niche to notch. Am J Pathol. 2010; 176(4):1577–1583

[90] Farrell MJ, Shin JI, Smith LJ, Mauck RL. Functional consequences of glucose and oxygen deprivation on engineered mesenchymal stem cell-based cartilage constructs. Osteoarthritis Cartilage. 2015; 23(1):134–142

[91] Razaq S, Wilkins RJ, Urban JP. The effect of extracellular pH on matrix turnover by cells of the bovine nucleus pulposus. Eur Spine J. 2003; 12(4):341–349

[92] Bibby SR, Jones DA, Ripley RM, Urban JP. Metabolism of the intervertebral disc: effects of low levels of oxygen, glucose, and pH on rates of energy metabolism of bovine nucleus pulposus cells. Spine. 2005; 30(5):487–496

[93] Tibiletti M, Kregar Velikonja N, Urban JP, Fairbank JC. Disc cell therapies: critical issues. Eur Spine J. 2014; 23 Suppl 3:S375–S384

[94] Risbud MV, Shapiro IM. Role of cytokines in intervertebral disc degeneration: pain and disc content. Nat Rev Rheumatol. 2014; 10(1):44–56

[95] Le Maitre CL, Freemont AJ, Hoyland JA. The role of interleukin-1 in the pathogenesis of human intervertebral disc degeneration. Arthritis Res Ther. 2005; 7(4):R732–R745

[96] Séguin CA, Pilliar RM, Roughley PJ, Kandel RA. Tumor necrosis factor-alpha modulates matrix production and catabolism in nucleus pulposus tissue. Spine. 2005; 30(17):1940–1948

[97] Sinclair SM, Shamji MF, Chen J, et al. Attenuation of inflammatory events in human intervertebral disc cells with a tumor necrosis factor antagonist. Spine. 2011; 36(15):1190–1196

[98] Shamji MF, Betre H, Kraus VB, et al. Development and characterization of a fusion protein between thermally responsive elastin-like polypeptide and interleukin-1 receptor antagonist: sustained release of a local antiinflammatory therapeutic. Arthritis Rheum. 2007; 56(11):3650–3661

[99] Nasto LA, Seo HY, Robinson AR, et al. ISSLS prize winner: inhibition of NF-κB activity ameliorates age-associated disc degeneration in a mouse model of accelerated aging. Spine. 2012; 37(21):1819–1825

[100] Iatridis JC, Mente PL, Stokes IA, Aronsson DD, Alini M. Compression-induced changes in intervertebral disc properties in a rat tail model. Spine. 1999; 24(10):996–1002

[101] Korecki CL, Kuo CK, Tuan RS, Iatridis JC. Intervertebral disc cell response to dynamic compression is age and frequency dependent. J Orthop Res. 2009; 27(6):800–806

[102] Barbir A, Godburn KE, Michalek AJ, Lai A, Monsey RD, Iatridis JC. Effects of torsion on intervertebral disc gene expression and biomechanics, using a rat tail model. Spine. 2011; 36(8):607–614

[103] Fernando HN, Czamanski J, Yuan TY, Gu W, Salahadin A, Huang CY. Mechanical loading affects the energy metabolism of intervertebral disc cells. J Orthop Res. 2011; 29(11):1634–1641

[104] Huang AH, Farrell MJ, Kim M, Mauck RL. Long-term dynamic loading improves the mechanical properties of chondrogenic mesenchymal stem cell-laden hydrogel. Eur Cell Mater. 2010; 19:72–85

[105] Sowa G, Agarwal S. Cyclic tensile stress exerts a protective effect on intervertebral disc cells. Am J Phys Med Rehabil. 2008; 87(7):537–544

[106] Baker BM, Shah RP, Huang AH, Mauck RL. Dynamic tensile loading improves the functional properties of mesenchymal stem cell-laden nanofiber-based fibrocartilage. Tissue Eng Part A. 2011; 17(9–10):1445–1455

[107] Hudson KD, Mozia RI, Bonassar LJ. Dose-dependent response of tissue-engineered intervertebral discs to dynamic unconfined compressive loading. Tissue Eng Part A. 2015; 21(3–4):564–572

[108] Tsai TL, Nelson BC, Anderson PA, Zdeblick TA, Li WJ. Intervertebral disc and stem cells cocultured in biomimetic extracellular matrix stimulated by cyclic compression in perfusion bioreactor. Spine J. 2014; 14(9):2127–2140

[109] Imai Y, Miyamoto K, An HS, Thonar EJ, Andersson GB, Masuda K. Recombinant human osteogenic protein-1 upregulates proteoglycan metabolism of human anulus fibrosus and nucleus pulposus cells. Spine. 2007; 32 (12):1303–1309, discussion 1310

[110] Zhang Y, Chee A, Thonar EJ, An HS. Intervertebral disk repair by protein, gene, or cell injection: a framework for rehabilitation-focused biologics in the spine. PM R. 2011; 3(6) Suppl 1:S88–S94

[111] Baker BM, Shah RP, Silverstein AM, Esterhai JL, Burdick JA, Mauck RL. Sacrificial nanofibrous composites provide instruction without impediment and enable functional tissue formation. Proc Natl AcadSci U S A. 2012; 109 (35):14176–14181

[112] Nathan AS, Baker BM, Nerurkar NL, Mauck RL. Mechano-topographic modulation of stem cell nuclear shape on nanofibrous scaffolds. Acta Biomater. 2011; 7(1):57–66

[113] Park SH, Gil ES, Cho H, et al. Intervertebral disk tissue engineering using biphasic silk composite scaffolds. Tissue Eng Part A. 2012; 18(5–6):447–458

[114] Mizuno H, Roy AK, Zaporojan V, Vacanti CA, Ueda M, Bonassar LJ. Biomechanical and biochemical characterization of composite tissue-engineered intervertebral discs. Biomaterials. 2006; 27(3):362–370

[115] Zhuang Y, Huang B, Li CQ, et al. Construction of tissue-engineered composite intervertebral disc and preliminary morphological and biochemical evaluation. Biochem Biophys Res Commun. 2011; 407(2):327–332

[116] Mizuno H, Roy AK, Vacanti CA, Kojima K, Ueda M, Bonassar LJ. Tissue-engineered composites of anulus fibrosus and nucleus pulposus for intervertebral disc replacement. Spine. 2004; 29(12):1290–1297, discussion 1297–1298

[117] Chan SC, Gantenbein-Ritter B. Preparation of intact bovine tail intervertebral discs for organ culture. J Vis Exp. 2012(60):3490

8 Intervertebral Disc Whole Organ Cultures

Marianna Peroglio, Zhen Li, Lorin Michael Benneker, Mauro Alini, and Sibylle Grad

Abstract

Whole intervertebral disc (IVD) organ cultures bridge the gap between in vitro and in vivo assays by offering a controlled environment where cells are kept in their native tissue. Applications of whole organ cultures include testing of tissue responses to novel surgical techniques and repair strategies for both the nucleus pulposus (NP) and the annulus fibrosus (AF). Importantly, whole organ cultures can be instrumental in deciphering the role of stem cells and therapeutic agents in a relevant and controlled environment. In this chapter, the historical perspective of whole organ cultures is presented and both unloaded whole organ cultures and loaded cultures implying the use of bioreactors are highlighted. This section is followed by evidence-based results obtained from whole organ cultures, which range from the evaluation of new surgical techniques and the damage and repair of both the AF and the NP, to the role of stem cells in IVD regeneration. Advantages and limitations of whole organ culture models are discussed. Finally, foreseen future applications are presented. Overall, whole organ cultures represent an alternative to preclinical models and help replace, or at least reduce, the need for animal research in line with the 3 R (replacement, reduction, and refinement) principles. Whole organ cultures promote a fast translation of new therapies from bench to bedside.

Keywords: 3 R principles, bioreactor, intervertebral disc, loading, whole organ culture

8.1 Introduction

The healthy state of an intervertebral disc (IVD) is ensured by a fine balance of biological and mechanical cues (see Chapter 1). During disc degeneration, there is a shift toward catabolism of the extracellular matrix (ECM) associated with structural changes that can finally lead to failure of the IVD (see Chapter 2).

Whole organ cultures can provide answers with respect to how changes in biological or mechanical signals can affect the biological and mechanical response of the IVD as a whole organ, as recently reviewed.[1,2] For instance, effects of needle puncture, discectomy, biomaterials, and biological therapies on whole IVD response have been investigated.[3,4,5,6]

Biomechanical questions can be answered by using thawed discs from a small- or large-animal frozen specimen collection (see Chapter 4). However, fresh tissue is required for biological evaluation and discs from large animal models are more representative of the human IVD as they involve high diffusional distances and, in some species, lack notochordal cells (see Chapter 5).

Clinicians can take advantage of whole organ cultures to evaluate new surgical approaches,[7] implants, and biological therapies (see Chapters 9–15), thereby collecting useful data for preclinical testing and for further applications in clinical trials.

In this respect, whole organ cultures can accelerate the translation from bench to bedside.[8]

Industry can also benefit from whole organ cultures given they provide a representative model of the targeted tissue that can be used for testing new therapies, compounds, and implants (see also Chapter 20). There is growing interest in the development of culture systems that better represent the in vivo situation. Indeed, there is a global shift from two-dimensional (2D) to three-dimensional (3D) cultures.[9] 3D cultures (e.g., alginate and agarose hydrogels) have been used for many years and have demonstrated a better maintenance of disc cell phenotype compared with 2D cultures on tissue-culture plastic. However, the hydrogel matrix surrounding the cells is very different from the native IVD tissue. In this respect, whole IVD organ cultures offer several advantages (summarized in ▸ Table 8.1); thus, there is an interest in whole organ culture to become an alternative method for testing new developments, provided that the method is standardized. Such standardization will allow more robust comparison of results among different institutions. Bioreactor-based culture systems represent a recent progress of 3D cultures that allow for reproduction of physiological processes such as perfusion or loading.[9]

Table 8.1 Advantages and limitations of whole organ cultures compared to in vitro and in vivo models

Advantages	Disadvantages
• Maintain the cells in their native niche and offer an ideal three-dimensional culture system.	• Do not reproduce the complex response (e.g., immune response) of a living organism.
• Represent a more robust setup compared with static two-dimensional cell cultures.	• Do not allow biocompatibility tests.
• Structural changes due to tissue damage or tissue repair are taken into account.	• Reaction of the structures surrounding the IVD is not taken into account (these include bone vertebrae, muscles, ligaments, spinal cord, and nerves).
• Better control of the culture conditions compared with in vivo studies (e.g., control of loading and nutrition parameters, reproducible degenerative models).	• Being more complex than traditional in vitro systems, whole organ cultures are less reproducible.
• In line with the 3 R principles of animal models, no animal needs to be sacrificed for research purposes if tissue is obtained from slaughterhouses.	• Application of multiple loading patterns (e.g., flexion/extension, lateral bending, axial rotation) not yet implemented.
• Do not require ethical approval when tissue is obtained from slaughterhouses because no animals are specifically sacrificed for research purposes.	
• Have low costs when using ovine or bovine coccygeal discs, given these can be obtained from slaughterhouses.	

Abbreviations: 3 R principles, replacement, reduction, and refinement; IVD, intervertebral disc.

In this chapter, whole organ cultures with and without external loading are described from a historical perspective. This section is followed by applications of whole organ cultures for the evaluation of new surgical techniques, as well as annulus fibrosus (AF), nucleus pulposus (NP), and end plate (EP) damage and repair. Recent developments in the use of mesenchymal stem cells (MSCs) are presented. A discussion about advantages and limitations of whole organ cultures compared with in vitro and in vivo models and future directions of whole organ cultures completes this chapter.

8.2 Historical perspective

8.2.1 Culture of Whole Intervertebral Discs without Loading

Since the 1970s, disc slices have been cultured in aqueous solutions. However, if no precautions are taken, such slices swell and lose proteoglycans. Urban and Maroudas demonstrated the prevention of swelling of disc slices cut from frozen human lumbar IVDs by adding polyethylene glycol to the culture medium, thus creating culture conditions iso-osmotic to the IVD environment.[10] Recently, Van Dijk et al applied a similar technique to maintain bovine NP explants viable for 42 days, although a downregulation of matrix protein expression was observed.[11]

Culture of whole IVDs was first performed by Chiba and colleagues using rabbit IVDs.[12] They found that embedding IVDs in alginate induced a higher proteoglycan synthesis rate and maintained higher matrix content compared with discs cultured without alginate during the 1-month time frame of the study. Fifteen years later, Risbud et al cultured whole rat IVDs using hyperosmotic medium supplemented with transforming growth factor β (TGF-β) and found that the vitality of the NP cells could be maintained for 1 week.[13] In another study, Le Maitre et al found that human IVD tissue structure and cell function could be maintained when the tissue was constrained in a plastic ring during the 3-week culture, whereas this was not the case in free-swelling culture conditions.[14]

Long-term cultures (49 days) were first reported by Haschtmann et al for rabbit IVDs comprising bony EPs. Cell viability was maintained, although a reduced metabolic activity and a degenerative gene expression profile was found.[15] Gawri et al improved the preparation of IVDs for whole organ culture by carefully removing the vertebral bone and only leaving the cartilage EPs.[16] This allowed whole human IVDs with intact cartilage EPs to be cultured under free-swelling conditions with preservation of cell viability and ECM homeostasis for 1 month. This was not the case when the IVDs were cultured without cartilage EPs or when vertebral bone was left. Using this technique, culture time was extended to 4 months under free-swelling conditions, with cell viability above 95% in both NP and AF tissues, independent of the concentration of glucose or fetal calf serum in the culture medium.

A model to study IVD regeneration was first introduced by Roberts and colleagues, who used bovine coccygeal discs to mimic disc degeneration by enzymatic digestion with trypsin or papain.[17] The enzymatic treatment produced a cavity (~12% of the volume of the disc), which could be used to test injectable biomaterials or biological therapies. One week after trypsin injection, Jim et al found an aggrecan loss of 60%, whereas cell viability was preserved.[18]

Recently, MSC migration into the disc in response to the chemoattractant stromal cell derived factor-1 (SDF-1) was investigated by Pereira et al using free-swelling whole IVD short-term cultures.[19] In this study, a nucleotomy was performed through the EP and the cavity was filled with SDF-1 in saline solution or in a thermoreversible hyaluronic acid grafted with poly(N-isopropylacrylamide) (HA-pNIPAM) hydrogel carrier. Intact discs, nucleotomized discs solely filled with the hydrogel, and empty nucleotomized discs were used as controls. It was found that the nucleotomy itself induced MSC migration and that this phenomenon was enhanced by the HA-pNIPAM hydrogel. The use of SDF-1 in combination with the HA-pNIPAM hydrogel had a synergic effect on MSC migration.[19]

Overall, these studies indicate that it is possible to maintain large whole IVDs that are viable for months and that these discs can be used to investigate both degenerative and regenerative processes. Key features for the success of such culture models include the prevention of excessive swelling by hyperosmotic medium, mechanical confinement, or preservation of the cartilage EP; maintenance of the EP represents the condition that is closest to the physiological situation. However, care needs to be taken to conserve the permeability of the EP to allow diffusion of nutrients and waste products into and from the central parts of the IVD during the entire culture period.

8.2.2 Culture of Intervertebral Discs under Loading

It is well-known that IVDs have a tendency to swell when immersed in aqueous solutions. The idea of using mechanical loading to avoid swelling of IVD tissue was introduced in 1981 by Urban and Maroudas.[10] By employing a pressure of 0.65 MPa, they could prevent swelling of IVD slices. Static load application to whole bovine coccygeal IVDs was reported by Ohshima et al in 1995.[20] They found that when static loads were applied for 8 hours, the matrix synthesis rate was highest under a pressure of 0.13 to 0.26 MPa, whereas both low static pressure (0.01 MPa) and high static pressure (0.4 MPa) decreased the matrix synthesis rate. With the goal to improve nutrient diffusion into the IVD, Lee et al compared IVD cultures with and without vertebral EPs under a static load of 0.25 MPa and medium perfusion for 1 week.[21] When IVDs were cultured without vertebral EPs, cell viability and biosynthetic responsiveness could be preserved.

Shifts between two static loads, simulating a diurnal load and a nocturnal rest, represent a progress toward physiological loading. Gantenbein et al used ovine coccygeal discs (systemically anticoagulated before death) perfused with culture medium and maintained them under static load (0.2 MPa) or "diurnal" load (0.8 MPa for 16 hours followed by 0.2 MPa for 8 hours) for 4 days.[22] It was found that solutes could diffuse deeper into the IVD when diurnal load was applied.

A more sophisticated development was represented by the introduction of air-controlled systems and the automated

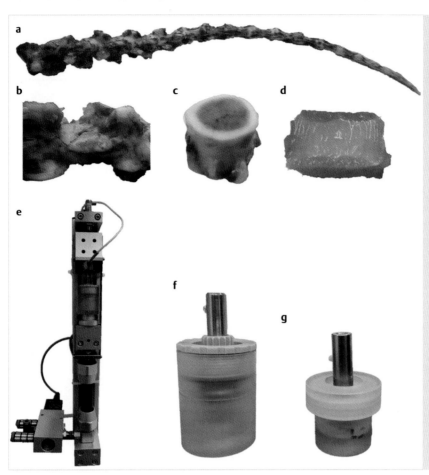

Fig. 8.1 Specimens and equipment for loaded whole organ culture of ovine or bovine discs. Images from a bovine model: **(a)** a whole tail, **(b)** a motion segment, **(c)** an intervertebral disc (IVD) with endplates (EPs), **(d)** a sagittal section of the IVD with bony EPs, **(e)** an IVD bioreactor, **(f)** a bioreactor chamber for large discs, **(g)** and a bioreactor chamber for small discs.

application of simulated physiological compressive loading cycles in medium-perfused chambers (▸ Fig. 8.1).[23] The simulated physiological loading comprised two periods of sinusoidal loading between 0.4 and 0.8 MPa at a frequency of 0.2 Hz separated by 2 hours of static load at 0.6 MPa, followed by a resting static load at 0.2 MPa for 14 hours. To mimic limited nutrition in the IVD, which is an important factor in disc degeneration, discs were cultured under simulated physiological loading in medium with either limited or sufficient glucose concentration for 21 days. Limited nutrition induced a cell viability decrease of ~50% within a few days and the surviving cells could not compensate matrix production during the time frame of the study. In a follow-up study, Illien-Jünger et al applied this loading pattern with a cyclic load at either 0.2 Hz or 10 Hz to IVDs cultured in medium with limited or sufficient glucose concentration for 1 week.[24] It was found that both combinations of limited glucose with low frequency loading and of high frequency loading with high glucose concentration resulted in cell death. Culture in limited glucose and under high frequency loading had an additive effect on cell death and induced gene expression upregulation of the matrix degrading enzyme matrix metalloproteinase 13 (MMP-13). This bioreactor system was also used to induce degeneration in a controlled manner in bovine coccygeal discs and to study regenerative therapies based on MSC homing.[25]

Such IVD bioreactor systems generating temporally controlled loading regimes opened the way to the development

of other bioreactors capable of applying simulated physiological compressive loading patterns in bovine[26] and caprine IVDs.[27] Haglund et al optimized the loading regime for coccygeal bovine IVDs and found that disc height loss occurred mainly during preconditioning (48 hours at 0.1 MPa static load) and during the first week of dynamic loading (0.1–0.3 MPa at 0.1 Hz).[26] Moreover, when comparing low (0.1–0.3 MPa), medium (0.1–0.6 MPa), and high (0.1–1.2 MPa) load at 1 Hz, cell viability was better preserved under low loading conditions for this type of discs. In another study, Paul et al cultured lumbar caprine discs without load, under low dynamic load (0.1–0.2 MPa, 1 Hz) or under simulated-physiological load (alternating every 30 minutes between 0.1–0.2 MPa at 1 Hz and 0.1–0.6 MPa at 1 Hz for 16 hours, followed by 8 hours of low dynamic load). They found that cell viability, density, and gene expression were best preserved when simulated physiological loading was applied. However, none of the loading regimes had an effect on the ECM content during the 21 days of culture.[27] In a follow-up study, it was found that both dynamic and static overloading induced pathological changes. Both types of loading induced an upregulation of catabolic and pro-inflammatory genes, as well as water and proteoglycan loss. Dynamic overloading caused cell death in all IVD regions, whereas static overloading mainly affected the outer AF.[28]

Recent advancements in the design of bioreactors allow the simultaneous loading of several human lumbar discs.[29] Walter et al cultured human lumbar discs under compressive loading (0.1 MPa for 12 hours followed by 0.2 MPa for 12 hours) for 21 days and reported a cell viability of ~ 80% for both the NP and AF regions.

The simulation of torsional movements has attracted interest from athletes who actively participate in sports involving torsional movement of the spine and are frequently diagnosed with disc prolapse. Therefore, bioreactors capable of applying torsion were developed by Chan et al.[30] Using bovine coccygeal discs, it was found that torsion (1 hour/day at 0.1 Hz during 4 days) at low amplitude (2 degrees) can improve cell viability compared with statically loaded discs, whereas high magnitude torsion (5 degrees) can induce a significant increase in cell apoptosis in the NP. Moreover, cell metabolic activity in the NP decreased with increasing torsion amplitude.

Simulation of complex loading patterns is one of the latest developments of IVD bioreactors. Walter et al studied the cellular and structural response of bovine coccygeal discs to low-magnitude asymmetric compressive loading (15-degree angle).[31] They found that asymmetric compression induced cell death, upregulation of catabolic and pro-inflammatory cytokines, and structural disruption. In another study, Chan et al applied compression (0.4–0.8 MPa at 0.2 Hz) and/or torsion (–2 degrees to 2 degrees at 0.2 Hz) to bovine coccygeal discs for 8 hours/day, followed by 16 hours of free swelling for a period of 15 days.[32] The effect of combined cyclic compression and torsion was region-specific, with a higher cell death in the NP compared with simple torsion or simple compression, whereas the AF responded with active matrix remodeling.

Taken together, bioreactors represent an ideal setup to study the link between loading and nutrition, two of the main factors considered to be implicated in IVD degeneration.

8.3 Evidence-based Results: Current Applications of Whole Organ Cultures

8.3.1 New Surgical Techniques

Whole organ cultures can provide useful insight when evaluating new surgical techniques. For instance, Vadalà et al recently developed a transpedicular approach to perform nucleotomies. Whereas the feasibility of the technique could be tested on cadaveric spines,[7] a whole organ culture model was required to assess the effect of this approach on the viability of the surrounding tissue (▶ Fig. 8.2a).[4] By using lactate dehydrogenase staining on cryosections, it was possible to identify which nucleotomy method (purely mechanic, purely enzymatic, or combined mechanic and enzymatic) yielded a reproducible defect while preserving the viability of the surrounding tissue.

8.3.2 Annulus Fibrosus Damage and Repair

In terms of AF damage, Korecki et al investigated the early effect of needle puncture injury on cell response using bovine coccygeal disc organ culture.[3] They found that even a small needle (25-gauge) initiates immediate alterations in disc height, stiffness, and viscoelastic properties that do not recover over time. Furthermore, localized structural disruption, loss of cell viability, and matrix remodeling were associated with needle puncture injury.

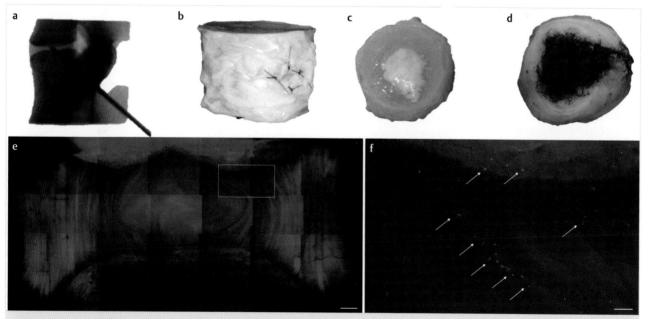

Fig. 8.2 Examples of applications of whole organ cultures: (a) X-ray image of the transpedicular approach; (b) whole intervertebral disc (IVD) with annulus fibrosus (AF) defect with 4-point suture; (c) whole IVD with end plate (EP) defect and bone cement sealing; (d) transversal section of an IVD with a 2% w/v agarose hydrogel (stained with methylene blue for better visualization) as nucleus pulposus (NP) filler; (e) fluorescence image of sagittal section of a degenerated IVD (scale bar = 1,000 μm) on which PKH26-labelled mesenchymal stem cells (MSCs) were applied to study cell homing; (f) magnified view of the region marked in image (e), with PKH26-labelled MSCs (red fluorescence) migrating through the EP and in the inner AF indicated with arrows (scale bar = 200 μm).

Concerning AF repair, a detailed description of repair strategies can be found in Chapter 15. Here, we focus on whole organ culture experiments of AF repair (an example is given in ► Fig. 8.2b). Schek et al reported on genipin cross-linked fibrin hydrogels with dynamic modulus similar to AF tissue, allowing the growth of human disc cells and good adhesion to the native AF tissue.[33] This material was later evaluated in a whole organ culture model by Likhitpanichkul et al, who found that the biomaterial remained well-integrated with native AF tissue for 14,000 cycles of compressive loading.[34] Moreover, in the presence of the hydrogel there was a better preservation of cell viability around the defect, lower nitric oxide release, and AF cell migration into the gel.

The potential of a poly(trimethylene carbonate) scaffold seeded with human bone marrow–derived stromal cells and covered with poly(ester-urethane) membrane for AF rupture repair has been evaluated in a whole disc organ culture model.[5] Following 14 days of dynamic loading (0–0.1 MPa, 0.1 Hz, 3 hours/day), implanted MSCs showed an upregulation of type V collagen (a potential AF marker) compared with MSCs before implantation in the AF defect. In the tissue surrounding the scaffold, there was an upregulation of anabolic markers and a downregulation of catabolic markers compared with tissue collected at the beginning of the experiment.

8.3.3 Nucleus Pulposus Damage and Repair

One way to induce degenerative changes in the organ-cultured IVD is the combined application of limited nutrition and high frequency loading.[24] However, if this model is used to further investigate regenerative approaches, the volume of therapeutics that can be injected in the IVD is very limited. In this respect, the use of enzymes will decrease the proteoglycan content in the NP and provide additional space for injection.

Detailed description of NP repair strategies can be found in Chapter 14. Here, we focus on whole organ culture experiments of NP repair (examples in ► Fig. 8.2c, d). Chen et al evaluated the combined application of platelet-rich plasma (PRP) and MSCs in a porcine model.[35] Using whole organ cultures where degeneration was induced by injection of chymopapain, MSCs in PRP were supplied to the disc. Following 4 weeks of culture, increased proteoglycan content was found in the MSC/PRP-treated group compared with control. Nonetheless, in vivo results indicated that the MSC/PRP combination induced an osteogenic response.

Link N, the peptide that stabilizes the proteoglycan aggregates, was extensively evaluated by Mwale et al. In vitro tests demonstrated that link N stimulated proteoglycan synthesis in degenerated human IVD cells,[36] enhanced chondrogenic differentiation, and downregulated hypertrophic and osteogenic markers of MSCs.[37] In a whole organ culture model both link N and MSCs restored the ECM (proteoglycan and collagen II) of bovine IVDs in which degeneration was induced by trypsin injection.[38] These results correlated well with in vivo findings, whereby link N increased the proteoglycan content and the anabolic response in rabbit IVDs where degeneration was induced by needle puncture.[39]

In another study, Malonzo et al used a papain-induced enzymatic disc degeneration model in bovine coccygeal discs to test a thermoreversible hydrogel (with or without NP cells or MSCs) under static load for 7 days.[40] Although the hydrogel's load-bearing capacity was limited, the cell viability could be maintained at > 70% following one week of organ culture. A trypsin digestion model was recently applied by Gawri et al to study the influence of dynamic loading on disc regeneration following enzymatic treatment.[41] They demonstrated that loading stimulated ECM synthesis (both aggrecan and type II collagen) and that the newly synthesized proteoglycans were in the same size range as in intact IVDs. Injection of TGF-β doubled proteoglycan synthesis rate compared with controls.

Li et al studied fibrinogen-hyaluronan conjugated hydrogels as NP cell carriers both in vitro and in whole organ culture.[42] In partially nucleotomized discs cultured under free-swelling conditions, a better integration with native NP tissue was observed for the conjugated gel compared with a fibrinogen-hyaluronan mixture with the same composition. The conjugate hydrogel also restored disc height and compressive stiffness under dynamic load.

Whole organ culture models have also been used to investigate the effect of anti-inflammatory compounds. Kim et al have found that the intradiscal injection of lactoferricin attenuates proteoglycan loss in mouse and rabbit discs where inflammation was induced by addition of interleukin (IL)-1 to the culture medium.[43]

8.3.4 Cartilage End Plate Damage and Repair

It has been shown that excessive loading and fracture induce cell death in the cartilaginous EP. Ariga et al investigated the effect of a 24-hour load (range: 0–1 MPa) on whole mouse coccygeal discs and found that the number of apoptotic cells was correlated to the amount of mechanical stress and that mitogen-activated protein kinase (MAPK) could counteract this apoptotic pathway.[44] The effect of EP fracture on the migration of EP chondrocytes into the NP was studied by Kim et al.[45] Following a 48-hour culture period of whole IVDs with fractured and with intact EPs, an extensive migration of EP chondrocytes was observed in the fractured group. As attested by immunohistochemistry, the migrating chondrocytes expressed membrane type I MMP and Ki-67 and deposited type II collagen.

To understand the link between acute trauma, inflammatory factors, neoinnervation, disc degeneration, and pain, Alkhatib et al induced EP fractures in human IVD. Following 3 days of culture, IVDs were collected for analysis and the conditioned culture medium was applied on neural cells.[46] A significantly higher cell death and increased aggrecan fragmentation were observed in injured IVDs versus intact IVDs. Conditioned medium from injured IVDs induced significant neurite sprouting compared with noninjured media.

8.3.5 Stem Cells: Trophic Factors, Differentiation and Migration

The exact role of MSCs in IVD repair is still unclear. In fact, the peculiar IVD environment (hypoxic, low glucose concentration, avascular) and especially the degenerated IVD environment (low pH, presence of inflammatory cytokines) can represent a challenge for the survival of MSCs. Nonetheless, there is evidence that MSCs and disc cells interact and that the trophic factors released by the degenerative disc cells trigger MSC differentiation toward the disc phenotype, whereas the factors released by the MSCs rescue the degenerative disc cells and induce a shift toward a healthier phenotype. Indeed, Strassburg et al co-cultured in direct contact human bone marrow–derived MSCs and NP cells from healthy or degenerated human NP tissue for 1 week.[47] They found that MSCs differentiated to the NP phenotype with both healthy and degenerated NP. On the other hand, MSCs had no effect on healthy NP cells, but enhanced matrix gene expression in degenerate NP cells. In another study, Le Maitre et al injected MSCs in bovine NP explants and found that they survived for 4 weeks inside the tissue and that MSCs from older subjects differentiated spontaneously into NP-like cells.[48]

Preconditioning of MSCs prior to implantation has been proposed as a way to improve their survival in the harsh degenerated disc environment. Stem cell differentiation into disc cells can be triggered by the use of appropriate growth factors and/or carriers, such as a thermoreversible hyaluronan hydrogel.[6] In this study, MSCs were preconditioned in thermoreversible hyaluronan hydrogel beads (3D culture) in the presence of growth factors such as TGF-β1 or growth and differentiation factor 5 (GDF-5). Following preconditioning, cells were recollected by simple cooling of the hydrogel and then supplied to nucleotomized discs. Nonetheless, it was found that the combination of the thermoreversible hydrogel and the disc environment induced a stronger differentiation of MSCs toward the disc phenotype than preconditioning followed by delivery to the discs.

Several recent studies report on the use of chemotactic agents to recruit stem/progenitor cells to a damaged area of the IVD (an example is given in ▶ Fig. 8.2e–f). The use of bioreactors for whole organ disc culture has demonstrated that degenerative discs release factors that attract bone marrow–derived MSCs.[25] In addition, the results suggest that the chemokine (C-C motif) ligand 5 (CCL5) is the main chemoattractant factor involved in this migration process.[49] This opens the way to new approaches, such as the combination of hydrogels inductive of MSC differentiation toward the disc phenotype with chemoattractants that enhance MSC migration toward the injured part of the IVD.[19] In this respect, the mobilization of endogenous/progenitor cells, whose presence in the IVD has been recently discovered,[50] represents a promising self-healing approach. Two very recent review articles cover the topics of cell-based therapies for IVD regeneration[51] and how such therapies may be influenced by the inflammatory environment of the degenerate disc.[52]

8.3.6 Advantages and Limitations of Whole Organ Cultures Compared to In Vitro and In Vivo

Advantages and limitations of whole organ cultures are presented in Table 1. The main advantage of whole organ cultures compared with in vitro cell culture systems (see Chapter 7) is that cells are kept in the IVD niche (characterized by abundant matrix, slow diffusion, hypoxia, and low glucose concentration), whereby their function and cell–cell interaction is preserved. Therefore, whole organ culture systems seem more appropriate to test new therapies. For instance, drug testing is strongly influenced by the diffusion properties of the drug, which is very different in a tissue versus in culture medium. Another advantage compared with in vitro cell culture is that structural changes due to tissue damage or tissue repair are taken into account. Finally, recent developments in the preparation and culture of whole IVDs make long-term cultures (i.e., several months) possible.[16] With that, long-term effects of a new treatment can be assessed, such as the potential of different drugs to induce repair in an adult human disc.

When compared with in vivo studies, organ culture experiments offer a better control of the mechanical and biochemical conditions. Furthermore, all current animal models have limitations in terms of size (rabbits, rodents), biomechanics (quadrupeds), and age of the animals, as well as the way to induce degeneration (posttraumatic degeneration after an injury compared with degenerative changes in human discs resulting from low nutrition, cell apoptosis, etc.).[53] In whole organ culture models involving the use of bovine and ovine tail discs, no animal needs to be sacrificed for research purposes, in line with the 3R (replacement, reduction, and refinement) principles of animal models[54] (for further information about the 3R principles: https://www.nc3rs.org.uk/the-3rs).

Whole organ cultures also have some limitations. Although they are more comprehensive than traditional in vitro cultures, whole organ cultures do not reproduce the complex response of a living organism and the reaction of the structures surrounding the IVD is not taken into account. These include bone vertebrae, muscles, ligaments, spinal cord, and nerves. The presence of the vertebra, which is a highly vascularized tissue, is very relevant for whole body responses given that this is not an immuno-privileged region such as the IVD. This means that biocompatibility and immune responses cannot be effectively determined using in vitro cultures. New biomaterials, such as scaffolds or hydrogels, and (allogeneic) cell therapies will therefore require additional preclinical in vivo tests before translation to clinical application. Last, the whole organ culture being more complex than a traditional in vitro system, is also more difficult to reproduce.

Taken together, whole organ culture models contribute to bridge the gap between in vitro and in vivo assays.

8.4 Future Directions of Whole Organ Cultures

IVD whole organ cultures have been used by various research groups around the world for the evaluation of new surgical techniques, biomaterials for NP and AF repair, and biological treatments. They have the potential for higher predictability than in vitro assays and, unlike in vivo models, they can be used for screening. In view of the wide range of promising biologics and delivery systems,[55] there is the need for a standardized whole organ culture testing method, such as an ASTM standard. Such a standard will further promote the use of whole organ cultures for preclinical investigations.

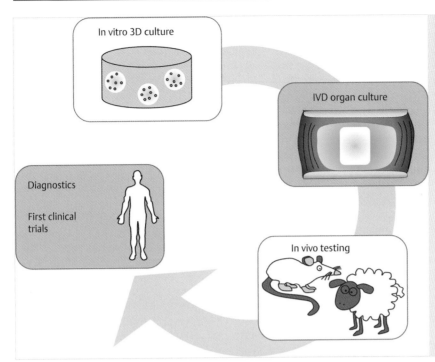

Fig. 8.3 Scheme representing the test of a new therapy starting from in vitro, moving to organ cultures, further in vivo testing, and finally applied to humans for diagnostics or first clinical trials. It is foreseen that in specific cases, in vitro three-dimensional (3D) cultures and in vivo testing may not be necessary and that intervertebral disc (IVD) organ cultures may provide the necessary information, for example, in the case of new diagnostic tools.

With a steadily increasing field of application for whole organ cultures, further replacement or at least reduction of animal use, in line with the 3 R principles, is expected (▶ Fig. 8.3). This will have strong ethical and economic implications and will foster the translation from bench to bedside. Indeed, results from whole organ culture studies[49] have already served as a basis for the screening of relevant markers for disc degeneration in human blood samples.[56] In addition, whole organ culture can provide insight into physiotherapeutic, pharmaceutical, and tissue engineering treatments.

With respect to local cell and matrix responses, whole organ cultures of human IVDs represent the closest model to the clinical situation and are essential in ensuring a successful translation. Successful implementation of long-term cultures (up to several months) allows for the testing of long-term effects of new treatments on human IVDs[16] and bioreactors capable of loading human discs have recently been established.[26,29]

More complex loading patterns, when successfully implemented in organ cultures, will bring further insight not only on pathogenesis of disc degeneration, but also on the challenges for regeneration.[57] More stringent test methods have already proven to be valuable in testing new implant designs.[58] The development of strict biological tests will also ease the evaluation of new biological therapies and finally facilitate the translation of the most effective therapies. The regenerative role of biological therapies (such as the application of MSCs) still requires further investigation, and whole organ cultures can serve to elucidate their functions in a relevant setting. Furthermore, questions about systemic reactions such as immune responses still cannot be answered by current in vitro models. Similarly, pain behavior is challenging to assess with organ cultures, although indirect measurements are possible by investigating markers of inflammation and pain, nociceptors, and neural ingrowth.[59]

A further development of 3D cultures is represented by organs-on-chip.[60] This new microfabrication technology bears the potential to reproduce multiorgan interactions, disease dynamics, and drug activity.[61] From a research perspective, organ-on-chip systems have not yet been applied to the IVD, but they could bring additional insights into immune responses, and vascular and neural ingrowth.

8.5 Conclusion

Whole organ culture models provide a useful link between in vitro and in vivo assays, offer a screening tool for novel treatments, and address some of the safety concerns associated with new procedures. When mimicking disc degenerative conditions, degeneration is generally induced rapidly (e.g., by needle puncture, excessive loading, injection of enzymes), although with the recent development of long-term whole organ cultures, it may be possible to better mimic the slow degenerative process occurring in human discs and to study the long-term regenerative responses.

Overall, it is expected that the number of animals used in research can be minimized by using whole organ cultures for preliminary testing, whereas large-animal in vivo models will be still required to take into account the whole body response and small animal models to elucidate and find ways to minimize pain associated with disc degeneration. If successful, well-designed clinical studies with a special focus on safety aspects will be needed to validate such new procedures on appropriately selected patients (see Chapter 3, Chapter 6).

Clinicians and researchers need to continue to work closely together to make whole organ culture models as representative as possible of specific clinical situations and types of disc diseases. This will certainly contribute to unveil hurdles for translation and, by a better understanding of the underlying causes, to surpass them.

8.6 References

[1] Illien-Junger S, Walter BA, Mayer JE, Hecht AC, Iatridis JC. Intervertebral disc culture models and their applications to study pathogenesis and repair. In: Shapiro IM, Risbud MV, eds. The Intervertebral Disc: Molecular and Structural Studies of the Disc in Health and Disease.Wien: Springer; 2014:353–372

[2] Gantenbein B, Illien-Jünger S, Chan SC, et al. Organ culture bioreactors—platforms to study human intervertebral disc degeneration and regenerative therapy. Curr Stem Cell Res Ther. 2015; 10(4):339–352

[3] Korecki CL, Costi JJ, Iatridis JC. Needle puncture injury affects intervertebral disc mechanics and biology in an organ culture model. Spine. 2008; 33(3):235–241

[4] Vadalà G, Russo F, Pattappa G, et al. A nucleotomy model with intact annulus fibrosus to test intervertebral disc regeneration strategies. Tissue Eng Part C Methods. 2015; 21(11):1117–1124

[5] Pirvu T, Blanquer SB, Benneker LM, et al. A combined biomaterial and cellular approach for annulus fibrosus rupture repair. Biomaterials. 2015; 42:11–19

[6] Peroglio M, Eglin D, Benneker LM, Alini M, Grad S. Thermoreversible hyaluronan-based hydrogel supports in vitro and ex vivo disc-like differentiation of human mesenchymal stem cells. Spine J. 2013; 13(11):1627–1639

[7] Vadalà G, Russo F, Pattappa G, et al. The transpedicular approach as an alternative route for intervertebral disc regeneration. Spine. 2013; 38(6): E319–E324

[8] Benneker LM, Andersson G, Iatridis JC, et al. Cell therapy for intervertebral disc repair: advancing cell therapy from bench to clinics. Eur Cell Mater. 2014; 27:5–11

[9] Naing MW, Williams DJ. Three-dimensional culture and bioreactors for cellular therapies. Cytotherapy. 2011; 13(4):391–399

[10] Urban JP, Maroudas A. Swelling of the intervertebral disc in vitro. Connect Tissue Res. 1981; 9(1):1–10

[11] van Dijk BG, Potier E, Ito K. Long-term culture of bovine nucleus pulposus explants in a native environment. Spine J. 2013; 13(4):454–463

[12] Chiba K, Andersson GB, Masuda K, Momohara S, Williams JM, Thonar EJ. A new culture system to study the metabolism of the intervertebral disc in vitro. Spine. 1998; 23(17):1821–1827, discussion 1828

[13] Risbud MV, Izzo MW, Adams CS, et al. An organ culture system for the study of the nucleus pulposus: description of the system and evaluation of the cells. Spine. 2003; 28(24):2652–2658, discussion 2658–2659

[14] Le Maitre CL, Hoyland JA, Freemont AJ. Studies of human intervertebral disc cell function in a constrained in vitro tissue culture system. Spine. 2004; 29(11):1187–1195

[15] Haschtmann D, Stoyanov JV, Ettinger L, Nolte LP, Ferguson SJ. Establishment of a novel intervertebral disc/endplate culture model: analysis of an ex vivo in vitro whole-organ rabbit culture system. Spine. 2006; 31(25):2918–2925

[16] Gawri R, Mwale F, Ouellet J, et al. Development of an organ culture system for long-term survival of the intact human intervertebral disc. Spine. 2011; 36(22):1835–1842

[17] Roberts S, Menage J, Sivan S, Urban JP. Bovine explant model of degeneration of the intervertebral disc. BMC Musculoskelet Disord. 2008; 9:24

[18] Jim B, Steffen T, Moir J, Roughley P, Haglund L. Development of an intact intervertebral disc organ culture system in which degeneration can be induced as a prelude to studying repair potential. Eur Spine J. 2011; 20(8):1244–1254

[19] Pereira CL, Gonçalves RM, Peroglio M, et al. The effect of hyaluronan-based delivery of stromal cell-derived factor-1 on the recruitment of MSCs in degenerating intervertebral discs. Biomaterials. 2014; 35(28):8144–8153

[20] Ohshima H, Urban JP, Bergel DH. Effect of static load on matrix synthesis rates in the intervertebral disc measured in vitro by a new perfusion technique. J Orthop Res. 1995; 13(1):22–29

[21] Lee CR, Iatridis JC, Poveda L, Alini M. In vitro organ culture of the bovine intervertebral disc: effects of vertebral endplate and potential for mechanobiology studies. Spine. 2006; 31(5):515–522

[22] Gantenbein B, Grünhagen T, Lee CR, van Donkelaar CC, Alini M, Ito K. An in vitro organ culturing system for intervertebral disc explants with vertebral endplates: a feasibility study with ovine caudal discs. Spine. 2006; 31(23):2665–2673

[23] Jünger S, Gantenbein-Ritter B, Lezuo P, Alini M, Ferguson SJ, Ito K. Effect of limited nutrition on in situ intervertebral disc cells under simulated-physiological loading. Spine. 2009; 34(12):1264–1271

[24] Illien-Jünger S, Gantenbein-Ritter B, Grad S, et al. The combined effects of limited nutrition and high-frequency loading on intervertebral discs with endplates. Spine. 2010; 35(19):1744–1752

[25] Illien-Jünger S, Pattappa G, Peroglio M, et al. Homing of mesenchymal stem cells in induced degenerative intervertebral discs in a whole organ culture system. Spine. 2012; 37(22):1865–1873

[26] Haglund L, Moir J, Beckman L, et al. Development of a bioreactor for axially loaded intervertebral disc organ culture. Tissue Eng Part C Methods. 2011; 17(10):1011–1019

[27] Paul CP, Zuiderbaan HA, Zandieh Doulabi B, et al. Simulated-physiological loading conditions preserve biological and mechanical properties of caprine lumbar intervertebral discs in ex vivo culture. PLoS One. 2012; 7(3):e33147

[28] Paul CP, Schoorl T, Zuiderbaan HA, et al. Dynamic and static overloading induce early degenerative processes in caprine lumbar intervertebral discs. PLoS One. 2013; 8(4):e62411

[29] Walter BA, Illien-Jünger S, Nasser PR, Hecht AC, Iatridis JC. Development and validation of a bioreactor system for dynamic loading and mechanical characterization of whole human intervertebral discs in organ culture. J Biomech. 2014; 47(9):2095–2101

[30] Chan SC, Ferguson SJ, Wuertz K, Gantenbein-Ritter B. Biological response of the intervertebral disc to repetitive short-term cyclic torsion. Spine. 2011; 36(24):2021–2030

[31] Walter BA, Korecki CL, Purmessur D, Roughley PJ, Michalek AJ, Iatridis JC. Complex loading affects intervertebral disc mechanics and biology. Osteoarthritis Cartilage. 2011; 19(8):1011–1018

[32] Chan SC, Walser J, Käppeli P, Shamsollahi MJ, Ferguson SJ, Gantenbein-Ritter B. Region specific response of intervertebral disc cells to complex dynamic loading: an organ culture study using a dynamic torsion-compression bioreactor. PLoS One. 2013; 8(8):e72489

[33] Schek RM, Michalek AJ, Iatridis JC. Genipin-crosslinked fibrin hydrogels as a potential adhesive to augment intervertebral disc annulus repair. Eur Cell Mater. 2011; 21:373–383

[34] Likhitpanichkul M, Dreischarf M, Illien-Junger S, et al. Fibrin-genipin adhesive hydrogel for annulus fibrosus repair: performance evaluation with large animal organ culture, in situ biomechanics, and in vivo degradation tests. Eur Cell Mater. 2014; 28:25–37, discussion 37–38

[35] Chen WH, Liu HY, Lo WC, et al. Intervertebral disc regeneration in an ex vivo culture system using mesenchymal stem cells and platelet-rich plasma. Biomaterials. 2009; 30(29):5523–5533

[36] Gawri R, Antoniou J, Ouellet J, et al. Best paper NASS 2013: link-N can stimulate proteoglycan synthesis in the degenerated human intervertebral discs. Eur Cell Mater. 2013; 26:107–119, discussion 119

[37] Antoniou J, Wang HT, Alaseem AM, Haglund L, Roughley PJ, Mwale F. The effect of Link N on differentiation of human bone marrow-derived mesenchymal stem cells. Arthritis Res Ther. 2012; 14(6):R267

[38] Mwale F, Wang HT, Roughley P, Antoniou J, Haglund L. Link N and mesenchymal stem cells can induce regeneration of the early degenerate intervertebral disc. Tissue Eng Part A. 2014; 20(21–22):2942–2949

[39] Mwale F, Masuda K, Pichika R, et al. The efficacy of Link N as a mediator of repair in a rabbit model of intervertebral disc degeneration. Arthritis Res Ther. 2011; 13(4):R120

[40] Malonzo C, Chan SC, Kabiri A, et al. A papain-induced disc degeneration model for the assessment of thermo-reversible hydrogel-cells therapeutic approach. J Tissue Eng Regen Med. 2015; 9(12):E167–E176

[41] Gawri R, Moir J, Ouellet J, et al. Physiological loading can restore the proteoglycan content in a model of early IVD degeneration. PLoS One. 2014; 9(7): e101233

[42] Li Z, Kaplan KM, Wertzel A, et al. Biomimetic fibrin-hyaluronan hydrogels for nucleus pulposus regeneration. Regen Med. 2014; 9(3):309–326

[43] Kim JS, Ellman MB, Yan D, et al. Lactoferricin mediates anti-inflammatory and anti-catabolic effects via inhibition of IL-1 and LPS activity in the intervertebral disc. J Cell Physiol. 2013; 228(9):1884–1896

[44] Ariga K, Yonenobu K, Nakase T, et al. Mechanical stress-induced apoptosis of endplate chondrocytes in organ-cultured mouse intervertebral discs: an ex vivo study. Spine. 2003; 28(14):1528–1533

[45] Kim KW, Ha KY, Park JB, Woo YK, Chung HN, An HS. Expressions of membrane-type I matrix metalloproteinase, Ki-67 protein, and type II collagen by chondrocytes migrating from cartilage endplate into nucleus pulposus in rat intervertebral discs: a cartilage endplate-fracture model using an intervertebral disc organ culture. Spine. 2005; 30(12):1373–1378

[46] Alkhatib B, Rosenzweig DH, Krock E, et al. Acute mechanical injury of the human intervertebral disc: link to degeneration and pain. Eur Cell Mater. 2014; 28:98–110, discussion 110–111

[47] Strassburg S, Richardson SM, Freemont AJ, Hoyland JA. Co-culture induces mesenchymal stem cell differentiation and modulation of the degenerate human nucleus pulposus cell phenotype. Regen Med. 2010; 5(5):701–711

[48] Le Maitre CL, Baird P, Freemont AJ, Hoyland JA. An in vitro study investigating the survival and phenotype of mesenchymal stem cells following injection into nucleus pulposus tissue. Arthritis Res Ther. 2009; 11(1):R20

[49] Pattappa G, Peroglio M, Sakai D, et al. CCL5/RANTES is a key chemoattractant released by degenerative intervertebral discs in organ culture. Eur Cell Mater. 2014; 27:124–136, discussion 136

[50] Sakai D, Nakamura Y, Nakai T, et al. Exhaustion of nucleus pulposus progenitor cells with ageing and degeneration of the intervertebral disc. Nat Commun. 2012; 3:1264

[51] Clarke LE, Richardson SM, Hoyland JA. Harnessing the potential of mesenchymal stem cells for IVD regeneration. Curr Stem Cell Res Ther. 2015; 10 (4):296–306

[52] Krock E, Rosenzweig DH, Haglund L. the inflammatory milieu of the degenerate disc: is mesenchymal stem cell-based therapy for intervertebral disc repair a feasible approach? Curr Stem Cell Res Ther. 2015; 10(4):317–328

[53] Alini M, Eisenstein SM, Ito K, et al. Are animal models useful for studying human disc disorders/degeneration? Eur Spine J. 2008; 17(1):2–19

[54] Walser J, Ferguson SJ, Gantenbein-Ritter B. Design of a mechanical loading device to culture intact bovine spinal motion segments under multiaxial motion. In: Davies J, ed. Replacing Animal Models: A Practical Guide to Creating and Using Culture-Based Biomimetic Alternatives. Chichester, UK: John Wiley & Sons, Ltd; 2012:89–105

[55] Fontana G, See E, Pandit A. Current trends in biologics delivery to restore intervertebral disc anabolism. Adv Drug Deliv Rev. 2015; 84:146–158

[56] Grad S, Bow C, Karppinen J, et al. Systemic blood plasma CCL5 and CXCL6: Potential biomarkers for human lumbar disc degeneration. Eur Cell Mater. 2016; 31:1–10

[57] Costi JJ, Stokes IA, Gardner-Morse MG, Iatridis JC. Frequency-dependent behavior of the intervertebral disc in response to each of six degree of freedom dynamic loading: solid phase and fluid phase contributions. Spine. 2008; 33(16):1731–1738

[58] Wilke HJ, Ressel L, Heuer F, Graf N, Rath S. Can prevention of a reherniation be investigated? Establishment of a herniation model and experiments with an anular closure device. Spine. 2013; 38(10):E587–E593

[59] Krock E, Rosenzweig DH, Chabot-Doré AJ, et al. Painful, degenerating intervertebral discs up-regulate neurite sprouting and CGRP through nociceptive factors. J Cell Mol Med. 2014; 18(6):1213–1225

[60] Huh D, Hamilton GA, Ingber DE. From 3D cell culture to organs-on-chips. Trends Cell Biol. 2011; 21(12):745–754

[61] Lee JB, Sung JH. Organ-on-a-chip technology and microfluidic whole-body models for pharmacokinetic drug toxicity screening. Biotechnol J. 2013; 8 (11):1258–1266

9 Biological Treatment Approaches: Basic Ideas and Principles

Victor Y. Leung and Kenneth M.C. Cheung

Abstract

Clinical studies indicate an association of intervertebral disc (IVD) degeneration severity with low back pain, implying that prevention or relief of the degeneration is relevant to the management of this global disease burden. Although the cause of disc degeneration remains to be fully elucidated, various biological approaches of reparation provide potential solutions as well as important insights into the nature of degeneration. These include the delivery of growth factors, stem cells, and other biologics, which aim to replenish or enhance the function of matrix-producing cells, or to control catabolism. Various lines of evidence suggest that the intervention relies on a proper control of inflammation, reconstructing the microenvironment in the disc, and ultimately rebuilding the disc mechanics. Stage of degeneration may also play a role. In this chapter, we discuss the principles as well as the strengths and weaknesses behind these biological approaches in the context of disc degeneration. Moreover, in view of the irreversible progression of disc degeneration, we discuss how a combination of screening to identify predisposed subjects and development of prophylactics may be critical to the effective treatment of degeneration.

Keywords: biologics, intervertebral disc, microenvironment, regeneration, stem cells

9.1 Historical Perspective

The cause of back pain is thought to be multifactorial. Over the last decade, there has been a dispute about the correlation between back pain and the dysfunction of spinal motion segments. However, with the advances in imaging techniques and refinement of study design and scale, recent reports have provided strong evidence to support a link between intervertebral disc (IVD) degeneration, possibly together with end plate anomalies, and a subset of low back pain cases.[1,2,3] Treatments that slow IVD degeneration progression may reduce the incidence and development of low back pain. The IVD is the largest cartilaginous unit in the body, and its degeneration is often progressive and irreversible by nature.[4] The IVD is constantly subject to mechanical load through the activity of spinal muscles, body weight, and various body postures and movements. Further mechanical insult can be caused by accidents and obesity. Age-related, environmental, and genetic factors also play roles in IVD function and health.[2,5,6] A thorough understanding of its causes is required to derive rational means to revive the spinal segment function. Because the etiology of disc degeneration is still not exactly clear to date, researchers have attempted to utilize the current knowledge in disc biology together with the experience and concepts from related systems and disorders to device plausible remedies. Although these remedies may not present a complete or ideal solution to treat IVD degeneration, such investigations have uncovered new insights into the degeneration mechanism, which may enhance future reparative strategies. A careful revisit of these investigations may shed light on the principles important to the success of disc engineering and regeneration in the future.

9.2 Goal of Intervention

The principles of current strategies or devices to intervene in IVD degeneration largely derive from the abnormalities and symptoms observed at moderate to severe stages of the degeneration. Current surgical interventions aim to treat the symptoms by removing the problematic motion segment, followed by immobilization of the joint, or otherwise replacement of the joint with a prosthetic disc. In the era of tissue engineering and regeneration, efforts have been made to develop minimally invasive biological or chemical means to preserve the native disc function and even to introduce prophylactic measures for high risk or predisposed subjects. Based on current understanding of IVD degeneration and technological advancement, a spectrum of interventions has been investigated in various labs. Some of them, in particular the cell-based therapies, have made their course into clinical trials.[7] Although it is not clear if the abnormalities observed in the IVD are part of the primary causes of the degeneration, many of them have been shown to correlate with the severity of degeneration. Dealing with these anomalies, in particular the molecular pathology, has been considered a relevant and rational approach to alleviate the degeneration, ultimately reducing the incidence of back pain and disability. These approaches may be divided into four categories based on principles of action: control of inflammation and catabolic events, conferring instant mechanical strength/function, stimulation of cell anabolism for matrix replenishment, and microenvironmental reconstruction.

9.2.1 Control of Inflammation and Catabolic Events

Disc degeneration initiation and progression is linked to inflammation. These include the findings of increased expression of pro-inflammatory mediators mediated by interleukin (IL)-1 signaling, and to a lesser extent, tumor necrosis factor-α (TNF-α) signaling.[8,9] Inflammation leads to elevated catabolism in IVD, especially the activity of matrix degradative enzyme, which degrades and remodels collagen and proteoglycans of the disc matrix.[10,11] Modulating inflammatory and catabolic factors is therefore considered critical to the inhibition of degeneration progression and hence supportive to intrinsic or assisted IVD repair.

9.2.2 Conferring Instant Mechanical Strength/Function

Although it is not entirely clear how IVD degeneration may cause back pain, perturbed stability and biomechanics of the spinal segment are proposed to play a major role. One school of thought to alleviate the degeneration-induced symptoms is to provide a direct immediate support to the mechanical function of the degenerated motion segment instead of dealing with the cause of degeneration. These treatments range from implementation of a scaffold to replace the nucleus pulposus (NP)[12] or patch the disrupted annulus,[13] to the bioengineering of whole disc constructs[14] and IVD allograft transplantation.[15]

9.2.3 Stimulation of Cell Anabolism for Matrix Replenishment

A major anabolic function of disc cells is to produce extracellular matrix (ECM) that contributes to the disc tissue mechanics. To balance the enhanced matrix degradation and restore the matrix content in a degenerated disc, strategies have been designed to directly augment the anabolism in the disc cells, or otherwise to increase the quantity of functional cells.[16] This can be achieved through directly delivering relevant matrix-producing cells, or stem cells that may differentiate in situ to produce matrices. Apart from cells, delivery of important genes and proteins that positively regulate matrix production and/or cell proliferation has also been investigated.

9.2.4 Microenvironment Reconstruction

The microenvironment that cells reside within is important to cell function and is therefore thought to be the potential rate limiting factor for disc regeneration. This microenvironment includes nutritional supply, oxygenation, osmolarity, the surrounding matrix meshwork, and the availability of the growth factor or cytokine reservoir. Strategies that modify nutrient diffusion, hypoxic stress, collagen fibril architecture, and other factors that have a role in the disc cell niche have been proposed to hold promise in promoting IVD repair.[17,18]

9.3 A Consideration of Disease Stage

Therapies often work within a window of disease severity. For IVD degeneration, the degenerative stage can be determined using different methods, such as evaluation of disc height, histological score, and various molecular markers. Clinically, IVD degeneration is graded under specific imaging techniques, which usually reflect the water content (which in turn correlates with proteoglycan level) and/or collagen integrity in disc matrix. On the other hand, studying the degeneration nature and progression at histological and molecular levels in animal models as well as clinical specimens has expanded our understanding of stage-specific characteristics. Such investigations also extend to cadaveric samples to interrogate age-related degeneration. Overall, studies have suggested that the IVD exhibits trends of changes ranging from nano- to macroscale levels (▶ Table 9.1) during the degeneration:

9.3.1 Nanoscale Anomalies

The IVD contains a high matrix-to-cell content. Collagens and proteoglycans form a meshwork of macromolecular structure

Table 9.1 Nano- to macroscale changes at different IVD degeneration stages

Mild	Moderate	Severe
Nanoscale changes	Microscale changes	Macroscale changes
• Matrix protein degradation • Inflammation cascade activation • Reduced cell anabolic activity	• Collagen fibril/PG disorganization • Compromised disc cell viability and function • Infiltration of inflammatory and fibroblast-like cells	• Mechanically compromised gross disc structures • Deformity in other supportive tissues, e.g., facet joints • Osteophyte formation

Abbreviations: PG, proteoglycan.

in the disc matrix. In addition to providing mechanical strength to the disc, this matrix meshwork also interacts with cytokines and growth factors and therefore provides a reservoir of inductive signals. Moreover, the matrix can directly regulate mechanotransduction signals to the adhered cells and regulate their activity. It is therefore believed that a disrupted matrix meshwork may not only impact on the mechanical properties of the disc, but also significantly influence disc cell behaviors. Injurious stimuli or other forms of stresses, such as excessive mechanical load, reduced nutritional supply, and hypoxia, may also compromise the cell anabolism and induce inflammatory cascades that lead to matrix breakdown. The damage in matrices is presumably the lead cause of the mechanical instability in the motion segment at early degeneration.[19,20]

9.3.2 Deterioration of Microscale Structures and Cell Activity

Under continual stresses, inflammation signals and damage of matrix elicit a tissue repair response. This is thought to be analogous to wound healing, involving a deposition of provisional matrices and subsequent remodeling. This process may include inflammatory cell and fibroblast-like cell infiltration. Cell death, possibly due to the inability to counter stresses, may amplify the inflammatory process. However, without removal of the stresses, the remodeling process is thought to remain dysfunctional. Consequently, the disc matrices become constituted by a fibrous meshwork with compromised function. Moreover, water content is reduced due to loss of proteoglycans. The sustained stimuli, as well as the abnormal matrices, further impact on cell function and phenotype. It is believed that resident disc stem/progenitor cell activity is also affected, thereby disabling the self-repair mechanism.[21]

9.3.3 Deformation of the Motion Segment Unit

At the late stage of degeneration, the abnormal disc matrix fails to provide the mechanical strength necessary to support the load in the spine, causing the IVD to deform.[22] This severely damages the compartmental structures that likely lead to major cell death in the IVD, in particular the NP. The collapse of the

IVD further causes the facet joints to be subjected to abnormal load and subsequent degeneration.[23] Osteophyte formation is also induced. As a result, the whole intervertebral motion unit becomes mechanically incompetent and grossly deformed in anatomical appearance.

9.4 Advantages and Disadvantages of Treatments

9.4.1 Long-term Effects

One of the targets of intervening in IVD degeneration is to inhibit or delay its progression. Intervention, especially those aiming to promote cell anabolism or inhibit catabolism, which may exert moderate to long-term effects, is therefore desirable. However, due to the relatively short half-lives of proteins, therapies involving use of gene and protein constructs may require multiple treatments or carefully designed delivery devices to obtain sustained results. It remains to be determined if cellular- or biomolecule-based interventions will generate an outcome comparable to total disc replacement.

9.4.2 On-shelf Availability and Consistency

Shelving and consistent efficacy is an important aspect for biologics. Gene and protein-based therapeutics are in general superior in on-shelf availability and activity consistency compared with other types of interventions. Cell- or plasma-derived products by nature tend to have more variation in therapeutic activity and therefore require an implementation of rigorous quality control. Allogenic cell transplantation may overcome the issues of on-shelf availability and may provide consistency in efficacy related to the use of autogeneic sources. In particular, mesenchymal stem cells (MSCs)/stromal cells can avoid allogenic recognition and may serve as a promising cell therapy in this aspect.[24]

9.4.3 Cost to Patients

Cost of therapy is determined by many factors. It depends not only on the type of intervention, but also the treatment regime.

Compared with recombinant protein and gene products, living tissue–derived cell and plasma products may be subject to more stringent regulation and quality control in preparation which in turn leads to higher costs. Moreover, intervention that requires local delivery such as intradiscal injection, as an essential feature of aforementioned therapies, also adds cost to treatment. Nonetheless, this becomes negligible if the delivery can be conducted along with discography. On the other hand, the recent realization of disc allograft transplantation may provide a less expensive alternative to total disc or nucleus replacement.[15,25] Although a long way to clinical practice, the cost of tissue engineered IVD or bioengineering of complete spinal segment is rather difficult to predict.

9.4.4 Repeatability

Apart from motion segment replacement, satisfactory control of IVD degeneration may likely necessitate repeated treatments, especially when the long-term effectiveness of therapies is not clear. In fact, due to the unclear etiology, degeneration progression may recur. Unlike systemic therapies or oral drugs, intradiscal regimes obviously do not favor multiple treatments.

9.5 Insights from Other Degenerative Diseases

9.5.1 A Historical View of the Therapies

Effective therapeutics often require a good understanding of the disease mechanism, in particular the molecular pathogenic events. Owing to the relatively limited understanding in IVD degeneration, the search for therapies leverages the knowledge from related tissues such as articular joints. Because of the similarities in the disease features and shared genetic components,[26] osteoarthritis has been a relevant model to facilitate generation of insights and development of therapeutics for IVD degeneration. Among the many options, gene/protein therapies and stem cell–based therapies/engineering have been widely explored (▶ Fig. 9.1).

The potential of gene therapies in disc repair has been reported in a number of in vivo or disc explant culture studies.[27,28,29] The driving force of such studies is in part because of the successful experience of such therapies in disease models

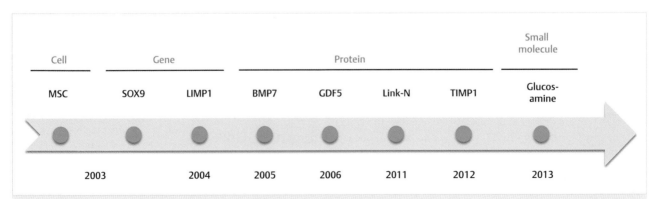

Fig. 9.1 A time line of major biologics being investigated for intervertebral disc repair. Abbreviations: BMP, bone morphogenetic protein; GDF, growth and differentiation factor; MSC, mesenchymal stem cell; TIMP, tissue inhibitor of mettaloproteinase.

that have a genetic basis, and that these approaches may provide prolonged therapeutic effects. Gene therapies have been tested in animal models or early clinical trials and are effective in treating tissue degeneration, in particular neural degeneration.[30] Classic examples include the use of virus-mediated gene therapy to treat retinal degeneration to restore vision[31] and reduce loss of neurons in Parkinson's disease,[32] or implanting genetically modified cells to treat Alzheimer's disease.[33] Gene therapy has also been getting increasing attention in orthopaedics.[34] Preclinical studies have demonstrated that gene therapy that enhances IL receptor antagonist (IL-RA) expression may modify osteoarthritis.[35,36] A similar use of the therapy to inhibit anti-inflammatory interleukins may reduce rheumatoid arthritis.[37,38]

Although gene-based therapies present an attractive approach to disease intervention, their safety is still controversial because of their power in genetic manipulation. Protein therapies, on the other hand, may be less versatile in comparison with gene therapies; however, they are likely to have fewer issues concerning safety while offering similar function. In fact, the IVD is virtually avascular and presents an enclosed tissue architecture. Theoretically, this enables therapeutic agents to be retained locally when applied through intradiscal delivery. Sustained action can be further achieved when combined with devices that allow controlled release. This encourages the development of growth factor (e.g., bone morphogenetic protein [BMP] and TGF-β) and other protein-based (e.g., platelet-rich plasma) therapies for treating IVD degeneration by augmenting the anabolic activity of the disc cells, especially the capacity of NP cells in the production of proteoglycans.

Stem cell–based intervention and tissue bioengineering are often regarded as promising, and perhaps the most attractive approaches to prevent degenerative diseases or even rebuild/repair the damaged tissues. In particular, the use of MSCs has been investigated in treating IVD degeneration. MSCs are originally identified as the stromal cells in the bone marrow, and have a preferential capacity to differentiate into cartilage and bone cells. They have been under active clinical investigation for treating various musculoskeletal conditions.[39] These include nonunions, bone defects, avascular necrosis, cartilage defects, and osteoarthritis, and even as a means to induce spinal fusion. The efficacy of MSC-based therapies in treating IVD degeneration has been established in preclinical settings. In addition to their stem-like properties, MSCs are known to possess immunomodulatory activities and have been widely adopted as immunotherapies, such as in graft-versus-host disease and Crohn's disease, without apparent safety issues. Because inflammation is a major contributing factor of IVD degeneration, MSC therapy is considered a promising approach for treatment. Additionally, MSCs have also been used to engineer tissue constructs, aiming to directly reconstruct the NP or annulus fibrosus (AF), such as in cases of disc herniation. Although there have been some successes in engineering whole IVD construct in small animals, how stem cell–based tissue engineering may derive complete spinal motion segments for transplantation in humans remains a question. This is considered to be the ultimate goal for treating the most severe forms of disc degeneration. Native IVD scaffolds derived from decellularization[40] can perhaps provide a template to assist the construction.

9.6 Roles of Biologics in Future IVD Degeneration Management

9.6.1 Designing Effective Therapies

Effective strategies for treating IVD degeneration, except for complete disc engineering and transplantation, would inevitably require clarifying and hence targeting the initiation and progression factors involved in the pathogenic mechanisms. Otherwise, the interventions are likely to result in simply delaying the degeneration progression instead of modifying the disease or even eliciting a repair.

Understanding the degeneration mechanisms may require sophisticated approaches, such as characterizing human IVD degeneration by genomics and proteomics techniques, to discover the risk factors and causative genes/proteins. Studying the roles of other nonbiological cues such as mechanical insults and specific lifestyles are also important. Whereas the use of cell culture or explant cultures may facilitate the search for influential factors, it is necessary, if not essential, to validate their actual roles in vivo. Regarding this aspect, various groups have placed efforts on seeking or generating animal models that present a phenotype resembling the human IVD degeneration,[41] or constructing bioreactor systems to culture whole human IVD long term under controlled mechanical stimulation that emulates physiological or pathological loading.[42]

IVD degeneration is thought to be multifactorial, and that genetic, mechanical and environmental factors are likely to interact to manifest the degeneration. Given the complex etiology, it is not yet clear if combining interventions that target the different factors may increase the effectiveness in modifying the degeneration or in fact be required for full repair or functional regeneration to happen. Clinically, this might implicate the need for controlled bed rest, carefully designed programs of physical therapy and rehabilitation, or even implantation of special biomedical devices (e.g., to reduce the mechanical load to the joint segment) in addition to the administration of biologics.

9.6.2 Suitability of Interventions

The targets of gene and protein therapies are IVD cells. Therefore, most biological therapies may have limited action at the severe degeneration stage due to very few cells remaining in the IVD. Cell-based therapies on the other hand aim to replenish matrix-producing cells to rebuild the disc mechanics. MSCs may modulate inflammation and catabolism in addition to differentiation into matrix producing cells. However, because severely degenerated IVD generally have largely deteriorated or abnormally remodeled structures, interventions that primarily aim to promote matrix production or control matrix degradation may have limited potential to recover the IVD function. In fact, at severe degeneration stage, treating the IVD may only have limited efficacy in recovering the motion segment function as a whole unless the degenerated facet joints is also effectively repaired or reconstructed. Total disc replacement with bioengineered constructs or disc allograft transplantation is considered to be a more effective approach for treating severe IVD degeneration. To this end, it is believed that most therapeutic interventions are likely be effective for treating IVD degeneration at moderate instead of severe stage, unless auxiliary measures are adopted in the regime (which remains to be revealed). Symptomatic subjects who are not at the final stage of IVD degeneration but who failed to respond to conservative treatments should consider the new interventions, which are considered less invasive and traumatic compared with spinal fusion or total disc replacement operations. Patients with severely degenerated IVD are likely to benefit from a transplantation of disc allograft or yet-to-be realized bioengineered IVD or motion segment constructs.

9.7 Prospect of Prophylactic Treatment

9.7.1 Are Prophylactics Necessary and Feasible?

Either trauma-induced or sporadic IVD degeneration takes time to develop and progress. A degenerated IVD with altered mechanics gradually becomes susceptible to prolapse and herniation. This implies that a control of the chronic degenerative changes, which can appear long before detection or manifestation of symptoms, may be critical to preempt IVD degeneration. Unless the etiology of IVD degeneration can be delineated, chances are that the degeneration may recur after treatments. When initiated, IVD degeneration is progressive and not irreversible by nature. Symptomatic subjects often have developed severe IVD degeneration where the motion units and possibly the nerve function (e.g., in sciatica and spondylomyelopathy) have been compromised. Therefore, there is a need to call for a prophylactic regime to prevent IVD degeneration to develop.

Although no prophylactic treatment has proven effective, avoiding obesity and inappropriate postures have been proposed to minimize IVD degeneration incidence. One reason for the lack of prophylactic measures is the inability to pinpoint the etiology of degeneration. Another reason may be that the IVD is virtually avascular, and therefore thought to be not readily accessible by oral or systemic medications. Attempt to deliver the therapeutics into the disc requires direct access into the disc by needle or catheter, which raises the worry of damaging the IVD and hence inducing degeneration. A third reason is that there has not been a consensus on which subjects should receive the prophylactics because of difficulty in the prognosis of IVD degeneration progression.

A repeatable and noninvasive regime is appealing to the prophylactic management of IVD degeneration. One example is the use of supplements such as glucosamine, which have been suggested to reduce joint pain related to cartilage degeneration. However, based on evidence from preclinical studies and clinical trials, the efficacy of glucosamine, and whether it can effectively repair cartilage is still controversial. A pilot study in induced IVD degeneration in a rabbit model on the other hand has suggested that oral supplementation of glucosamine may exert negative effects.[43] The potential of various supplements would therefore need to be carefully investigated in the future.

9.7.2 Screening and Monitoring

With the development of sophisticated techniques in screening and monitoring IVD degeneration, there are opportunities for developing prophylactics to control IVD degeneration progression or even disc repair at early stages. Advances in the understanding of IVD degeneration etiology and risk factors, population screening strategies, and biomarker/imaging are paramount, if not a prerequisite, for effective application of prophylactics. Various research groups have made significant efforts in seeking the genetic factors that may predispose IVD degeneration.[5] Genetic risk factors may provide means to identify and hence screen for susceptible subjects for opportunities of treating the degeneration at its onset or before it reaches irreversible stages. Development of sensitive and minimally invasive assays for biomarker analysis[44] and imaging techniques[45] that enable detection of early IVD degeneration are of equal importance to effective monitoring and treatment.

9.8 References

[1] Cheung KM, Samartzis D, Karppinen J, Luk KD. Are "patterns" of lumbar disc degeneration associated with low back pain?: new insights based on skipped level disc pathology. Spine. 2012; 37(7):E430–E438

[2] Cheung KM, Karppinen J, Chan D, et al. Prevalence and pattern of lumbar magnetic resonance imaging changes in a population study of one thousand forty-three individuals. Spine. 2009; 34(9):934–940

[3] Teraguchi M, Yoshimura N, Hashizume H, et al. The association of combination of disc degeneration, end plate signal change, and Schmorl node with low back pain in a large population study: the Wakayama Spine Study. Spine J. 2015; 15(4):622–628

[4] Buirski G. Magnetic resonance signal patterns of lumbar discs in patients with low back pain. A prospective study with discographic correlation. Spine. 1992; 17(10):1199–1204

[5] Eskola PJ, Lemmelä S, Kjaer P, et al. Genetic association studies in lumbar disc degeneration: a systematic review. PLoS One. 2012; 7(11):e49995

[6] Battié MC, Videman T, Kaprio J, et al. The Twin Spine Study: contributions to a changing view of disc degeneration. Spine J. 2009; 9(1):47–59

[7] Sakai D, Andersson GB. Stem cell therapy for intervertebral disc regeneration: obstacles and solutions. Nat Rev Rheumatol. 2015; 11(4):243–256

[8] Shamji MF, Setton LA, Jarvis W, et al. Proinflammatory cytokine expression profile in degenerated and herniated human intervertebral disc tissues. Arthritis Rheum. 2010; 62(7):1974–1982

[9] Le Maitre CL, Hoyland JA, Freemont AJ. Catabolic cytokine expression in degenerate and herniated human intervertebral discs: IL-1beta and TNFalpha expression profile. Arthritis Res Ther. 2007; 9(4):R77

[10] Millward-Sadler SJ, Costello PW, Freemont AJ, Hoyland JA. Regulation of catabolic gene expression in normal and degenerate human intervertebral disc cells: implications for the pathogenesis of intervertebral disc degeneration. Arthritis Res Ther. 2009; 11(3):R65

[11] Hoyland JA, Le Maitre C, Freemont AJ. Investigation of the role of IL-1 and TNF in matrix degradation in the intervertebral disc. Rheumatology (Oxford). 2008; 47(6):809–814

[12] Halloran DO, Grad S, Stoddart M, Dockery P, Alini M, Pandit AS. An injectable cross-linked scaffold for nucleus pulposus regeneration. Biomaterials. 2008; 29(4):438–447

[13] Likhitpanichkul M, Dreischarf M, Illien-Junger S, et al. Fibrin-genipin adhesive hydrogel for annulus fibrosus repair: performance evaluation with large animal organ culture, in situ biomechanics, and in vivo degradation tests. Eur Cell Mater. 2014; 28:25–37, discussion 37–38

[14] Bowles RD, Gebhard HH, Härtl R, Bonassar LJ. Tissue-engineered intervertebral discs produce new matrix, maintain disc height, and restore biomechanical function to the rodent spine. Proc Natl Acad Sci U S A. 2011; 108 (32):13106–13111

[15] Huang YC, Xiao J, Lu WW, Leung VY, Hu Y, Luk KD. Lumbar intervertebral disc allograft transplantation: long-term mobility and impact on the adjacent segments. Eur Spine J. 2016

[16] Fontana G, See E, Pandit A. Current trends in biologics delivery to restore intervertebral disc anabolism. Adv Drug Deliv Rev. 2015; 84:146–158

[17] Huang YC, Leung VY, Lu WW, Luk KD. The effects of microenvironment in mesenchymal stem cell-based regeneration of intervertebral disc. Spine J. 2013; 13(3):352–362

[18] Tam WK, Cheung KM, Leung VY. intervertebral disc engineering through exploiting mesenchymal stem cells: progress and perspective. Curr Stem Cell Res Ther. 2016; 11(6):505–512

[19] Aladin DM, Cheung KM, Ngan AH, et al. Nanostructure of collagen fibrils in human nucleus pulposus and its correlation with macroscale tissue mechanics. J Orthop Res. 2010; 28(4):497–502

[20] Aladin DM, Cheung KM, Chan D, et al. Expression of the Trp2 allele of COL9A2 is associated with alterations in the mechanical properties of human intervertebral discs. Spine. 2007; 32(25):2820–2826

[21] Huang S, Leung VY, Long D, et al. Coupling of small leucine-rich proteoglycans to hypoxic survival of a progenitor cell-like subpopulation in Rhesus Macaque intervertebral disc. Biomaterials. 2013; 34(28):6548–6558

[22] Inoue N, Espinoza Orías AA. Biomechanics of intervertebral disk degeneration. Orthop Clin North Am. 2011; 42(4):487–499, vii

[23] Fujiwara A, Tamai K, Yamato M, et al. The relationship between facet joint osteoarthritis and disc degeneration of the lumbar spine: an MRI study. Eur Spine J. 1999; 8(5):396–401

[24] Ryan JM, Barry FP, Murphy JM, Mahon BP. Mesenchymal stem cells avoid allogeneic rejection. J Inflamm (Lond). 2005; 2:8

[25] Ruan D, He Q, Ding Y, Hou L, Li J, Luk KD. Intervertebral disc transplantation in the treatment of degenerative spine disease: a preliminary study. Lancet. 2007; 369(9566):993–999

[26] Ikegawa S. The genetics of common degenerative skeletal disorders: osteoarthritis and degenerative disc disease. Annu Rev Genomics Hum Genet. 2013; 14:245–256

[27] Le Maitre CL, Hoyland JA, Freemont AJ. Interleukin-1 receptor antagonist delivered directly and by gene therapy inhibits matrix degradation in the intact degenerate human intervertebral disc: an in situ zymographic and gene therapy study. Arthritis Res Ther. 2007; 9(4):R83

[28] Leckie SK, Bechara BP, Hartman RA, et al. Injection of AAV2-BMP2 and AAV2-TIMP1 into the nucleus pulposus slows the course of intervertebral disc degeneration in an in vivo rabbit model. Spine J. 2012; 12(1):7–20

[29] Paul R, Haydon RC, Cheng H, et al. Potential use of Sox9 gene therapy for intervertebral degenerative disc disease. Spine. 2003; 28(8):755–763

[30] Tuszynski MH. Growth-factor gene therapy for neurodegenerative disorders. Lancet Neurol. 2002; 1(1):51–57

[31] Acland GM, Aguirre GD, Ray J, et al. Gene therapy restores vision in a canine model of childhood blindness. Nat Genet. 2001; 28(1):92–95

[32] Choi-Lundberg DL, Lin Q, Chang YN, et al. Dopaminergic neurons protected from degeneration by GDNF gene therapy. Science. 1997; 275(5301):838–841

[33] Tuszynski MH, Thal L, Pay M, et al. A phase 1 clinical trial of nerve growth factor gene therapy for Alzheimer disease. Nat Med. 2005; 11(5):551–555

[34] Kang R, Ghivizzani SC, Muzzonigro TS, Herndon JH, Robbins PD, Evans CH. The Marshall R. Urist Young Investigator Award. Orthopaedic applications of gene therapy. From concept to clinic. Clin Orthop Relat Res. 2000(375):324–337

[35] Goodrich LR, Grieger JC, Phillips JN, et al. scAAVIL-1ra dosing trial in a large animal model and validation of long-term expression with repeat administration for osteoarthritis therapy. Gene Ther. 2015; 22(7):536–545

[36] Fernandes J, Tardif G, Martel-Pelletier J, et al. In vivo transfer of interleukin-1 receptor antagonist gene in osteoarthritic rabbit knee joints: prevention of osteoarthritis progression. Am J Pathol. 1999; 154(4):1159–1169

[37] Woods JM, Katschke KJ, Volin MV, et al. IL-4 adenoviral gene therapy reduces inflammation, proinflammatory cytokines, vascularization, and bony destruction in rat adjuvant-induced arthritis. J Immunol. 2001; 166(2):1214–1222

[38] Woods JM, Amin MA, Katschke KJ, Jr, et al. Interleukin-13 gene therapy reduces inflammation, vascularization, and bony destruction in rat adjuvant-induced arthritis. Hum Gene Ther. 2002; 13(3):381–393

[39] Steinert AF, Rackwitz L, Gilbert F, Nöth U, Tuan RS. Concise review: the clinical application of mesenchymal stem cells for musculoskeletal regeneration: current status and perspectives. Stem Cells Transl Med. 2012; 1(3):237–247

[40] Chan LK, Leung VY, Tam V, Lu WW, Sze KY, Cheung KM. Decellularized bovine intervertebral disc as a natural scaffold for xenogenic cell studies. Acta Biomater. 2013; 9(2):5262–5272

[41] Alini M, Eisenstein SM, Ito K, et al. Are animal models useful for studying human disc disorders/degeneration? Eur Spine J. 2008; 17(1):2–19

[42] Gantenbein B, Illien-Jünger S, Chan SC, et al. Organ culture bioreactors–platforms to study human intervertebral disc degeneration and regenerative therapy. Curr Stem Cell Res Ther. 2015; 10(4):339–352

[43] Jacobs L, Vo N, Coelho JP, et al. Glucosamine supplementation demonstrates a negative effect on intervertebral disc matrix in an animal model of disc degeneration. Spine. 2013; 38(12):984–990

[44] Poole AR. Biologic markers and disc degeneration. J Bone Joint Surg Am. 2006; 88 Suppl 2:72–75

[45] Farshad-Amacker NA, Farshad M, Winklehner A, Andreisek G. MR imaging of degenerative disc disease. Eur J Radiol. 2015; 84(9):1768–1776

10 Learning from Successes of Tissue Engineering Strategies for Cartilaginous Disorders

Stephen R. Sloan, Jr. and Lawrence J. Bonassar

Abstract

The design of biological and tissue engineered approaches for treating intervertebral disc (IVD) pathologies should not be an entirely novel progression; there are numerous examples of clinically successful treatments in medical fields bearing similarity to the spine. Tissue engineered implants have been US Food and Drug Administration (FDA) approved to treat a variety of musculoskeletal disorders in the clinic since the 1990s, providing ample time for long-term studies and design alterations.[1,2,3,4,5,6] Autologous chondrocyte implantation (ACI) is one example of a clinically successful intervention in an orthopaedic field with great relevance to the spine that garnered success in thousands of patients.[3,6,7,8] Although treating the spine has its own complexities and unique challenges facing biological repair, important lessons can be learned from clinical triumphs in related fields.

Keywords: articular cartilage, auricular cartilage, autologous chondrocyte implantation, meniscus, nasal cartilage

10.1 Historical Perspective

Three types of biologics used clinically to treat pathological cartilage are biomolecule-, cell-, and scaffold-based approaches, which may be used independently or in combination with each other.[2,9,10] The strategy of biomolecule therapies is to augment natural tissue healing processes through invigorating cells with signals to proliferate, migrate, or assemble proteins necessary for repair. There are a whole host of cytokines, growth factors, and enzymes used clinically to treat cartilaginous disorders including fibrin, transforming growth factor (TGF-β), bone morphogenetic proteins (BMP), platelet-derived growth factor (PDGF) and insulin-like growth factor (IGF), to name a few. The strategy of cellular therapies with or without scaffold material is to induce cellular proliferation and the production of extracellular matrix (ECM) proteins as well as other signal biomolecules. Scaffold-based approaches comprise cytocompatible biomaterials that replace native tissue and/or function as carriers for cells producing native proteins and cytokines. This chapter primarily focuses on interventions involving tissue scaffolds, as there are already biomolecule- and cell-based biologics for intervertebral disc (IVD) in the clinical setting.[11,12,13]

10.1.1 Relevant Cartilaginous Tissues

The IVD is by no means identical to other cartilaginous tissues; however, there are many anatomical, pathological, and macroenvironmental similarities between the tissues. There are multiple types of cartilage found in the human body bearing semblances to the IVD that are worth discussing, such as meniscus, articular, ear, and nose cartilage. Just like the IVD, most types of cartilage, when healthy, are avascular and lack nerves.[14,15] Whereas chondrocytes, native cartilage cells, are at homeostasis under hypoxic conditions, avascular tissues do not receive the cocktail of growth factors and proteins necessary to proliferate and self-heal after injury. Degenerative disc disease (DDD) is a progressive disease that becomes more prevalent with increasing age and may be induced by traumatic injury, much akin to the degeneration of articular cartilage and meniscus.[16,17,18,19] Degenerated cartilage and IVD are chronic pathologies due to their inability to self-heal, and are difficult to treat without the introduction of biological material such as cells, biomolecules, and tissues.

Every cartilaginous tissue has a unique mechanical environment, but many mirror both the static and cyclic loading states experienced by the IVD during standing and walking/exercising.[20,21] Articular cartilage and menisci are most similar to IVDs given they are sandwiched between bones and function to absorb shock, transmit loads, and stabilize joints.[22] Articular cartilage in the knee is thoroughly discussed in this chapter because the cyclic compressive loading in the knee is the most analogous to the spine.[23] The ECM of cartilaginous tissues including IVDs are compositionally dense in collagen, proteoglycans, elastin, and water, with varying content in each tissue yielding excellent mechanical properties, flexibility, or structural integrity.[17,24,25,26,27,28,29,30] The cellular composition of IVDs is similar to other cartilage cell populations given that native annulus fibrosus (AF) cells are chondrocyte-like and native nucleus pulposus (NP) cells are fibroblast-like.[31] Tissue engineered biologics used in the clinic to treat cartilage pathologies are composed of identical biomaterials and cells used in preclinical IVD studies, hence the necessity to look toward fields to promote translation of IVD biologics.[1,13,32,33]

10.2 Status of Successful Products

Orthopaedics and other surgical fields treating cartilage have seen a plethora of US Food and Drug Administration (FDA)-approved biologics enter clinical trials and the marketplace since the 1990s, and have much to offer IVD biologics in terms of strategy and design. The following sections discuss various FDA-approved products and those currently in clinical trials to offer guidance and motivation for IVD biologics.

10.2.1 Articular Cartilage

By the numbers, there are more commercially available and clinically tested products for treating and repairing articular cartilage than any other cartilaginous tissue (▶ Table 10.1). This could stem from the fact that focal chondral defects are present in up to 63% of patients undergoing arthroscopy of the knee; however, DDD has been shown to be present in up to 90% of older adults.[34,35] Articular cartilage lesions resulting from traumatic injury or degenerative diseases lead to chronic pain and decreased mobility, hindering patients from enjoying physical

Table 10.1 Ongoing and completed FDA-approved clinical trials regarding biologics for repairing and replacing articular cartilage

Clinical trial name	Product	Clinical trial phase	FDA status	Minimum # of patients	Scaffold material	Cell type	Seeding density (10^6/cm^2)	Reference
Study of the Treatment of Articular Repair	Carticel	IV	Completed	>10,000	Tibial periosteum	Autologous chondrocytes	≥2.0	6
Novocart® 3D for Treatment of Articular Cartilage of the Knee	Novocart 3D	III	Recruiting	6,000	Type I collagen	Autologous chondrocytes	0.5–3.0	42
Neocartilage Implant to Treat Cartilage Lesions of the Knee	RevaFlex	III	Active, not recruiting	12	N/A	Juvenile chondrocytes	N/A	44
A Comparison between the Performance of Chondrocytes versus Microfracture Technique on Knee Symptoms	MACI	III	Completed	295	Porcine type I/III collagen	Autologous chondrocytes	0.5–1.0	36
Confirmatory Study of NeoCart in Knee Cartilage Repair	NeoCart	III	Recruiting	170	Bovine type I Collagen	Autologous Chondrocytes	N/A	40,63
Clinical Trial for the Regeneration of Cartilage Lesions in the Knee	Nose2Knee	II	Recruiting	7	Porcine type I/III collagen	Autologous nasal chondrocytes	N/A	45,46
Comparison of BioCart™ II with Microfracture for Treatment of Cartilage Defects of the Femoral Condyle	BioCart II	II	Unknown	40	Fibrin	Autologous chondrocytes	0.5	41
DeNovo NT Natural Tissue Graft Stratified Knee Study	DeNovo NT	Unknown	Recruiting	>10,000	Minced allograft cartilage	Juvenile chondrocytes	N/A	43

activities and a high quality of life.[36] Although translation of successful interventions from the laboratory to the clinic is notoriously difficult due to the FDA approval process, novel technologies for articular cartilage repair have had years of clinical success.

Autologous Chondrocyte Implantation—First Generation

Autologous chondrocyte implantation (ACI) and its stepwise iterations are great examples of clinically successful interventions to motivate the progression of IVD biologics (▶ Fig. 10.1, ▶ Table 10.2). Used to treat symptomatic cartilage defects of the femoral condyle, ACI treatments replaced interventions such as microfracture, abrasion chondroplasty, and osteochondral grafting. The aforementioned treatments are inadequate to restore native cartilage function and structure due to their lack of long-term stability and inability to treat large defect areas.[37,38] Carticel® (Vericel Corp.) is the shining star of the articular cartilage biologics, implanted in over 10,000 (and counting) patients since its introduction in 1995 and subsequent FDA approval in 1997.[6] The two-step ACI procedure involves taking a cartilage biopsy upon first arthroscopy to harvest autologous chondrocytes from trivial knee cartilage, culturing cells in vitro to expand the population while maintaining correct phenotype, and then implanting the cells in a defect site under a periosteal membrane during the second arthroscopy.[6] The strength of the procedures lies in the use of autologous chondrocytes, which decreases the risk of an immune response to the implanted cells and also ensures a phenotype similar to native cells. Carticel is considered the "first generation" of ACI, from which other procedures evolved with more complex treatment strategies involving scaffolds and biomolecules.[37]

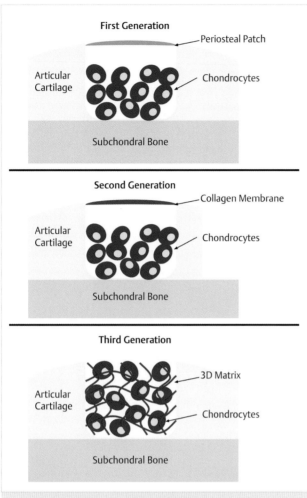

Fig. 10.1 Cartoon representation of the first three generations of autologous chondrocyte implantation.

biomaterials to promote autologous chondrocyte expansion, such as NeoCart (Histogenics Inc.), BioCart II (ProChon Biotech Ltd.), and Novocart 3D (Aesculap Inc.).[40,41,42] The third generation also introduced new methods for culturing the autologous chondrocytes. NeoCart, for example, seeds chondrocytes onto a bovine type-I collagen matrix, which is mechanically stimulated in a hypoxic bioreactor to condition the matrix for optimal function in the body.[40] Second and third generation treatments show similar clinical outcomes to the first generation; however, there are surgical advantages such as reduced operative time, reduced tourniquet time, and ability to use minimally invasive techniques.[36]

More recent advances in the ACI procedure aim to reduce ACI to a single operation and minimize the morbidity of autologous cartilage harvest.[37] Products such as RevaFlex (ISTO Technologies Inc.), Nose2Knee, and DeNovo NT (Zimmer Inc.) are still in the earlier stages of clinical trials; however, they offer novel technologies that may improve clinical outcomes compared with the earlier generations of ACI. DeNovo NT and RevaFlex substitute the autologous chondrocyte population for human juvenile chondrocytes, whereas DeNovo NT uses minced allograft cartilage as a scaffold biomaterial, and RevaFlex is scaffold-free.[43,44] Using allogenic chondrocytes enables cell implantation to be performed in a single operation; however, there are patient risks associated with histocompatibility and disease transmission. Nose2Knee attempts to reduce knee cartilage morbidity by harvesting autologous nasal septum cartilage for chondrocytes.[45,46] The Nose2Knee ACI procedure is similar to MACI due to the use of a collagen membrane; however, the use of nasal chondrocytes removes the necessity of additional knee cartilage damage during cell harvesting. IVD biologics can benefit from many ACI clinical trials; however, the need to refrain from multiple operations and progressing disc degeneration during cell harvest makes Nose2Knee a future-oriented product.

Cases involving patients receiving Carticel ACI result in more successful outcomes over long periods of time than with contemporary nonbiological interventions. While there is debate whether ACI results in a greater percent of hyaline cartilage versus fibrocartilage, the failure rate for Carticel ACI at a 10-year follow-up was 17% versus 55% for mosaicplasty.[7] Other studies have noted greater success rates in younger patients who presented sooner for surgery, demonstrating the value of prophylactic intervention before cartilage succumbs to degeneration.[39]

Autologous Chondrocyte Implantation – Second and Third Generation

As Carticel ACI was performed in more patients, the "second generation" of ACI treatments substituted collagen membranes for the periosteal flap to avoid in situ patch hypertrophy and periosteal harvest morbidity.[37] Matrix-induced autologous chondrocyte implantation (MACI) employs a bovine type-I/III collagen patch on which to seed chondrocytes, reducing implant hypertrophy and the need for revision surgery.[36] The further classification of progressing generations of ACI are somewhat unclear; however, the "third generation" of products are characterized by the use of three-dimensional (3D) scaffold

10.2.2 Meniscus—Autologous Concentrates

The menisci are fibrocartilaginous structures that transmit loads and reduce friction in many articulating joints, with the most prominent being the crescent-shaped lateral and medial menisci of the knee. Originally thought to be vestigial muscles of the knee, menisci were commonly completely removed when damaged, until biomechanical studies in the 1980s elucidated their role of reducing joint contact stresses.[47] Meniscal tears require surgical intervention in about 85% of the cases, and repair strategies involving sutures, staples, and anchors merely preserve function instead of healing the damaged tissue.[48,49] Meniscal allografts have been implanted in patients and studied in 10-year longitudinal clinical trials, which reportedly improved knee pain and function in most patients.[4] Allografts appear to be decent options to preserve knee function and prevent further cartilage degradation, but they fail at a rate of 55% upon second-look surgery. Current standard-of-care procedures to treat torn and damaged menisci have not proven long-term effectiveness, motivating novel biological treatments with the hopes of improving knee pain and function over decades of use.

Biologics used to treat meniscal tears have not developed as quickly as those for articular cartilage, with clinical trials only

Table 10.2 Representative images of articular cartilage repair products with FDA approval for clinical use and trials

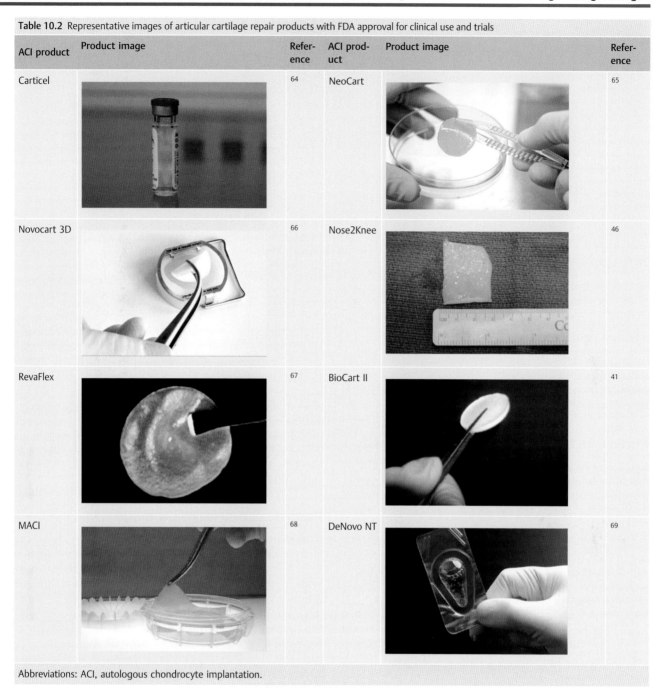

ACI product	Product image	Reference	ACI product	Product image	Reference
Carticel		64	NeoCart		65
Novocart 3D		66	Nose2Knee		46
RevaFlex		67	BioCart II		41
MACI		68	DeNovo NT		69

Abbreviations: ACI, autologous chondrocyte implantation.

involving autologous blood concentrates composed of growth factors and cells (▶ Table 10.3). A second generation of platelet rich plasma (PRP) known as platelet rich fibrin (PRF) is currently in clinical trials to treat meniscal tears in a one-step operation.[50] PRF is neither a classic platelet concentrate nor a fibrin glue, and uses a less complex preparation method than PRP to provide a similar cocktail of growth factors to promote healing and tissue regeneration.[51] Surgical outcomes for patients treated with PRF have not yet been reported; however, animal studies have shown that PRF increases healing capabilities in avascular tissues.[52] Bone marrow aspirate concentrate (BMAC) is another autologous product that is obtained and administered in a single operation, and contains mesenchymal stem cells (MSCs) in addition to growth factors.[53] Bone marrow-derived MSCs are well studied for their condrogenic potential, ease of recruitment, low neoplastic differentiation, and lack of ethical controversy unlike other sources of stem cells. Bone marrow is also rich in components that lead to tissue healing, with platelets and growth factors such as TGF-β, PDGF, and vascular endothelial growth factor (VEGF). BMAC was found to improve the healing of meniscal tears in a sheep model, with significantly more neovascularization and formation of cartilage plaques.[53]Although not as complex as tissue engineered biologics with scaffolds and cultured cells, autologous concentrates enable relatively simple operations with promising preclinical outcomes.

Table 10.3 Ongoing and completed FDA-approved clinical trials regarding biologics for repairing and replacing meniscus and nasal cartilage

	Clinical trial name	Product	Clinical trial phase	FDA status	Minimum # of patients	Scaffold material	Cell type	Seeding density ($10^6/cm^2$)	Reference
Meniscus	Novel One-step Repair of Knee Meniscal Tear Using Platelet Rich Fibrin	N/A	Unknown	Enrolling by invitation	N/A	Platelet rich fibrin	N/A	N/A	50,52
	Autologous Bone Marrow Aspirate Concentrate in Patients Undergoing Meniscectomy	N/A	Unknown	Active, not yet recruiting	N/A	Bone marrow aspirate concentrate	Bone marrow–derived mesenchymal stem cells	N/A	53
Nose	Tissue Engineered Nasal Cartilage for Reconstruction of the Alar Lobule	N/A	1	Completed	5	Porcine type I/III collagen	Autologous nasal chondrocytes	4.0	57

10.2.3 Ear and Nose Cartilage

Ear and nose cartilage is not subject to substantial mechanical loading like the IVD or articular cartilage, but the challenge of finding optimal scaffold biomaterials and cell sources for biological therapeutics yields insight for IVD biologics.

Reconstructing and Replacing the Outer Ear

A difficulty in plastic surgery is reconstructing or replacing the auricular cartilage of the ear after traumatic injury or congenital defect. The current standard of care relies on hand carving autologous costal cartilage or high-density polyethylene to form ear-like structures, which requires extreme surgical skill yet will not likely match the aesthetic appearance of native tissue.[30] Tissue engineered whole auricle constructs have been implanted in animals dating back to 1992, typically composed of human, bovine, or porcine chondrocytes seeded onto synthetic or fibrin scaffolds.[30,54] Animal studies have demonstrated the ability of tissue engineered constructs to mimic the anatomical appearance and cartilaginous composition of the human ear.[54] Molds are typically used to form the correct human ear shape, although nascent studies have developed methods of laser scanning and 3D printing to better duplicate anatomical shapes and personalize interventions.[55]

Tissue engineered constructs for reconstructing and replacing the ear are not without flaws, and still have areas that need improving. Preclinical studies employing synthetic scaffold materials, such as polyglycolic acid and polylactic acid, have shown synthetic materials are subject to extrusion, inflammation, and foreign body reactions.[30] In vivo host responses to implanted constructs lead to scaffold shrinkage and distortion, a poor outcome for an aesthetic structure such as the ear.[30] Autologous cartilage grafts from the nose or ribs are recognized as superior scaffold biomaterials, but the ambition of tissue engineering is to reduce donor-site morbidity and avoid multiple operations. Composite materials composed of both degradable and nondegradable biomaterials overcome geometric changes in vivo, and will likely be critical to the success of tissue

engineering whole auricles.[56] Lastly, tissue engineered whole auricles require 100 to 150 million chondrocytes depending on the size and porosity of the construct.[30] Further complicating the massive cellular requirement is the fact that chondrocytes lose their cartilaginous phenotype when passaged multiple times in vitro, and will lack necessary histological and biochemical characteristics if implanted in vivo. The shortcomings mentioned above are shared by many fields employing tissue engineering for biological interventions, and will be hurdles to overcome before tissue engineered constructs are readily available in the clinic.

Reconstructing Nasal Cartilage

Nasal cartilage is replaced or reconstructed in the clinic after traumatic injury or resection of skin cancer tumors. Unlike biologics for ear cartilage reconstruction, there are biological interventions for nasal cartilage with ongoing clinical trials. A clinical trial studying the use of tissue engineering to reconstruct alar lobules, the cartilaginous ridges that flare out laterally around the nostrils, used autologous chondrocytes harvested from the nasal septum as the cell population.[57] The harvested chondrocytes were expanded for 2 weeks in two-dimensional (2D) culture prior to seeding onto a porcine type I/III collagen membrane and implantation into the body. One year after implantation, the alar cartilage was structurally stable, had adequate respiratory function, pleased patients aesthetically, and displayed tissue composition typical of native alar cartilage. This intervention was only performed in five individuals; however, the study demonstrated the safety and efficacy of tissue engineered cartilage for nasal reconstruction, and managed to generate cartilage 40 times larger than the original biopsy.

10.3 Challenges Specific to the Spine

While biological treatments used in the clinic to treat cartilaginous pathologies have direct relevance to treating IVDs, there are challenges specific to the spine to keep in mind when engineering and studying biologics for the spine. The anatomy of the IVD is compositionally more complex than other cartilages, with three distinct tissues. The AF, NP, and vertebral end plates are three interdependent structures, with unique cell populations, biochemical compositions, and functions.[58] Although other cartilaginous structures are not entirely homogeneous, the IVD is less gradated and more heterogeneous. The biomechanical environment of the IVD is also less well understood than cartilage counterparts. Little is known about the role of facet joints in spine biomechanics, there are controversies regarding the three column model, and load distribution within the IVD is not well characterized.[59,60] Simply analyzing clinical outcomes is much more difficult in the spine, as multifactorial statistics need to address multiple spinal levels.

The structure of the cartilaginous structures of the spine involve complexities that are absent in other cartilaginous tissues. Notably, the presence of two distinct tissues, the NP and AF, make tissue engineering of the IVD more akin to engineering an organ than a single tissue. Whereas other types of cartilage have smooth spatial gradients of phenotypes (e.g., surface to deep zone in articular cartilage or white to red zone in the meniscus), the IVD has a distinct boundary between the NP and AF, as well as gradients between the inner and outer AF. Engineering of an IVD requires the generation of a network of large, organized fibers in the AF, similar to the meniscus, as well as the development of a proteoglycan-rich network in the NP, similar to articular cartilage. Thus, although the task of assembling a tissue engineered IVD (TE-IVD) presents unique challenges, lessons can be learned from successes at engineering other types of cartilage.

Regarding the treatments themselves, a donor site for autologous disc cells is an obstacle, as creating a lesion in the IVD destabilizes the disc and leads to degeneration.[61] Cartilage repair treatments such as ACI are able to biopsy cartilage from trivial non–weight-bearing locations such as the intercondylar notch, where minimal morbidity is caused to the patient.[62] Fixation is another primary concern when implanting scaffolds or biomaterials, as material could potentially displace out of the disc space and impinge nerves or compress the spinal cord. The process of anchoring a TE-IVD also presents a distinct challenge compared with other cartilaginous tissues, in that such an implant would be required to integrate with yet another type of cartilage of the vertebral end plate, whereas anchoring of the meniscus or articular cartilage takes place directly to bone. Although prolapses of implanted meniscus scaffolds may be uncomfortable and require revision surgery, prolapsed disc implants can compress the spinal cord or cause severe neurological damage. Lastly, operating on the spine is a relatively new field with virtually no commercial biological products and studies. Even other fields with similar amounts of biological innovation have a better grasp of the body's response to repair, as in the case with total hip replacement, with the first total hip surgery performed over 50 years ago. Total disc replacement has only been performed in unique case studies, with little longitudinal data to perform biomedical analyses or draw substantial conclusions.

10.4 Conclusion

Designing biologics for the repair, replacement, and regeneration of the IVD is a difficult task; however, there is motivation to be found in the plethora of products available to treat cartilaginous disorders in other parts of the body. ACI products such as Carticel have been studied for more than 2 decades in thousands of human patients, providing the tissue engineering community with a wealth of knowledge of how biologics interact with the human body. Although the spine has its own unique challenges to overcome, many similar hurdles were presented to the investigators who developed clinically successful products to repair cartilage in the knee, ear, and nose. Cartilage biologics have a proven track record in the clinic, paving the way for the IVD to reap the benefits in the near future.

10.5 References

[1] McNickle AG, Provencher MT, Cole BJ. Overview of existing cartilage repair technology. Sports Med Arthrosc Rev. 2008; 16(4):196–201

[2] McGowan KB, Stiegman G. Regulatory challenges for cartilage repair technologies. Cartilage. 2013; 4(1):4–11

[3] Bartlett W, Skinner JA, Gooding CR, et al. Autologous chondrocyte implantation versus matrix-induced autologous chondrocyte implantation for osteochondral defects of the knee: a prospective, randomised study. J Bone Joint Surg Br. 2005; 87(5):640–645

[4] Hommen JP, Applegate GR, Del Pizzo W. Meniscus allograft transplantation: ten-year results of cryopreserved allografts. Arthroscopy. 2007; 23(4):388–393

[5] Browne JE, Anderson AF, Arciero R, et al. Clinical outcome of autologous chondrocyte implantation at 5 years in US subjects. Clin OrthopRelat Res. 2005(436):237–245

[6] Zaslav K, Cole B, Brewster R, et al. STAR Study Principal Investigators. A prospective study of autologous chondrocyte implantation in patients with failed prior treatment for articular cartilage defect of the knee: results of the Study of the Treatment of Articular Repair (STAR) clinical trial. Am J Sports Med. 2009; 37(1):42–55

[7] Bentley G, Biant LC, Carrington RW, et al. A prospective, randomised comparison of autologous chondrocyte implantation versus mosaicplasty for osteochondral defects in the knee. J Bone Joint Surg Br. 2003; 85(2):223–230

[8] Knutsen, G, Engebretsen, L, Ludvigsen, TC, et al. Autologous chondrocyte implantation compared with microfracture in the knee. A randomized trial. J Bone Joint Surg Am. 2004; 86-A(3):455–464

[9] Anz A W, Hackel JG, Nilssen EC, Andrews JR. Application of biologics in the treatment of the rotator cuff, meniscus, cartilage, and osteoarthritis. J Am Acad Orthop Surg. 2014; 22(2):68–79

[10] Moran CJ, Busilacchi A, Lee CA, Athanasiou KA, Verdonk PC. Biological augmentation and tissue engineering approaches in meniscus surgery. Arthroscopy. 2015; 31(5):944–955

[11] Akeda K, Imanishi T, Ohishi K. Intradiscal injection of autologous platelet-rich-plasma for the treatment of lumbar disc degeneration—preliminary prospective clinical trial for discogenic low back pain patients. Paper presented at: Orthopaedic Research Society Annual Meeting. San Francisco 2012

[12] Han I. Autologous adipose derived stem cell therapy for intervertebral disc degeneration. https://ClinicalTrials.gov/show/NCT02338271; 2015. Accessed October 13, 2016

[13] Moriguchi Y, Alimi M, Khair T, et al. biological treatment approaches for degenerative disk disease: A literature review of in vivo animal and clinical data. Global Spine J. 2016; 6(5):497–518

[14] Malda J, Martens DE, Tramper J, van Blitterswijk CA, Riesle J. Cartilage tissue engineering: controversy in the effect of oxygen. Crit Rev Biotechnol. 2003; 23(3):175–194

[15] Laurencin CT, Ambrosio AM, Borden MD, Cooper JA, Jr. Tissue engineering: orthopedic applications. Annu Rev Biomed Eng. 1999; 1(1):19–46

[16] Buirski G. Magnetic resonance signal patterns of lumbar discs in patients with low back pain. A prospective study with discographic correlation. Spine. 1992; 17(10):1199–1204

[17] Howell R, Kumar NS, Patel N, Tom J. Degenerative meniscus: pathogenesis, diagnosis, and treatment options. World J Orthop. 2014; 5(5):597–602

[18] Buckwalter JA, Mankin HJ. Articular cartilage: degeneration and osteoarthritis, repair, regeneration, and transplantation. Instr Course Lect. 1998; 47:487–504

[19] Urban JP, Roberts S. Degeneration of the intervertebral disc. Arthritis Res Ther. 2003; 5(3):120–130

[20] Adams MA, Freeman BJ, Morrison HP, Nelson IW, Dolan P. Mechanical initiation of intervertebral disc degeneration. Spine. 2000; 25(13):1625–1636

[21] Palmoski MJ, Brandt KD. Effects of static and cyclic compressive loading on articular cartilage plugs in vitro. Arthritis Rheum. 1984; 27(6):675–681

[22] Mow VC, Huiskes R. Basic Orthopaedic Biomechanics & Mechano-biology. Lippincott Williams & Wilkins; 2005

[23] Buckwalter JA. Osteoarthritis and articular cartilage use, disuse, and abuse: experimental studies. J Rheumatol Suppl. 1995; 43:13–15

[24] Valentin JE, Badylak JS, McCabe GP, Badylak SF. Extracellular matrix bioscaffolds for orthopaedic applications. A comparative histologic study. J Bone Joint Surg Am. 2006; 88(12):2673–2686

[25] Dahl JP, Caballero M, Pappa AK, Madan G, Shockley WW, van Aalst JA. Analysis of human auricular cartilage to guide tissue-engineered nanofiber-based chondrogenesis: implications for microtia reconstruction. Otolaryngol Head Neck Surg. 2011; 145(6):915–923

[26] Sandmann GH, Eichhorn S, Vogt S, et al. Generation and characterization of a human acellular meniscus scaffold for tissue engineering. J Biomed Mater Res A. 2009; 91(2):567–574

[27] Iatridis JC, Kumar S, Foster RJ, Weidenbaum M, Mow VC. Shear mechanical properties of human lumbar annulus fibrosus. J Orthop Res. 1999; 17(5):732–737

[28] Iatridis JC, Nicoll SB, Michalek AJ, Walter BA, Gupta MS. Role of biomechanics in intervertebral disc degeneration and regenerative therapies: what needs repairing in the disc and what are promising biomaterials for its repair? Spine J. 2013; 13(3):243–262

[29] Griffin DJ, Bonnevie ED, Lachowsky DJ, et al. Mechanical characterization of matrix-induced autologous chondrocyte implantation (MACI®) grafts in an equine model at 53 weeks. J Biomech. 2015; 48(10):1944–1949

[30] Bichara DA, O'Sullivan NA, Pomerantseva I, et al. The tissue-engineered auricle: past, present, and future. Tissue Eng Part B Rev. 2012; 18(1):51–61

[31] Henriksson HB, Hagman M, Horn M, Lindahl A, Brisby H. Investigation of different cell types and gel carriers for cell-based intervertebral disc therapy, in vitro and in vivo studies. J Tissue Eng Regen Med. 2012; 6(9):738–747

[32] Tatara AM, Mikos AG. Tissue Engineering in Orthopaedics. J Bone Joint Surg Am. 2016; 98(13):1132–1139

[33] Hudson KD, Alimi M, Grunert P, Härtl R, Bonassar LJ. Recent advances in biological therapies for disc degeneration: tissue engineering of the annulus fibrosus, nucleus pulposus and whole intervertebral discs. CurrOpinBiotechnol. 2013; 24(5):872–879

[34] Curl WW, Krome J, Gordon ES, Rushing J, Smith BP, Poehling GG. Cartilage injuries: a review of 31,516 knee arthroscopies. Arthroscopy. 1997; 13(4):456–460

[35] Hicks GE, Morone N, Weiner DK. Degenerative lumbar disc and facet disease in older adults: prevalence and clinical correlates. Spine. 2009; 34(12):1301–1306

[36] Basad E, Ishaque B, Bachmann G, Stürz H, Steinmeyer J. Matrix-induced autologous chondrocyte implantation versus microfracture in the treatment of cartilage defects of the knee: a 2-year randomised study. Knee Surg Sports Traumatol Arthrosc. 2010; 18(4):519–527

[37] Dewan AK, Gibson MA, Elisseeff JH, Trice ME. Evolution of autologous chondrocyte repair and comparison to other cartilage repair techniques. BioMed Res Int. 2014; 2014:272481

[38] Huang BJ, Hu JC, Athanasiou KA. Cell-based tissue engineering strategies used in the clinical repair of articular cartilage. Biomaterials. 2016; 98:1–22

[39] Mithöfer K, Peterson L, Mandelbaum BR, Minas T. Articular cartilage repair in soccer players with autologous chondrocyte transplantation: functional outcome and return to competition. Am J Sports Med. 2005; 33(11):1639–1646

[40] Crawford DC, DeBerardino TM, Williams RJ, III. NeoCart, an autologous cartilage tissue implant, compared with microfracture for treatment of distal femoral cartilage lesions: an FDA phase-II prospective, randomized clinical trial after two years. J Bone Joint Surg Am. 2012; 94(11):979–989

[41] Nehrer S, Chiari C, Domayer S, Barkay H, Yayon A. Results of chondrocyte implantation with a fibrin-hyaluronan matrix: a preliminary study. Clin OrthopRelat Res. 2008; 466(8):1849–1855

[42] Zak L, Albrecht C, Wondrasch B, et al. Results 2 years after matrix-associated autologous chondrocyte transplantation using the Novocart 3D Scaffold: an analysis of clinical and radiological data. Am J Sports Med. 2014; 42(7):1618–1627

[43] Yanke AB, Tilton AK, Wetters NG, Merkow DB, Cole BJ. DeNovo NT particulated juvenile cartilage implant. Sports Med Arthrosc Rev. 2015; 23(3):125–129

[44] McCormick F, Cole BJ, Nwachukwu B, Harris JD, Adkisson HD, Farr J. Treatment of focal cartilage defects with a juvenile allogeneic 3-dimensional articular cartilage graft. Oper Tech Sports Med. 2013; 21(2):95–99

[45] Pelttari K, Pippenger B, Mumme M, et al. Adult human neural crest-derived cells for articular cartilage repair. SciTransl Med. 2014; 6(251):251ra119

[46] Mumme M, Miot S, et al. Nasal chondrocyte-based engineered autologous cartilage tissue for repair of articular cartilage defects: an observational first-in-human trial. Lancet. 2016; 388(10055):1985–1994

[47] Ahmed AM, Burke DL. In-vitro measurement of static pressure distribution in synovial joints–Part I: Tibial surface of the knee. J BiomechEng. 1983; 105(3):216–225

[48] Majewski M, Susanne H, Klaus S. Epidemiology of athletic knee injuries: a 10-year study. Knee. 2006; 13(3):184–188

[49] Vrancken ACT, Buma P, van Tienen TG. Synthetic meniscus replacement: a review. IntOrthop. 2013; 37(2):291–299

[50] Chan WP. Novel one-step repair of knee meniscal tear using platelet-rich fibrin. https://ClinicalTrials.gov/show/NCT01211119; 2011

[51] Dohan DM, Choukroun J, Diss A, et al. Platelet-rich fibrin (PRF): a second-generation platelet concentrate. Part I: technological concepts and evolution. Oral Surg Oral Med Oral Pathol Oral Radiol Endod. 2006; 101(3):e37–e44

[52] Kuo, T-F, Lin, M-F, Lin, Y-H, et al. Implantation of platelet-rich fibrin and cartilage granules facilitates cartilage repair in the injured rabbit knee: preliminary report. Clinics (Sao Paulo). 2011; 66(10):1835–1838

[53] Duygulu F, Demirel M, Atalan G, et al. Effects of intra-articular administration of autologous bone marrow aspirate on healing of full-thickness meniscal tear: an experimental study on sheep. Acta OrthopTraumatol Turc. 2012; 46(1):61–67

[54] Vacanti C, Cima L, Ratkowski D, Upton J, Vacanti J. Tissue engineering of new cartilage in the shape of a human ear employing specially configured synthetic polymers seeded with chondrocytes. Paper presented at: Materials Research Society Symposium Proceedings 1992

[55] Cohen DL, Malone E, Lipson H, Bonassar LJ. Direct freeform fabrication of seeded hydrogels in arbitrary geometries. Tissue Eng. 2006; 12(5):1325–1335

[56] Zhou L, Pomerantseva I, Bassett EK, et al. Engineering ear constructs with a composite scaffold to maintain dimensions. Tissue Eng Part A. 2011; 17(11–12):1573–1581

[57] Fulco I, Miot S, Haug MD, et al. Engineered autologous cartilage tissue for nasal reconstruction after tumour resection: an observational first-in-human trial. Lancet. 2014; 384(9940):337–346

[58] Raj PP. Intervertebral disc: anatomy-physiology-pathophysiology-treatment. Pain Pract. 2008; 8(1):18–44

[59] Denis F. The three column spine and its significance in the classification of acute thoracolumbar spinal injuries. Spine. 1983; 8(8):817–831

[60] Cavanaugh JM, Ozaktay AC, Yamashita HT, King AI. Lumbar facet pain: biomechanics, neuroanatomy and neurophysiology. J Biomech. 1996; 29(9):1117–1129

[61] Osti OL, Vernon-Roberts B, Moore R, Fraser RD. Annular tears and disc degeneration in the lumbar spine. A post-mortem study of 135 discs. J Bone Joint Surg Br. 1992; 74(5):678–682

[62] Niemeyer P, Pestka JM, Kreuz PC, et al. Standardized cartilage biopsies from the intercondylar notch for autologous chondrocyte implantation (ACI). Knee Surg Sports Traumatol Arthrosc. 2010; 18(8):1122–1127

[63] Histogenics Corporation announces financial and operating results for the fourth quarter and year ended December 31, 2015 [press release]. Waltham, Mass: Investor Relations, March 10, 2016

[64] Maffet M. Cartilage Restoration Procedures - Autologous Chondrocyte Implantation. https://www.drmaffet.com/knee-surgery-houston/cartilage-restoration-procedures-autologous-chondrocyte-implantation/#lightbox[gallery-1]/9/. Accessed January 3, 2017

[65] Histogenics. NeoCart. 2016; http://www.histogenics.com/products-platform/neocart. Accessed October 13, 2016

[66] TETEC. Novocart. 2016; http://www.tetec-ag.com/cps/rde/xchg/cw-tetec-en-int/hs.xsl/7232.html. Accessed October 13, 2016

[67] Adkisson HD , IV, Gillis MP, Davis EC, Maloney W, Hruska K A. In vitro generation of scaffold independent neocartilage. Clin OrthopRelat Res. 2001(391) Suppl:S280–S294

[68] Halpin M. US regulatory environment for cell therapy products: Industry case studies. Genzyme. http://www.mfds.go.kr/jsp/common/download.jsp?fileinfo=S*5*%B9%CC%20FDA%20%C7%E3%B0%A1%BB%E7%B7%CA%20%B0%F8%C0%AF%20(Case%20I)_Dr_Halpin.pdf*0aa6f2a7186c4e9

cd6a08770133f0b4b*pdf*/files/upload/1/TB_F_INFODATA/12018/ 0aa6f2a7186c4e9 cd6a08770133f0b4b*545333*2011:11:07%2010:36:10. Accessed October 13, 2016

[69] Zimmer. DeNovo NT Natural Tissue Graft: Surgical Technique. 2009; http:// www.zimmer.com/content/dam/zimmer-web/documents/en-US/pdf/surgical-techniques/knee/zimmer-denovo-nt-natural-tissue-graft-surgical-technique.pdf. Accessed October 13, 2016

11 Treatment of Degenerative Disc Disease and Disc Regeneration: Proteins and Genes

Daisuke Sakai and Jordy Schol

Abstract

Treatment of degenerative disc disease (DDD) and disc regeneration by administration of proteins and genes has been studied for the past 2 decades. To facilitate treatment of DDD and disc regeneration, the agents need to possess anabolic effects, which promotes cell proliferation, enhance production of matrix, or inhibit catabolic pathways. Various peptides, proteins, and compounds derived synthetically or from natural herbs have been analyzed to possess an effect on IVD cell metabolism. Additionally, enhancements of specific genes by gene transduction have also been assessed to facilitate anabolic and anticatabolic responses in IVD cells. Despite abounding amounts of basic research published, very few proteins are found in the market as an actual medicinal product. One reason for this may be due to the character of the disease being affected by multiple factors that makes it difficult to prove the products' efficacy in clinical trials.

Keywords: annulus fibrosus, gene therapy, intervertebral disc, nucleus pulposus, protein injections, regenerative medicine

11.1 Overview and Historical Perspective of Peptides, Proteins, and Compound Injection Therapy or Gene Therapy for Intervertebral Repair

Degeneration of the intervertebral disc (IVD) is the primary cause of degenerative disc disease (DDD) that is frequently associated with low back and neck pain.[1,2] For the past 2 decades, there has been plenty of ongoing research to develop biological treatment strategies for IVD repair. The fundamental strategy behind biological IVD repair is to facilitate endogenous cell survival, viability, and function. The main functional role of IVD cells is to produce and remodel appropriate extracellular matrix (ECM). Among the biological treatment strategies, this chapter covers two major areas that have been reported in the literature: (1) to inject peptides, proteins, and compounds (excluding growth factors and growth factor-related proteins) and (2) IVD cell gene therapy. Numerous proteins and compounds have been shown to promote nucleus pulposus (NP) cell proliferation and stimulate ECM synthesis. Some assessed factors also exhibit anti-inflammatory effects or downregulate catabolic responses. Because the IVD consists of a compartment-like anatomy and is secluded from the vasculature, localized injections of agents are easier compared with

other organs. Additionally, administration can be achieved by discography approaches, which makes it easier for the clinicians to deliver the agents compared with open surgery approaches often used in, for example, articular cartilage regeneration. However, it has been suggested that IVD puncture can induce degeneration.[3] Systemic approaches to deliver agents to the IVD may not be optimal due to the avascular nature of the IVD, resulting in low efficiency and high dose requirements.

Another option to stimulate cells is by gene transfer, also known as gene therapy. (▶ Fig. 11.1) Gene therapy allows for the introduction of new or overexpressed genes into a cell population. Although very promising, gene therapy has for a long time been an undesirable field of research due to a failed gene therapy clinical trial in 1999 that resulted in the death of an 18-year-old patient with ornithine transcarbamylase deficiency. In the past few years, gene therapy has regained interest and has been investigated as a treatment option for a variety of musculoskeletal diseases. The genes tested include morphogens, growth factors, and anti-inflammatory agents. Proteins produced endogenously as a result of gene therapy are nascent molecules that have undergone posttranslational modification. Gene transfer also has the advantage that it can deliver products with an intracellular site of action, such as transcription factors, noncoding ribonucleic acid (RNA), and proteins that need to be inserted into a cell compartment or membrane.[4] After an initial experimental feasibility study using adenovirus vector to deliver *LacZ* gene into rabbit IVDs, many genes have been transferred to IVD cells in in vitro and in vivo experimental models.[5,6] However, gene therapy has not been performed in humans to treat DDD due to the fact that vectors with high gene transfection efficiency are primarily viral, which may induce serious side effects. Gene therapy may become more prominent with the development of safer, more efficient and controllable gene transfer methods.

11.2 Strategies Using Peptides, Proteins, and Compounds

Injection of peptides, proteins, and compounds is a common practice in the clinic. Proteins are biomolecules or macromolecules composed of long chain amino acid residues. Peptides on the other hand are also composed of amino acid chains, but are by definition up to 50 amino acids long. Both constitute the building blocks and machinery of the cells and are capable of stimulating cells by activating or inhibiting cell receptor activity or by resulting in ECM alterations (▶ Fig. 11.1; ▶ Table 11.1).

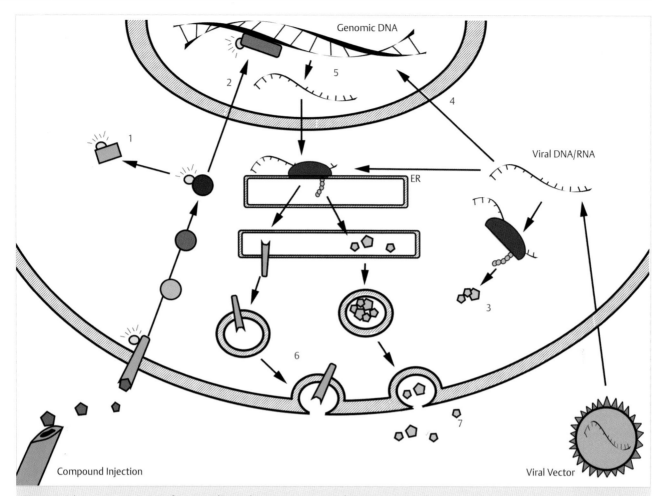

Fig. 11.1 Schematic presentation of agent and gene therapy treatment mechanism. Injection of agents or viral vector to target cell in order to alter cell behavior or phenotype. **(1)** Receptor-pathway activation by injected agent. **(2)** Agent-receptor–mediated transcription activation of regenerative genes. **(3)** Translation of viral deoxyribonucleic acid (DNA) or ribonucleic acid (RNA) either in cytosol or at the endoplasmic reticulum. **(4)** Incorporation of viral DNA or RNA into the host genome. **(5)** Activated transcription of regenerative genes by transcription vectors translated from transfected genetic material. **(6)** Introduced genetic material resulted in membrane receptors on cell membrane. **(7)** Secretion of proteins and compounds encoded by the introduced DNA or RNA.

Table 11.1 Overview of assessed proteins, peptides, and compounds for IVD regeneration

Name	Type	Researcher	Year	Species	Vitro/Vivo	Findings
Alendronate	Compound	Luo et al	2013	Rat	Vivo	Increased COL2 and ACAN expression
						Decreased MMP-1, -3, and -13 expression
						Decreased MMP-1, -3, and -13 protein levels
						Maintained imaging features
Lactoferricin	Peptide	Kim et al	2012	Bovine	Vitro	Increased expression of TIMP-1, -2, and -3
						Decreased expression of ADMATS-4 and -5, MMP-1 and -3
						Increased protein level of TIMP-1, -2, and -3
						Decreased protein level of ADMATS-4 and -5, MMP-1 and -3
						Increased PG deposition
		Kim et al	2013	Human	Vitro	Limited IL-1 and LPS–mediated PG deterioration

Table 11.1 (continued)

Name	Type	Researcher	Year	Species	Vitro/Vivo	Findings
						Decreased MMP-1, -3, and -13, ADAMTS-4, -5 expression
						Decreased MMP-1, -3, and -13, and ADAMTS-4, -5 production
				Bovine	Vitro	Limited IL-1 and LPS–mediated PG deterioration
						Decreased MMP-1, -3, and -13, and ADAMTS-4 and -5 expression
						Decreased MMP-1, -3, and -13, and ADAMTS-4 and -5 production
				Murine	Ex vivo	Attenuated IL-6 and LPS–mediated matrix deterioration
				Rabbit	Ex vivo	Attenuated IL-6 and LPS–mediated matrix deterioration
		Ellman et al	2013	Bovine	Vitro	Increased ACAN expression
						Increased ACAN deposition when combined with BMP-7
Link-N	Protein	Mwale et al	2003	Bovine	Vitro	Increased PG, type II and IX collagen production
						Increased cell number
						Decreased MMP production
		Wang et al	2013	Human	Vitro	Increased COL2 and ACAN expression
						Decreased of MMP-1 expression
						Decreased of MMP-1 production
		Wang et al	2013	Rabbit	Vitro	Increased ACAN, COL2, BMP-4, BMP-7 and SOX9 expression
						Increased aggrecan, type II collagen, SOX9 and BMP7 production
Lovastatin	Compound	Hu et al	2011	Human	Vitro	Increased COL2 and SOX9 expression
						Decreased COL1 expression
						Increased BMP2 and BMP7 expression
		Hu et al	2014	Rat	Vivo	Increased ACAN, COL2 and SOX9 expression
						Decreased COL1 expression
						Increased BMP-2 and type 2 collagen production
Paeoniflorin	Compound	Lijun et al	2015	Rabit	Vivo	Reduced apoptotic cell number
Peniel 2000	Peptide	Kwon et al	2013	Bovine	Vitro	Increased type 2 COL and aggrecan production with TGF-β
				Rabbit	Vivo	Improved imaging features
						Increased PG deposition
Resveratol	Compound	Li et al	2010	Bovine	Vitro	Reduced IL-1 or bFGF induced MMP-13 and ADAMTS-4 expression
						Increased PG deposition
		Wuertz et al	2011	Human	Vitro	Reduced MMP-1, -3, -13, and IL-6 and IL-8 expression
						Reduced MMP-1, -3, -13, and IL-6 and IL-8 production

Table 11.1 (continued)

Name	Type	Researcher	Year	Species	Vitro/Vivo	Findings
				Rat	Vivo	Reduced pain behavior
Simvastatin	Compound	Zhang et al	2008	Rat	Vitro	Increased BMP-2, COL2, and ACAN expression
						Increased PG deposition
		Than et al	2014	Rat	Vivo	Increased COL2 and ACAN expression
						Increased PG deposition
						Retarded disc degeneration

Abbreviations: BMP, bone morphogenetic protein; COL, collagen; IL, interleukin; LPS, lipopolysaccharide; MMP, matrix metalloproteinase; PG, proteoglycan; SOX9, SRY (sex determining region Y) box 9; TGF, transforming growth factor; TIMP, tissue inhibitor of metalloproteinase.

11.2.1 Statins

Statins or 3-hydroxy-3-methylglutaryl-coenzyme A (HMG-CoA) reductase inhibitors are highly effective cholesterol-lowering drugs that are believed to reduce the morbidity associated with coronary artery disease. In 1999, through an examination of 30,000 compounds in a search for a bone morphogenetic (BMP)-2 inducing stimulant, investigators found that HMG-CoA reductase inhibitor statin was the only compound that specifically increased BMP-2 messenger RNA (mRNA) levels in osteoblasts.[7] This finding confirmed BMP's capacity to enhance matrix production by IVD cells.[8] These findings led to the work of Zhang and Lin in 2008, which tested the stimulatory effect of simvastatin on IVD cell metabolism.[9] The results of this study showed that simvastatin significantly upregulated BMP-2 mRNA expression, followed by aggrecan and type II collagen gene expression and proteoglycan deposition by IVD cells. This effect was mediated through the inhibition of the mevalonate pathway. The same group further reported an in vivo study using a rattail IVD puncture model to test whether simvastatin can facilitate IVD regeneration. In this study, simvastatin was loaded in poly(ethylene glycol)-poly(lactic acid-co-glycolic acid)-poly(ethylene glycol) gel and injected in the injured IVD. Results showed that this treatment increased aggrecan expression and sulfated glycosaminoglycan (sGAG) content, and significantly increased mRNA levels of BMP-2 and type II collagen in the IVD. Magnetic resonance imaging (MRI) findings and histology also demonstrated milder degeneration in the IVDs receiving treatment, which suggested that single injection of simvastatin possesses the potential to retard or regenerate the degenerative IVD. Other research groups looked into lovastatin, the first statin in the market. It was tested in vitro and showed upregulation of genes encoding type II collagen and transcription factor SRY (sex determining region Y) box 9 (SOX9) in human degenerative NP cells, while suppressing the expression of type I collagen.[10] Subsequently, by in vivo examination, it was confirmed that intradiscal administration of lovastatin solution upregulated the expressions of BMP-2 and SOX9 and promoted chondrogenesis of rat caudal discs after needle puncture and substance injection.[11] These results demonstrate potential regenerative effects of statins in IVD degeneration. Where we are now with the application for IVD regeneration or associated back pain still remains to be clarified. Although a large-scale animal study has been reported to determine dose and effect, no clinical trials or study in humans has been found to date and this potential treatment awaits investigation.[12]

11.2.2 Bisphosphonates

Bisphosphonates are drugs reported to be effective in conditions with bone fragility, and commonly are prescribed to elderly patients for the treatment of osteoporosis. A previous study on correlation of bone mineral density and lumbar IVD degeneration has shown that bone mineral density of not only the lumbar vertebrae but also the calcaneus and radius was mutually related to lumbar IVD degeneration from an early stage of degeneration.[13] A laboratory investigation using ovariectomized (OVX) rats has shown strong association between osteopenia and disc degeneration.[14] These facts led the experiment to test whether alendronate, one of the most common bisphosphonates in the market, has any effect on the progression of IVD degeneration. Results demonstrated that subcutaneous injections of alendronate in OVX rats helped in preserving the anatomical structure and function of the adjacent vertebrae and motion segments. Also retarded progression of IVD degeneration and maintained matrix metabolism was observed compared with the saline control.[15] Up until now no clinical investigation has been reported.

11.2.3 Lactoferricin

Lactoferricin is an iron- and heparin-binding glycoprotein from the transferrin family, which is synthesized by epithelial cells and is present in most mammalian exocrine secretions. Lactoferricin has been isolated from bovine milk by pepsin digestion as LfcinB[16] and has been shown to possess anti-inflammatory, antioxidative, anticatabolic, and anabolic effects on bovine disc cells in vitro.[17,18] Furthermore, a recent report indicates that LfcinB synergistically stimulates anabolic effect in IVD cells with BMP-7. This effect results from LfcinB-mediated activation of Sp1 and SMAD signaling pathways by (1) phosphorylation of SMAD1/5/8; (2) downregulation of SMAD inhibitory factors (i.e., noggin [BMP receptor antagonist] and SMAD6 [inhibitory SMAD]); and (3) upregulation of SMAD4 (universal co-SMAD). (▶ Fig. 11.2) These data indicate that LfcinB suppression of noggin may eliminate the negative feedback of BMP-7, thereby maximizing biological activity of BMP-7 and ultimately shifting homeostasis to a proanabolic state in disc cells.[19] No clinical investigations are available.

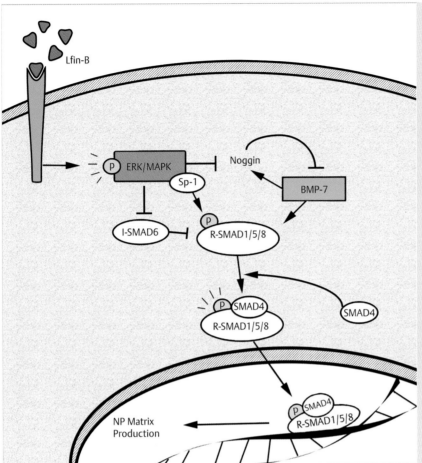

Fig. 11.2 ERK/MAPK and SMAD mediated pathway by lactoferricin activation. LfcinB stimulates ERK/MAPK pathway resulting activation of R-SMAD1/5/8 allowing for SMAD4-SMAD1/5/8 combination for matrix component and SOX9 expression. Moreover, noggin and SMAD6 are inhibited by ERK/MAPK activation. (Adapted with permission from Ellman et al 2013.[19]) Abbreviations: BMP, bone morphogenetic protein; NP, nucleus pulposus; Sp-1, specificity protein 1; Lfin-B, lactoferricin.

11.2.4 Peniel 2000

A novel peptide named Peniel 2000 (P2K) with a binding activity to transforming growth factor (TGF)-β1 was discovered using a knowledge-based in silico drug discovery strategy from biglycan, an ECM component of the IVD. TGF-β1 stimulation can demonstrate an anabolic effect in IVD cells. TGF-β1 is able to signal through type I receptors ALK1 and ALK5 with opposing effects (▶ Fig. 11.3). ALK1 dependent pathway activates through phosphorylation of SMAD1/5/8 and ALK5 dependent pathway activates through SMAD2/3 phosphorylation. A study has shown that regulation of TGF-β signaling through these two independent pathways is a key mechanism in the degenerative process of IVDs. TGF-β1 could stimulate the synthesis of ECM components by the SMAD2 pathway via ALK5 and inhibit the regeneration of IVD tissue by the SMAD1/5/8 pathway via ALK1. It was reported that TGF-β1 activates both anabolic SMAD2 and antianabolic SMAD1/5/8 pathways, and a tight balance between the two pathways inhibits the regeneration of degenerative IVDs. P2K treatment blocks the antianabolic pathway by SMAD1/5/8, but allows a minimal activation of anabolic pathway by SMAD2, thus induces the expression of ECM in IVDs and stimulates regeneration of IVDs.[20] No clinical application of P2K has been reported.

11.2.5 Link Protein Peptide

Link protein is a glycoprotein that stabilizes the interaction between major matrix structural components: aggrecan and hyaluronan[21] (▶ Fig. 11.4). In human articular cartilage, link protein binds aggrecan along the hyaluronan chain. The resulting aggregates are trapped within the meshlike network of type II collagen fibrils, producing a large, stable macromolecular structure that contributes to water retention, compression resistance, and shock absorption in the cartilage.[22] Link protein exists in three isoforms, LP1, LP2, and LP3, all derived from the same structural gene. LP1 and LP2 are different glycosylated forms of the same intact protein core. LP3 is proteolytically derived from either LP1 or LP2 and formed by proteolytic cleavage between His16-Ile17 residues, resulting in the loss of the N-terminal 16 amino acids. This amino terminal peptide of link protein (link N) has been reported to possess anabolic effects in IVD cells.[23] Link N can further stimulate proteoglycan production in vivo in both the NP and annulus fibrosus (AF) when it is administered to the degenerate disc. In addition to stimulating the synthesis of aggrecan, link N is also able to downregulate metalloproteinase expression in the degenerate disc. Another study has shown that (1) link N upregulates mRNA expression of aggrecan and type II collagen and the protein level of type II collagen as well as sGAG; (2) the full length of link N is required

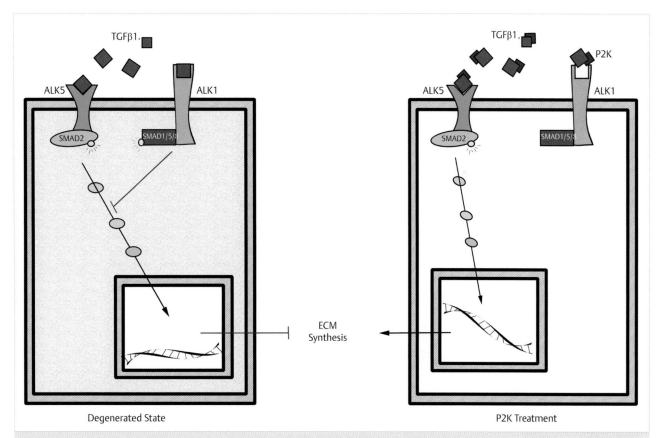

Fig. 11.3 Mechanism of TGFβ1-ALK1 activation inhibited by P2K. P2K inhibits binding of TGFβ1 to ALK1, resulting in decreased inhibition of the ALK5-mediated pathway. (Adapted with permission from Kwon et al 2013.[20]) Abbreviations: ECM, extracellular matrix; TGF, transforming growth factor.

for this upregulation—neither the reverse sequences of link N nor the truncated link Ns have shown the same beneficial effect as the full-length link N; and (3) link N has a much lesser osteoinductive effect compared to BMP-2 and BMP-7 as measured by osteocalcin mRNA and alkaline phosphatase activity. Taken together, these results suggest that link N could have value in stimulating the growth and regeneration of degenerated discs with less concern of forming unwanted bone-like tissue.[24] The same group further revealed that link N promotes disc matrix production, which was evidenced by increased expression of the chondrocyte-specific transcription factor SOX9 and the ECM macromolecules aggrecan and type II collagen. Using colocalization and pulldown studies they further document a noggin-insensitive direct peptide–protein association between link N and BMP-RII. This association mediated SMAD signaling converges on BMP genes leading to expression of BMP-4 and BMP-7. Furthermore, through a cell-autonomous loop BMP-4 and BMP-7 intensified SMAD1/5 signaling though a feed forward circuit involving BMP-RI, ultimately promoting expression of SOX9 and downstream aggrecan and type II collagen genes.[25] No clinical application has been reported.

11.2.6 Paeoniflorin

Paeoniflorin is an active component isolated from the Chinese medicinal herb, Paeoniae Radix. It has been reported to exhibit anti-inflammatory, analgesic, and antioxidative properties. One study has explored the effect of intragastric injection of paeoniflorin in a rabbit annular stab model and investigated its effect on apoptosis within the IVD. Results of the study indicated that the expression levels of Bax and caspase-9 in the paeoniflorin groups were significantly reduced compared with the control group, whereas the expression of Bcl-2 was significantly increased, which suggested that paeoniflorin may prevent NP cell apoptosis during IVD degeneration.[26] No further study has been reported for human IVDs.

11.2.7 Resveratol

The natural compound phytoestrogen resveratrol (RSV) isolated from red wines has been known to possess chondroprotective effects in joint arthritis and IVD cells. RSV can promote cell proliferation, antagonize catabolic factors, and enhance anabolic factors for ECM production in chondrocytes.[27]In the IVD cells, it has been reported that catabolic factors matrix metalloproteinase (MMP)-13 and the disintegrin-like and metalloprotease with thrombospondin motifs (ADAMTS)-4 induced by bFGF or interleukin (IL)-1 stimulation was blocked with RSV at the transcription level in cultured bovine IVD cells. RSV also promoted ECM synthesis and rescued ECM degradation induced by catabolic agents.[28] Another study further looked into the anti-inflammatory effects of RSV for treating pain using human IVD cells. In vitro results of this study showed that IL-1β induced upregulation of IL-6 and IL-8, whereas MMP-1, MMP-3, and MMP-13 mRNA levels were

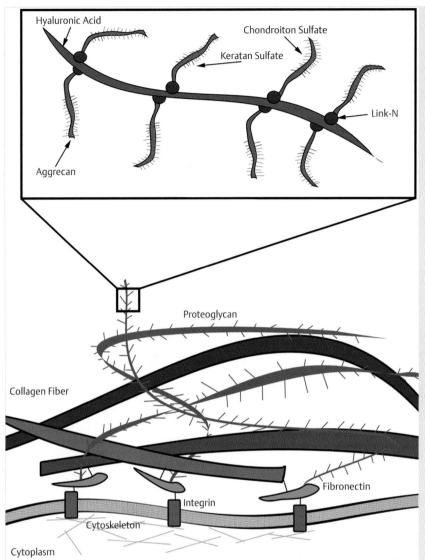

Fig. 11.4 Link N protein connecting ACAN to the hyaluronic acid (HA) backbone. A schematic representation of the extracellular matrix (ECM), zooming in on Link N as the linker between ACAN and HA.

reduced with RSV treatment. This effect appeared to not be mediated by mitogen-activated protein (MAP) kinase pathways or the NF-kappaB/SIRT1 pathway. Finally, in vivo administration in rats demonstrated that RSV treatment reduced IVD degenerative associated pain using a von Frey behavioral assessment in a rodent model of radiculopathy.[29] No clinical study has been performed to verify these effects in humans.

11.3 Strategies Using Gene Therapy

Gene therapy is an experimental technique that introduces genetic information to diseased cell populations to treat or prevent disease. For example, mutated genes can be inactivated, replaced, or removed. Also, new genes can be introduced. At present, research is focused on treating diseases brought about by a single-gene defect, such as cystic fibrosis or sickle cell anemia. However, the approaches discussed

below (▶ Table 11.2) utilize a gene construct with a promoter that allows for overexpression of the desired genes. Proteins constructed from the introduced gene can be post-translationally modified, such as glycosylation, as well as integrated into membranes or specific cell compartments. The genetic material, either deoxyribonucleic acid (DNA) or RNA, can be introduced into the host cell by viral or nonviral methods. Viral methods apply viruses, such as adenovirus or lentivirus, to introduce their genetic product into the cell. Depending on the virus, the DNA or RNA is then either temporally transcribed or permanently integrated into the host's chromosomal DNA (▶ Fig. 11.1). The second method uses naked DNA or complexes and is transferred into the cell by, for example, electroporation or nanoparticles. The advantage of the nonviral approach is the low host immunogenicity and potential of scalability; however, transfection efficiency remains low and most approaches are not applicable in situ.

Table 11.2 Overview of assessed gene transfers for IVD regeneration

Name	Type	Researcher	Year	Vector	Species	Vitro/Vivo	Findings
BMP-2	Protein	Moon et al	2012	Adenovirus	Human	Vitro	Increased PG production
		Wallach et al	2003	Adenovirus	Human	Vitro	Increased PG deposition
		Leckie et al	2012	AAV2	Rabbit	Vivo	Improved imaging features compared to degenerative model
							Retained type II collagen
							Retained matrix stiffness
							Increased elastic parameters
BMP-7	Protein	Gu et al	2015	AAV2	Canine	Vivo	Enhanced DHI maintenance
							Increased type II collagen and PG content
							Decreased type I collagen content
		Ren et al	2015	Adenovirus	Human	Vitro	Increased COL2 expression
GDF-5	Protein	Luo et al	2015	Adenovirus	Human	Vitro	Increased ACAN and COL2 expression
							Increased PG and type II collagen production
							Promoted cell proliferation
IGF-1	Protein	Moon et al	2012	Adenovirus	Human	Vitro	Increased PG production
		Zhang et al	2013	Adenovirus	Rabbit	Vitro	Decreased apoptotic cell number
LMP-1	Protein	Liu et al	2014	Lentivirus	Rat	Vitro	Increased COL2, ACAN, and versican expression
							Decreased MMP-3 and -13 expression
							Increased PG deposition
		Yoon et al	2004	Adenovirus	Rat	Vitro	Increased BMP-2, BMP-7, and ACAN expression
							Increased BMP2 and BMP7 production
							Increased PG deposition
		Kuh et al	2008	Adenovirus	Rabbit	Vitro	Increased ACAN, COL2, COL1, BMP-2, and BMP-7 expression by AF cells
							Increased ACAN, COL2, COL1, BMP-2, and BMP-7 production by AF cells
SOX9	Protein	Paul et al	2003	Adenovirus	Human	Vitro	Increased COL2 expression
							Increased type II collagen production
					Rabbit	Vivo	Preserved NP matrix architecture
		Ren et al	2015	Adenovirus	Human	Vitro	Increased COL2 expression
TGF-β1	Protein	Nishida et al	1999	AD/CMV	Rabbit	Vivo	Increased PG production

Table 11.2 (continued)

Name	Type	Researcher	Year	Vector	Species	Vitro/Vivo	Findings
		Moon et al	2012	Adenovirus	Human	Vitro	Increased PG production
TIMP-1	Protein	Wallach et al	2003	Adenovirus	Human	Vitro	Increased PG deposition
		Leckie et al	2012	AAV2	Rabbit	Vivo	Improved imaging features compared with degenerative model
							Retained type II collagen
							Unable to retain matrix stiffness

Abbreviations: AAV2, adeno-associated virus serotype 2; AF, annulus fibrosus; AV/CMV adenovirus/cytomegalovirus vector; BMP, bone morphogenetic protein; COL, collagen; DHI, disc height index; DGF, growth and differentiation factor; IGF, insulin-like growth factor; LMP, LIM mineralization protein; NP, nucleus pulposus; PG, proteoglycan; SOX9, SRY (sex determining region Y) box 9; TGF, transforming growth factor; TIMP, tissue inhibitor of metalloproteinase

11.3.1 TGF-β Superfamily Genes and IGF-1

There are many genes in the TGF-β superfamily that have been explored in research to affect IVD cell metabolism. TGF-β1 was the first gene tested for IVD regeneration. Adenovirus/cytomegalovirus vector containing human TGF-β1 complementary DNA (cDNA) (Ad/CMV-TGF-β1) was injected in rabbit IVDs. Results demonstrated an approximately 30-fold increase in active TGF-β1 synthesis and a 5-fold increase in total TGF-β1 production in rabbit IVDs receiving treatment. Consequently, a 2-fold increase of total proteoglycan in the IVDs receiving treatment was demonstrated.[30] In a later study by the same group, an identical approach was applied to assess the transduction of a TGF-β1 gene in human IVD cells. The result in vitro showed that similar to the study in rabbits, Ad/CMV-TGF-β1 also succeeded in transduction of TGF-β1 genes regardless of age, sex, surgical indication, disc level, and disc degeneration grade in 15 patients undergoing surgery.[31] In the same study, BMP-2 and insulin-like growth factor 1 (IGF-1) gene transfer was also assessed alone or in various combinations. Results showed that all treatment groups demonstrated significant upregulation of proteoglycan synthesis, suggesting that a cocktail of genes might also be applicable as treatment for DDD. Another study examined an adeno-associated virus serotype 2 (AAV2) vector used in a rabbit annular puncture model of disc degeneration to transfer BMP-2 gene. The result of this in vivo study showed that progression of IVD degeneration was retarded in the IVDs receiving AAV2-BMP-2, -IGF-1, and -TGFβ-1 injections by MRI findings and histology. The serum biochemical marker C-telopeptide of type II collagen increased in the degenerative control group but was recovered in the treated groups.[32] In a different study, human BMP-7 was also transduced by AAV2 to allogenic IVD cells of canines and transplanted to an IVD degeneration model. Results of this large animal study demonstrated that IVDs receiving allogenic NP cells transduced with AAV2-BMP-7 showed superior stability of the motion segment, and milder progression of degenerative changes detected by histology and enzyme-linked immunosorbent assay (ELISA).[33] Another study assessed the effect of overexpressing IGF-1 in rabbit NP cells and found that IGF-1 overexpression strongly inhibited apoptosis.[34] Finally, gene transduction of human growth and differentiation factor-5 (GDF-5) was tested using human degenerated NP cell cultures in vitro using adenoviral vector. Results showed that only NP cells that received treatment achieved upregulated proteoglycan and type II collagen synthesis at both protein and mRNA levels while promoting cell proliferation.[35]

11.3.2 TIMP-1

Tissue inhibitor metalloproteinase-1 (TIMP-1) acts to antagonize the catabolic effect of MMPs. Adenoviral vector mediated transduction of TIMP-1 was investigated in vitro using cultured human NP cells. Despite the fact that TIMP-1 acts as to oppose the degradation of newly synthesized proteoglycans, the results showed an increase in measured proteoglycans, which suggested that by activating TIMP-1, newly synthesized proteoglycans were allowed to accumulate in culture.[36]

11.3.3 LMP-1

LIM mineralization protein-1 (LMP-1) is a regulatory protein during osteogenesis and chondrogenesis. Its effects are accomplished via different mechanisms, including induction of cell proliferation and secretion of multiple different BMPs, as well as enhancement of BMP responsiveness by interaction with Smurf1 and Jab1.[37,38] It has been reported that genetic transduction of LMP-1 in vitro and in vivo is correlated with ECM synthesis in IVD cells. A study further investigated the effect of LMP-1 on IVD ECM production or degradation induced by inflammatory stimulation in a tumor necrosis factor (TNF)-α–induced cell model in vitro. The results of this study found that when lentivirus encoding LMP-1 was transfected, increased type II collagen, aggrecan, versican expression, and sGAG production could be observed. When short heparin LMP-1 was transfected, this was decreased. Lentivirus encoding LMP-1 abolished, whereas short heparin LMP-1 aggravated, TNF-α–mediated downregulation of the above matrix genes via ERK1/2 activation. Moreover, lentivirus encoding LMP-1 abrogated TNF-α–induced MMP-3 and MMP-13 expression via inhibiting p65 translocation and MMP-3 and MMP-13 promoter activity. LMP-1 had an ECM production maintenance effect under inflammatory stimulation. This effect was via upregulation of matrix gene expression at least partially through ERK1/2 activation, and downregulation of MMP expression through NF-kB inhibition.[39] LMP-1 transduced to AF cells by adenoviral vector in culture demonstrated increased sGAG production and increased mRNA expression of aggrecan, type I collagen, type II collagen, LMP-1, BMP-2, and BMP-7.[40]

11.3.4 SOX9

SOX9 is a pivotal transcription factor capable of induced chondorgenesis and crucial for chondrogenic phenotype maintenance.[41,42,43] Overexpression by adenoviral vector containing SOX9 in human degenerated IVD cells showed a strong increase in collagen type II production and mRNA expression.[44] Thereafter, an identical vector was introduced to degenerated rabbit IVDs. Compared with degenerated and green fluorescent protein (GFP)-transfected IVDs, the SOX9 transfected IVDs exhibited retention of ECM architecture and the NP cell morphology resembled more the healthy disc cell morphology, demonstrating the potential of SOX9 overexpression for disc degeneration attenuation. A different study also found increased COL2A1 expression when SOX9 was overexpressed by an adeno-associated viral vector in human NP cells.[45] Moreover, the investigators found that SOX9 cotransfected with BMP-7, resulting in significantly increased COL2A1 expression.

11.4 Future Perspectives

The development of peptide, protein, and compound injection therapies or gene therapies relies on the development of safe, efficient, cost-effective strategies that aim for real-market approval. Various agents and genes such as the ones listed above have been reported on in the literature. However, no human studies have been attempted to assess the effects or complications in humans. However, some products, such as BMPs and statins, are already widely used in the clinic for a variety of other musculoskeletal disorders and systemic diseases. One reason that we do not find these in the market for treatment in IVD diseases is due to the multifactorial nature of IVD degeneration, which makes it challenging to induce regeneration by single or even several factors. Identification of patients and their optimal treatment strategy is another difficult and elusive concern. Gene therapy approaches have shown promising results. Conceivably, new approaches and other targets, such as microRNA (miRNA) and small (or short) interfering RNA (siRNA), could give new insights and potential therapies for IVD degeneration. At present, only two gene therapy products have been approved by the US Food and Drug Administration and the European Medicines Agency for clinical use for patients with specific and severe indications. Ethical and safety issues need to be overcome in order to receive rational for in-human use of gene therapy for nonfatal diseases such as DDD.

In short, in vitro and in vivo studies show promising results to induce regeneration by implementing proteins or introducing gene constructs. However, a clear focus toward market application and market potentials is required when designing new studies, in order to advance the IVD regenerative medicine field.

11.5 References

[1] Chou D, Samartzis D, Bellabarba C, et al. Degenerative magnetic resonance imaging changes in patients with chronic low back pain: a systematic review. Spine. 2011; 36(21) Suppl:S43–S53

[2] Sakai D, Andersson GB. Stem cell therapy for intervertebral disc regeneration: obstacles and solutions. Nat Rev Rheumatol. 2015; 11(4):243–256

[3] Martin JT, Gorth DJ, Beattie EE, Harfe BD, Smith LJ, Elliott DM. Needle puncture injury causes acute and long-term mechanical deficiency in a mouse model of intervertebral disc degeneration. J Orthop Res. 2013; 31(8):1276–1282

[4] Evans CH, Huard J. Gene therapy approaches to regenerating the musculoskeletal system. Nat Rev Rheumatol. 2015; 11(4):234–242

[5] Nishida K, Kang JD, Suh JK, Robbins PD, Evans CH, Gilbertson LG. Adenovirus-mediated gene transfer to nucleus pulposus cells. Implications for the treatment of intervertebral disc degeneration. Spine. 1998; 23(22):2437–2442, discussion 2443

[6] Nishida K, Suzuki T, Kakutani K, et al. Gene therapy approach for disc degeneration and associated spinal disorders. Eur Spine J. 2008; 17 Suppl 4:459–466

[7] Mundy G, Garrett R, Harris S, et al. Stimulation of bone formation in vitro and in rodents by statins. Science. 1999; 286(5446):1946–1949

[8] Li J, Yoon ST, Hutton WC. Effect of bone morphogenetic protein-2 (BMP-2) on matrix production, other BMPs, and BMP receptors in rat intervertebral disc cells. J Spinal Disord Tech. 2004; 17(5):423–428

[9] Zhang H, Lin CY. Simvastatin stimulates chondrogenic phenotype of intervertebral disc cells partially through BMP-2 pathway. Spine. 2008; 33(16):E525–E531

[10] Hu MH, Hung LW, Yang SH, Sun YH, Shih TT, Lin FH. Lovastatin promotes redifferentiation of human nucleus pulposus cells during expansion in monolayer culture. Artif Organs. 2011; 35(4):411–416

[11] Hu MH, Yang KC, Chen YJ, Sun YH, Yang SH. Lovastatin prevents discography-associated degeneration and maintains the functional morphology of intervertebral discs. Spine J. 2014; 14(10):2459–2466

[12] Than KD, Rahman SU, Wang L, et al. Intradiscal injection of simvastatin results in radiologic, histologic, and genetic evidence of disc regeneration in a rat model of degenerative disc disease. Spine J. 2014; 14(6):1017–1028

[13] Nanjo Y, Morio Y, Nagashima H, Hagino H, Teshima R. Correlation between bone mineral density and intervertebral disk degeneration in pre- and postmenopausal women. J Bone Miner Metab. 2003; 21(1):22–27

[14] Wang T, Zhang L, Huang C, Cheng AG, Dang GT. Relationship between osteopenia and lumbar intervertebral disc degeneration in ovariectomized rats. Calcif Tissue Int. 2004; 75(3):205–213

[15] Luo Y, Zhang L, Wang WY, et al. Alendronate retards the progression of lumbar intervertebral disc degeneration in ovariectomized rats. Bone. 2013; 55(2):439–448

[16] Tsuda H, Sekine K, Fujita K, Ligo M. Cancer prevention by bovine lactoferrin and underlying mechanisms–a review of experimental and clinical studies. Biochem Cell Biol. 2002; 80(1):131–136

[17] Kim JS, Ellman MB, An HS, et al. Lactoferricin mediates anabolic and anti-catabolic effects in the intervertebral disc. J Cell Physiol. 2012; 227(4):1512–1520

[18] Kim JS, Ellman MB, Yan D, et al. Lactoferricin mediates anti-inflammatory and anti-catabolic effects via inhibition of IL-1 and LPS activity in the intervertebral disc. J Cell Physiol. 2013; 228(9):1884–1896

[19] Ellman MB, Kim J, An HS, et al. Lactoferricin enhances BMP7-stimulated anabolic pathways in intervertebral disc cells. Gene. 2013; 524(2):282–291

[20] Kwon YJ, Lee JW, Moon EJ, Chung YG, Kim OS, Kim HJ. Anabolic effects of Peniel 2000, a peptide that regulates TGF-β1 signaling on intervertebral disc degeneration. Spine. 2013; 38(2):E49–E58

[21] Hardingham, TE. The role of link-protein in the structure of cartilage proteoglycan aggregates. Biochem J. 1979; 177(1):237–247

[22] Seyfried NT, McVey GF, Almond A, Mahoney DJ, Dudhia J, Day AJ. Expression and purification of functionally active hyaluronan-binding domains from human cartilage link protein, aggrecan and versican: formation of ternary complexes with defined hyaluronan oligosaccharides. J Biol Chem. 2005; 280(7):5435–5448

[23] Mwale F, Demers CN, Petit A, et al. A synthetic peptide of link protein stimulates the biosynthesis of collagens II, IX and proteoglycan by cells of the intervertebral disc. J Cell Biochem. 2003; 88(6):1202–1213

[24] Wang Z, Hutton WC, Yoon ST. ISSLS Prize winner: effect of link protein peptide on human intervertebral disc cells. Spine. 2013; 38(17):1501–1507

[25] Wang Z, Weitzmann MN, Sangadala S, Hutton WC, Yoon ST. Link protein N-terminal peptide binds to bone morphogenetic protein (BMP) type II receptor and drives matrix protein expression in rabbit intervertebral disc cells. J Biol Chem. 2013; 288(39):28243–28253

[26] Shi L, Teng H, Zhu M, et al. Paeoniflorin inhibits nucleus pulposus cell apoptosis by regulating the expression of Bcl-2 family proteins and caspase-9 in a rabbit model of intervertebral disc degeneration. ExpTher Med. 2015; 10(1):257–262

[27] Im HJ, Li X, Chen D, et al. Biological effects of the plant-derived polyphenol resveratrol in human articular cartilage and chondrosarcoma cells. J Cell Physiol. 2012; 227(10):3488–3497

[28] Li X, Phillips FM, An HS, et al. The action of resveratrol, a phytoestrogen found in grapes, on the intervertebral disc. Spine. 2008; 33(24):2586–2595

[29] Wuertz K, Quero L, Sekiguchi M, et al. The red wine polyphenol resveratrol shows promising potential for the treatment of nucleus pulposus-mediated pain in vitro and in vivo. Spine. 2011; 36(21):E1373–E1384

[30] Nishida K, Kang JD, Gilbertson LG, et al. Modulation of the biologic activity of the rabbit intervertebral disc by gene therapy: an in vivo study of adenovirus-mediated transfer of the human transforming growth factor beta 1 encoding gene. Spine. 1999; 24(23):2419–2425

[31] Moon SH, Nishida K, Gilbertson LG, et al. Biologic response of human intervertebral disc cells to gene therapy cocktail. Spine. 2008; 33(17):1850–1855

[32] Leckie SK, Bechara BP, Hartman RA, et al. Injection of AAV2-BMP2 and AAV2-TIMP1 into the nucleus pulposus slows the course of intervertebral disc degeneration in an in vivo rabbit model. Spine J. 2012; 12(1):7–20

[33] Gu T, Shi Z, Wang C, et al. Human bone morphogenetic protein 7 transfected nucleus pulposus cells delay the degeneration of intervertebral disc in dogs. J Orthop Res. 2015. DOI: doi:10.1002/jor.22995

[34] Zhang CC, Cui GP, Hu JG, et al. Effects of adenoviral vector expressing hIGF-1 on apoptosis in nucleus pulposus cells in vitro. Int J Mol Med. 2014; 33(2):401–405

[35] Luo XW, Liu K, Chen Z, et al. Adenovirus-mediated GDF-5 promotes the extracellular matrix expression in degenerative nucleus pulposus cells. J Zhejiang UnivSci B. 2016; 17(1):30–42

[36] Wallach CJ, Sobajima S, Watanabe Y, et al. Gene transfer of the catabolic inhibitor TIMP-1 increases measured proteoglycans in cells from degenerated human intervertebral discs. Spine. 2003; 28(20):2331–2337

[37] Boden SD, Liu Y, Hair GA, et al. LMP-1, a LIM-domain protein, mediates BMP-6 effects on bone formation. Endocrinology. 1998; 139(12):5125–5134

[38] Sangadala S, Boden SD, Viggeswarapu M, Liu Y, Titus L. LIM mineralization protein-1 potentiates bone morphogenetic protein responsiveness via a novel interaction with Smurf1 resulting in decreased ubiquitination of Smads. J Biol Chem. 2006; 281(25):17212–17219

[39] Liu H, Pan H, Yang H, et al. LIM mineralization protein-1 suppresses TNF-α induced intervertebral disc degeneration by maintaining nucleus pulposus extracellular matrix production and inhibiting matrix metalloproteinases expression. J Orthop Res. 2015; 33(3):294–303

[40] Kuh SU, Zhu Y, Li J, et al. The AdLMP-1 transfection in two different cells; AF cells, chondrocytes as potential cell therapy candidates for disc degeneration. Acta Neurochir (Wien). 2008; 150(8):803–810

[41] Bell DM, Leung KK, Wheatley SC, et al. SOX9 directly regulates the type-II collagen gene. Nat Genet. 1997; 16(2):174–178

[42] Lefebvre V, de Crombrugghe B. Toward understanding SOX9 function in chondrocyte differentiation. Matrix Biol. 1998; 16(9):529–540

[43] de Crombrugghe B, Lefebvre V, Behringer RR, Bi W, Murakami S, Huang W. Transcriptional mechanisms of chondrocyte differentiation. Matrix Biol. 2000; 19(5):389–394

[44] Paul R, Haydon RC, Cheng H, et al. Potential use of Sox9 gene therapy for intervertebral degenerative disc disease. Spine. 2003; 28(8):755–763

[45] Ren XF, Diao ZZ, Xi YM, et al. Adeno-associated virus-mediated BMP-7 and SOX9 in vitro co-transfection of human degenerative intervertebral disc cells. Genet Mol Res. 2015; 14(2):3736–3744

12 Treatment of Degenerative Disc Disease/Disc Regeneration: Growth Factors and Platelet Rich Plasma

Koichi Masuda and Kenji Kato

Abstract

Homeostasis of the intervertebral disc (IVD) is tightly regulated by a biological balance between anabolic and catabolic activities of disc cells. Various growth factors that stimulate disc cell matrix synthesis have been evaluated preclinically using animal and human disc cells in vitro. Effective growth factors have also been tested for intradiscal injection therapy in a variety of animal species with promising structural modification results. Some growth factors have been evaluated for safety in humans; however, further studies are needed for human applications. Because most primary outcome measures in clinical trials have had pain-related outcomes, to achieve future successful development of growth factor therapies it is essential to develop animal models that provide evidence for pain relief and to establish pharmacokinetic models.

As a point-of-care product, platelet rich plasma (PRP) has gained clinical attention in the orthopaedic field. A prospective, double-blind, randomized controlled study has been published showing encouraging results; future large-scale multicenter trials should reveal its clinical usefulness for patients with discogenic pain. Although limitations of growth factor therapy, including the lack of nutrients and hypoxic and acidic conditions, are well recognized, it can be anticipated that its application to meticulously selected patients will be beneficial for pain relief and prevention of the progression of disc degeneration.

Keywords: animal model, disc degeneration, disc injection, growth factor, platelet rich plasma

12.1 Introduction

Degenerative disc diseases (DDDs) consist of various pathologies, such as intervertebral disc (IVD) herniation and discogenic low back pain, which cause various clinical symptoms. Generally, degenerated discs are characterized clinically by a reduction of disc height or IVD herniation as demonstrated by magnetic resonance imaging (MRI) or computed tomography (CT). These changes are considered to be caused by an imbalance of anabolism and catabolism, or homeostasis, of the disc cells residing in the nucleus pulposus (NP) and annulus fibrosus (AF).[1] The modulation of disc cell metabolism involves a variety of molecules, including cytokines, enzymes, enzyme inhibitors, and growth factors.[2] Although the pathogenesis of DDD is not yet fully understood, DDDs are characterized by a progressive process involving a combination of several factors, such as genetic background, aging, and mechanical stress. These changes result in the reduction of water content associated with the depletion of proteoglycans in the NP and structural changes or fissures in the AF. Genetic studies have shown relationships between DDDs and polymorphisms[3] in genes encoding collagen type I,[4] collagen type X,[5,6] aggrecan,[7] matrix metalloprotease-2 (MMP-2),[8] MMP-3,[9] interleukin-1 α (IL-1 α),[10] IL-6,[11] asporin,[12] and cartilage intermediate layer protein, otherwise known as CILP.[13,14]

Considering these characteristics, to treat DDDs, many efforts have investigated therapeutic strategies that stimulate matrix synthesis by growth factors or inhibit inflammatory cytokines, such as IL-1 and tumor necrosis factor- α (TNF- α).[15,16,17] Some efforts have developed therapeutic approaches to suppress disc degeneration by regulating the effects of proteolytic enzymes, such as MMP-1, MMP-3, and members of the disintegrin-like and metalloprotease with thrombospondin motifs (ADAMTS) family.[18,19,20] However, if treatment is aimed at recovering disc structure damage, the direct stimulation of cells contributing to matrix metabolism may be required. Since the pioneering work by Thompson et al,[21] the effects of a variety of growth factors have been tested (see reviews[3,22,23]) and have been shown to include an inhibitory effect on matrix degradation or cytokine expression.[3,24,25]

12.2 The Injection of Growth Factors into Intervertebral Discs (▶ Table 12.1)

Table 12.1 The in vivo effects of intradiscal injection treatments

Agent	Reference	Species	Site	Model	Effect
IGF-1	Walsh 2004[26]	Mice	Tail	Static compression 1 W, Tx 3 wk later	Clustering of inner annulus cells after single injection
GDF-5	Walsh 2004[26]	Mice	Tail	Static compression 1 W, Tx 3 wk later	Clustering of cells, increase in disc height (single injection)
TFG- β	Walsh 2004[26]	Mice	Tail	Static compression 1 W, Tx 3 wk later	Proliferation of cells (multiple injections)
bFGF	Walsh 2004[26]	Mice	Tail	Static compression 1 W, Tx 3 wk later	No response

Table 12.1 *(continued)*

Agent	Reference	Species	Site	Model	Effect
OP-1	An 2005[31]	Rabbit	Lumbar	None (normal)	Increased disc height and PG content in NP
OP-1	Imai 2003[34]	Rabbit	Lumbar	C-ABC: co-injection	Increased disc height and PG content in NP
OP-1	Masuda 2006[32]	Rabbit	Lumbar	Needle puncture: Tx 4 wk later	Increased disc height and PG content in NP and AF, improvement of MRI and histology grades
OP-1	Miyamoto 2006[33]	Rabbit	Lumbar	Needle puncture: Tx 4 wk later	Increased disc height and viscoelastic properties
OP-1	Imai 2007[35]	Rabbit	Lumbar	C-ABC: Tx 4 wks later	Increased disc height, PG content in NP and AF
GDF-5	Chujo 2006[41]	Rabbit	Lumbar	Needle puncture: Tx 4 wk later	Increased disc height, improvement of MRI and histology grades
GDF-5	Yan 2013[42]	Rat	Tail	Needle puncture: Tx 4 wk later	Increased height and GAG content and type II collagen gene in polylactic glycolic acid (PLGA) GDF-5 group
PRP	Nagae 2007[48]	Rabbit	Lumbar	Nucleotomy: immediate Tx	PRP + GHM group had less degeneration and increased PG; PRP + PBS group showed no differences
PRP	Sawamura 2009[49]	Rabbit	Lumbar	Nucleotomy: immediate Tx	PRP + GHM had greater disc height, water content, mRNA for PG core protein and type II collagen; fewer apoptotic cells in NP
PRP	Chen 2009[50]	Pig	Thoracic lumbar	Chymopapain: Tx 2 wk later	Increased aggrecan, type II collagen gene expression, histological improvement, disc height increase
PRP	Gullung 2011[51]	Rat	Lumbar	Needle puncture: Tx 2, 4 wk later	Disc height increase in the immediate injection group; histological improvement
PRP	Obata 2012[52]	Rabbit	Lumbar	Needle puncture: Tx 4 wk later	Disc height increase; no significant MRI T2-weighted signal
GDF-6 (BMP-13, CDMP-2)	Wei 2009[56]	Sheep	Lumbar	Annular stab (3 × 6 mm): immediate Tx	GDF-6 maintained disc height, MRI and histology scores, NP cell density; increased PG and collagen synthesis
BMP-2	Huang 2007[57]	Rabbit	Lumbar	Annular stab: intended for fusion	More degeneration, vascularity, and fibroblast (some fused with and without coral)

Table 12.1 *(continued)*

Agent	Reference	Species	Site	Model	Effect
BMP2/7 heterodimer	Peeters 2015[58]	Goat	Lumbar	C-ABC: Tx 12 wk later	No adverse effect, no significant improvement in disc height, GAG and hydroxyproline contents, and MRI
HGF	Zou 2013[59]	Rat	Tail	Needle puncture: Tx 12 wk later	Increased disc height T2-weighted value in MRI and improved histology
Link N protein	Mwale 2011[61]	Rabbit	Lumbar	Needle puncture: Tx 2 wk later	Increased aggrecan gene expression and decreased proteinase gene expression
INDIRECT BMP STIMULATION					
Lovastatin	Hu 2014[64]	Rat	Tail	Needle puncture: immediate Tx	Upregulation of BMP-2, type II collagen, and SOX9 expression; higher GAG and cell number; BMP-2
Simvastatin	Zhang 2009[63]	Rat	Tail	Needle puncture: Tx 4 wk later	Aggrecan, BMP-2, type II collagen gene expression; MRI improvement and histology
Simvastatin	Than 2014[62]	Rat	Tail	Needle puncture: Tx 6 wk later	BMP-2, aggrecan, and type II collagen gene expression; improved x-ray, MRI, and histology

Abbreviations: AF, annulus fibrosus; bFGF, basic fibroblast growth factor; BMP, bone morphogenetic protein; C-ABC, chondroitinase-ABC; CDMP, cartilage morphogenetic protein; GAG, glycosaminoglycan; GDF-5, -6, growth differentiation factor-5, -6; GHM, gelatin hydrogel microspheres; HGF, hepatocyte growth factor; IGF-1, insulin-like growth factor-1; Link N, amino terminal peptide of link protein (DHLSDNYTLDHDRAIH); MRI, magnetic resonance imaging; NP, nucleus pulposus; OP-1, osteogenic protein-1; PBS, phosphate-buffered saline; PG, proteoglycan; PRP, platelet rich plasma; mRNA, messenger ribonucleic acid; TGF-β, transforming growth factor-β; Tx: treatment.

The injection of growth factors was, for the first time, attempted in a mouse caudal disc degeneration model induced by static compression.[26] Walsh et al[26] reported that a single injection of growth and differentiation factor-5 (GDF-5), but not that of insulin-like growth factor-1 (IGF-1), transforming growth factor-β (TGF-β), or basic fibroblast growth factor (bFGF) was effective in stimulating disc regeneration. Furthermore, multiple injections (four injections, one per week) of TGF-β showed a stimulatory effect, although multiple injections of IGF-1, GDF-5, and bFGF did not significantly enhance their single dose effects.[26] The discussion by Walsh et al[26] suggested that a sustained delivery system, or a combined approach with a mechanical or cell-based device, might be essential to gain a beneficial therapeutic effect. Since the pioneering studies, a variety of growth factors have been studied in vitro and in vivo for disc regeneration (see reviews[3,22]). Osteogenic protein-1 (OP-1) and recombinant human GDF-5 (rhGDF-5) have been applied to patients as Phase Ib–II clinical trials following various preclinical safety and efficacy studies. Some evidence of efficacy of PRP has been shown in animal studies and has recently gained the attention of clinicians.

12.2.1 Injection of OP-1 into Intervertebral Discs

OP-1, also designated as bone morphogenetic protein-7 (BMP-7), was originally found to stimulate bone formation and is now known to also stimulate proteoglycan and collagen synthesis in chondrocytes[27] and IVD cells.[28,29,30,31] Therefore, we investigated the safety and efficacy of a single injection of OP-1 in the treatment of DDD, first using healthy rabbit IVDs[31] and then degenerated IVDs in the annular-puncture disc degeneration rabbit model.[32] A single injection of OP-1 into the NP of a disc 4 weeks after puncture resulted in a significant restoration of disc height and an increased signal intensity of the NP in T2-weighted MRIs at the 6-week time point after the OP-1 injection; these effects were sustained for the entire experimental period, up to 24 weeks. The degeneration grades of the punctured discs in the OP-1-injected group were significantly lower than those of the control lactose-injected group with a higher proteoglycan (PG) content of the NP and AF.[32] Biomechanical studies using similar conditions revealed that the injection of

OP-1 restored dynamic viscoelastic biomechanical properties, such as elastic and viscous moduli, of puncture-degenerated IVDs.[33] Similar reparative effects on disc structures were observed in the chondroitinase-ABC (C-ABC) and OP-1 co-injected model[34] and in the C-ABC-induced matrix depletion model of disc degeneration in the rabbit.[35] A clinical trial of OP-1 was initiated in 2007, but the results of the Phase I trial have not been published due to the withdrawal of the trial.

12.2.2 Injection of GDF-5 into Intervertebral Discs

GDF-5, originally found as a factor responsible for skeletal alternations in brachypodism mice,[36] is a member of the BMP family known for its role in bone formation. The gene-deletion of GDF-5 is reported to be associated with chondro-dysplasia in humans[37,38] and IVD degeneration in mice.[39] rhGDF-5 is another promising growth factor whose efficacy has been evaluated in in vitro and in animal models.[26,40,41] In a preclinical study, an injection of rhGDF-5 in the rabbit annular-puncture model resulted in a restoration of disc height and improvements in MRI and histological grading scores with statistical significance for 12 weeks (▶ Fig. 12.1).[41] In the rat tail disc puncture model, an injection of rhGDF-5 encapsulated in polylactic glycolic acid (PLGA) microspheres restored disc height, improved glycosaminoglycan (GAG) content, and increased collagen type II messenger ribonucleic acid (mRNA) levels.[42]

Since 2009, several Phase Ib and Phase II studies have been conducted (ClinicalTrials.gov, NCT00813813, United States; NCT01158924, Australia; NCT01182337, Korea) including a double-blinded study (NCT01124006, United States). The inclusion and exclusion criteria and outcome measures are listed in ▶ Table 12.2 and detailed results can be obtained at trials website.

Table 12.2 A multicenter, randomized, double-blind, placebo-controlled, clinical trial to evaluate the safety, tolerability, and preliminary effectiveness of two doses of intradiscal rhGDF-5 (single administration) for the treatment of early-stage lumbar disc degeneration (summary of the protocol, NCT01124006)

Study type: Interventional

Study design: Phase I, Phase II
- Allocation: Randomized
- Endpoint classification: Safety/Efficacy study
- Intervention model: Parallel assignment
- Masking: Double-blind (subject, investigator)
- Primary purpose: Treatment
- 24 patients

Inclusion criteria:
- Persistent low back pain with at least 3 months of nonsurgical therapy at one suspected symptomatic lumbar level (L3/L4–L5/S1) confirmed using a standardized provocative discography protocol
- Oswestry Disability Index of ≥ 30
- Low back pain score ≥ 4 cm as measured by Visual Analog Scale (VAS), at Visit 1 baseline

Exclusion criteria:
- Persons unable to have a discogram, CT, or MRI
- Abnormal neurological exam at baseline (e.g., chronic radiculopathy)
- Active radicular pain due to anatomical compression
- Extravasation of contrast agent into the epidural space during discography
- Suspected symptomatic facet joints and/or severe facet joint degeneration at the index level or adjacent segments

Primary outcome measures (12 mo):
- Neurological assessment for motor function and reflexes/sensory
- Treatment-emergent adverse events: Relationship to study drug

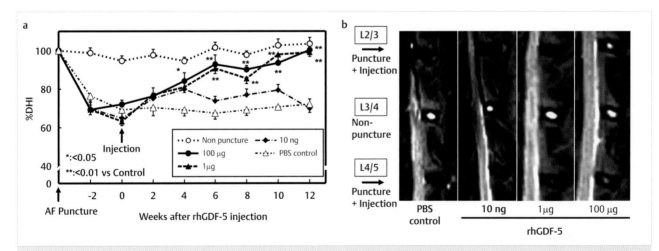

Fig. 12.1 Changes in the intervertebral disc (IVD) disc height index (DHI) after annular puncture and recombinant human growth and differentiation factor-5 (rhGDF-5) injection. **(a)** In a needle-puncture model of disc degeneration in adolescent (5–6 month-old) rabbits, a single injection of rhGDF-5 restored disc height after 4 weeks. Four weeks after an annular needle puncture in New Zealand White rabbits (weighing 3.5–4 kg), the rabbits received an injection of phosphate-buffered saline (PBS; 10 µL) or rhGDF-5 (10 ng, 1 or 100 µg, in 10 µL PBS) and were monitored radiographically for up to 12 weeks after the injections. By 4 weeks after the rhGDF-5 injection, the mean %DHI of injected discs in the rhGDF-5 group (100 µg) was significantly higher than that in the PBS group ($p < 0.05$). **(b)** After sacrifice, the spines were assessed by magnetic resonance imaging (MRI). The MRI of the nucleus pulposus (NP) in the rhGDF-5 group showed increased T2 signal intensity compared with that of the control group. (Modified with permission from Chujo et al.[41])

Table 12.2 (continued)

Study type: Interventional

Secondary Outcomes (changes at 12 mo from baseline):
- Oswestry Disability Index (ODI) change
- Pain VAS
- Physical component summary of quality-of-life-measure assessed by SF-36
- Mental component summary quality-of-life measure assessed by SF-36

Abbreviations: CT, computerized tomography; MRI, magnetic resonance imaging; rhGDF-5, recombinant human growth and differentiation factor-5; SF-36, 36-item Short Form Health Survey.

*Additional follow-up by telephone at 24 and 36 months. Full description and results are at https://clinicaltrials.gov/ct2/show/NCT01124006.

12.2.3 Injection of Platelet Rich Plasma into Intervertebral Discs

PRP, a plasma fraction containing multiple growth factors concentrated at high levels, can be produced by centrifugal separation of whole blood in the operating room. However, there are several methods to activate platelets and some publications lack descriptions about the activation method used; therefore, differences in biological activities can be expected. A detailed review of in vitro and in vivo effects of PRP on the IVD has been published.[43] Akeda et al[44] first reported that PRP is an effective stimulator of cell proliferation and PG and collagen synthesis, as well as PG accumulation, by porcine NP and AF cells cultured in alginate beads. Kim et al,[45] Liu et al,[46] and Cho et al[47] have reported the anti-inflammatory effects of PRP on various cytokines and metalloproteinases under inflammatory conditions.

In vivo experiments using rabbits have shown PRP prepared in gelatin hydrogel microspheres to be effective in the suppression of the progression of IVD degeneration induced by the partial removal of the NP.[48,49] Chen et al[50] showed an increased expression of aggrecan and collagen II mRNA 2 months after an injection of PRP. Gullung et al[51] showed that the immediate injection of PRP retained normal morphological features and high fluid content, as well as disc height, in the rat lumbar-disc needle-puncture model. Moreover, using the rabbit annular-puncture model, the active soluble releasate isolated following platelet activation of PRP (PRP-releasate) induced a reparative effect on rabbit degenerated IVDs.[52] Gui et al[53] reported similar results in the rabbit annular-puncture model at both 2 and 4 weeks postinjury.

Clinically, a prospective randomized study[54] showed that the intradiscal PRP-injection group showed a significant improvement in pain (only in the numerical rating scale [NRS] best pain score), function, and patient satisfaction compared with the control group at the 8-week time point. Because this was a relatively small study with only 47 patients, and not all pain parameters were improved and pain relieve was modest, further large-scale studies may be required to confirm the long-term efficacy of PRP for low back pain due to DDD as a point-of-care treatment.

12.2.4 Other Growth Factors or Growth Factor-related Molecules at Preclinical Stages

GDF-6 (BMP-13; also known as cartilage morphogenetic protein-2 [CDMP2]) is another member of the BMP family that is important for disc development[55]; it is expressed in human NP cells and induced discogenic differentiation of mesenchymal stem cells (MSCs).[56] The injection of BMP-13 at the time of surgery in an ovine annular-stab model prevented or retarded disc degeneration with higher cell numbers and matrix retention 12 months after the injection.[57] An injection of BMP-2 in the rabbit disc degeneration annular-stab model induced more degeneration and an increased vascularity; however, this study was intended to obtain fusion with and without coral and no clear quantitative outcome measures were presented.[58] Recent studies on BMP-2 or BMP-2/-7 heterodimers in the C-ABC–induced goat disc degeneration model showed no adverse effects, but also no significant improvement.[59] An injection of PLGA-polyethylene glycol (PEG)-PLGA loaded with hepatocyte growth factor (HGF) in the rat tail disc puncture model showed retardation of disc degeneration confirmed by increased MRI T2-weighted signal and the maintenance of disc height in the treatment group.[60] Thus, the effect of BMP-2 remains to be revealed in in vivo studies. Link N peptide, which stimulates matrix synthesis similar to that of growth factors,[61] was effective in recovering disc height with elevated expression of matrix genes in a rabbit disc degeneration model.[62] Instead of the direct application of growth factors into IVDs, the intradiscal administration of simvastatin[63,64] or lovastatin[65] in a rat disc degeneration model has been shown to stimulate BMP-2 or SRY (sex determining region Y) box 9 (SOX9) and shows some promise.

12.3 Limitations of the Therapeutic Application of the Injection of Growth Factors into Intervertebral Discs

12.3.1 The Half-Life of Growth Factors Injected into Intervertebral Discs

It is still not well known how long injected compounds are retained in the disc space after a single injection. Some authors have suggested a short half-life in the order of minutes,[66] and stressed the requirement for a drug delivery mechanism to provide the prolonged retention of injected drugs; however, a study of the half-life of OP-1 using radiolabeling indicated much greater times, likely more than 1 month (▶ Fig. 12.2).[67] This long elimination of substances from discs may be due to the enclosed structure by the AF and slow diffusion from the NP to the end plate, as well as their specific binding to collagen molecules.[68] The elimination time of injected growth factors depends on the binding capacity to the extracellular matrix (ECM), various

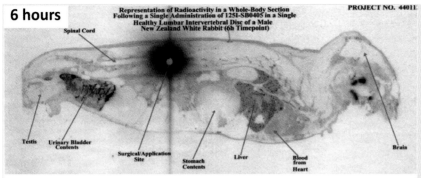

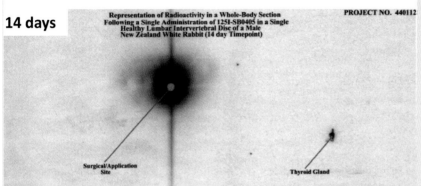

Fig. 12.2 Retention of radiolabeled bone morphogenetic protein 7 (BMP-7) in a rabbit disc. ^{125}I-labeled BMP-7 (otherwise known as osteogenic protein-1) was injected into the L3–4 disc of normal rabbits. The rabbits were subjected to whole body quantitative autoradiography (WBQA). At 6 hours after injection (**top**), ^{125}I-labeled BMP-7 was detected at the injection site, and in several organs, including the bladder and thyroid. The signal from the radiolabeled BMP-7 is prominent even after 14 days (**bottom**). The results of quantification of autography images indicated that the half-life of ^{125}I-labeled BMP-7 was longer than 1 month. (Modified with permission from Pierce et al.[67])

conditions of the disc, (i.e., the degree of disc degeneration and/or vascularization), the injection procedure itself (i.e., needle size, injection location, and volume), and characteristics of the vehicle or carrier. In addition, the effect of growth factor on cells is dependent on how long activity is retained after binding to their receptors. Further research to determine the mechanism of elimination using in vitro modeling analysis may be helpful.

12.3.2 Patient Selection: Stage of Disc Degeneration

Because the action of growth factors requires the presence of viable and metabolically active IVD cells, the application of growth factors to degenerated discs that have few viable cells[69] or poor response to growth factors[70] may be clinically irrelevant. It is also anticipated that oxygen consumption increases with stimulated metabolic activity and that anaerobic metabolism increases, resulting in a high concentration of lactic acid and low pH[71]; this may cause cell death and lead to treatment failure.

12.3.3 Nutritional Supply into Intervertebral Discs

The nutritional conditions of degenerated IVDs are often very limited because the end plates of IVDs are often calcified and sclerotic.[3,72] The enhancement of metabolic activities may result in the further depletion of nutrients and oxygen and the accumulation of metabolic waste. MRI technology has made it possible to evaluate the condition of end plates in detail[73] and the perfusion rate of solutes from the vertebral body into the IVD.[74, 75] The further development of noninvasive methods using MRI

may help in the selection of patients targeted for an injection of growth factor and the long-term changes after an injection.

12.3.4 Induction of Disc Degeneration by an Injection

Recent publications have revealed that discography induced disc degeneration of punctured IVDs[76] and that the injection of local analgesics and contrast agents negatively affected cell metabolism.[77,78,79,80,81] However, it is essential to identify the disc responsible for pain generation when patients have degeneration of multiple discs. The indications for discography to identify the cause of discogenic pain should be carefully considered based on a risk/benefit assessment; this also includes a vehicle injection into the control level that was performed in discography in clinical practice. The injection procedure for the control vehicle in a double-blinded clinical trial is another important point to take into account. In addition, the local toxicity assessment of injected molecules and pharmacokinetics analyses are essential even for those proven to be safe for systemic administration, especially considering the possible exposure to high concentrations of the injected molecule.

12.3.5 Limitations of Animal Models for Evaluating Pain

Many efforts have attempted to establish animal models to investigate degenerated IVDs[82]; these models have been used to evaluate the structural-modifying effects of treatment. In most clinical trials of intradiscal injection therapy, the primary outcome measures are pain assessment and safety. However, the quantitative assessment of pain reduction using a properly scaled dose injection produced in a preclinical model is not well established. Even positive results of imaging analyses, such as MRI and X-ray, and histological assessments indicating favorable structural changes, do not guarantee that the therapy will provide pain relief. Some research attempts to target aspects of pain, addressing the above points, have been made. Kawakami et al[83] showed that the autologous transplantation of NP tissues obtained from the rattail disc compression model into the dorsal root ganglion induced significant allodynia and that the injection of OP-1 into the disc abrogated the pain induction. Olmarker et al[84] also reported behavioral changes due to pain from disc degeneration by disc puncture in the rat. These studies may provide additional clinically relevant evidence in animal models for the development of an injection therapy.

12.3.6 Placebo Effects of an Injection Procedure

A recent clinical trial for fibrin sealant[85] and the preliminary results of the GDF-5 clinical trial (see ClinicalTrials.gov) indicate that the placebo effect for pain or spontaneous relief of pain are substantial. The further understanding of placebo effects and the selection of a patient population for an injection treatment are essential.

12.4 Conclusion

Various studies have shown the effectiveness of growth factor injections in preclinical models. Although some clinical trials have been performed, the clinical effect of growth factor injection treatment is not conclusive. Although the patient number was relatively small, a recent double-blinded study for PRP suggested short-term efficacy.[54] Further research on pain aspects after growth factor administration may fill the gap between preclinical results and clinical efficacy. One key component is the careful selection of appropriate patients for the stimulation of matrix production and to avoid further disease stage advancement due to depletion of nutrients. Multidisciplinary efforts by physicians, biologists, and radiologists may be a key to advance science in this field and to provide clinical benefits to a billion back pain patients.

12.5 References

[1] Masuda K, An HS. Prevention of disc degeneration with growth factors. Eur Spine J. 2006; 15 Suppl 3:S422–S432

[2] Risbud MV, Shapiro IM. Role of cytokines in intervertebral disc degeneration: pain and disc content. Nat Rev Rheumatol. 2014; 10(1):44–56

[3] Bae W, Masuda K. enhancing disc repair by growth factors and other modalities. In: Shapiro IM, Risbud MV, eds. The Intervertebral Disc: Molecular and Structural Studies of the Disc in Health and Disease. Springer-Verlag Wien; 2013:401–416

[4] Tilkeridis C, Bei T, Garantziotis S, Stratakis CA. Association of a COL1A1 polymorphism with lumbar disc disease in young military recruits. J Med Genet. 2005; 42(7):e44

[5] Annunen S, Paassilta P, Lohiniva J, et al. An allele of COL9A2 associated with intervertebral disc disease. Science. 1999; 285(5426):409–412

[6] Solovieva S, Lohiniva J, Leino-Arjas P, et al. Intervertebral disc degeneration in relation to the COL9A3 and the IL-1ss gene polymorphisms. Eur Spine J. 2006; 15(5):613–619

[7] Kawaguchi Y, Osada R, Kanamori M, et al. Association between an aggrecan gene polymorphism and lumbar disc degeneration. Spine. 1999; 24 (23):2456–2460

[8] Dong DM, Yao M, Liu B, Sun CY, Jiang YQ, Wang YS. Association between the -1306C/T polymorphism of matrix metalloproteinase-2 gene and lumbar disc disease in Chinese young adults. Eur Spine J. 2007; 16(11):1958–1961

[9] Takahashi M, Haro H, Wakabayashi Y, Kawa-uchi T, Komori H, Shinomiya K. The association of degeneration of the intervertebral disc with 5a/6a polymorphism in the promoter of the human matrix metalloproteinase-3 gene. J Bone Joint Surg Br. 2001; 83(4):491–495

[10] Solovieva S, Kouhia S, Leino-Arjas P, et al. Interleukin 1 polymorphisms and intervertebral disc degeneration. Epidemiology. 2004; 15(5):626–633

[11] Noponen-Hietala N, Virtanen I, Karttunen R, et al. Genetic variations in IL6 associate with intervertebral disc disease characterized by sciatica. Pain. 2005; 114(1–2):186–194

[12] Song YQ, Cheung KM, Ho DW, et al. Association of the asporin D14 allele with lumbar-disc degeneration in Asians. Am J Hum Genet. 2008; 82(3):744–747

[13] Virtanen IM, Song YQ, Cheung KM, et al. Phenotypic and population differences in the association between CILP and lumbar disc disease. J Med Genet. 2007; 44(4):285–288

[14] Seki S, Kawaguchi Y, Chiba K, et al. A functional SNP in CILP, encoding cartilage intermediate layer protein, is associated with susceptibility to lumbar disc disease. Nat Genet. 2005; 37(6):607–612

[15] Le Maitre CL, Freemont AJ, Hoyland JA. The role of interleukin-1 in the pathogenesis of human intervertebral disc degeneration. Arthritis Res Ther. 2005; 7(4):R732–R745

[16] Burke JG, G Watson RW, Conhyea D, et al. Human nucleus pulposis can respond to a pro-inflammatory stimulus. Spine. 2003; 28(24):2685–2693

[17] Weiler C, Nerlich AG, Bachmeier BE, Boos N. Expression and distribution of tumor necrosis factor alpha in human lumbar intervertebral discs: a study in surgical specimen and autopsy controls. Spine. 2005; 30(1):44–53, discussion 54

[18] Le Maitre CL, Freemont AJ, Hoyland JA. Localization of degradative enzymes and their inhibitors in the degenerate human intervertebral disc. J Pathol. 2004; 204(1):47–54

[19] Roberts S, Caterson B, Menage J, Evans EH, Jaffray DC, Eisenstein SM. Matrix metalloproteinases and aggrecanase: their role in disorders of the human intervertebral disc. Spine. 2000; 25(23):3005–3013

[20] Seki S, Asanuma-Abe Y, Masuda K, et al. Effect of small interference RNA (siRNA) for ADAMTS5 on intervertebral disc degeneration in the rabbit anular needle-puncture model. Arthritis Res Ther. 2009; 11(6):R166

[21] Thompson JP, Oegema TR , Jr, Bradford DS. Stimulation of mature canine intervertebral disc by growth factors. Spine. 1991; 16(3):253–260

[22] Bae WC, Masuda K. Emerging technologies for molecular therapy for intervertebral disk degeneration. Orthop Clin North Am. 2011; 42(4):585–601, ix

[23] Masuda K. Biological repair of the degenerated intervertebral disc by the injection of growth factors. Eur Spine J. 2008; 17 Suppl 4:441–451

[24] Chubinskaya S, Otten L, Soeder S, et al. Regulation of chondrocyte gene expression by osteogenic protein-1. Arthritis Res Ther. 2011; 13(2):R55

[25] Aigner T, Soeder S, Haag J. IL-1beta and BMPs–interactive players of cartilage matrix degradation and regeneration. Eur Cell Mater. 2006; 12:49–56, discussion 56

[26] Walsh AJ, Bradford DS, Lotz JC. In vivo growth factor treatment of degenerated intervertebral discs. Spine. 2004; 29(2):156–163

[27] Flechtenmacher J, Huch K, Thonar EJ, et al. Recombinant human osteogenic protein 1 is a potent stimulator of the synthesis of cartilage proteoglycans and collagens by human articular chondrocytes. Arthritis Rheum. 1996; 39 (11):1896–1904

[28] Masuda K, Takegami K, An H, et al. Recombinant osteogenic protein-1 upregulates extracellular matrix metabolism by rabbit annulus fibrosus and nucleus pulposus cells cultured in alginate beads. J Orthop Res. 2003; 21 (5):922–930

[29] Imai Y, Miyamoto K, An HS, Thonar EJ, Andersson GB, Masuda K. Recombinant human osteogenic protein-1 upregulates proteoglycan metabolism of human anulus fibrosus and nucleus pulposus cells. Spine. 2007; 32 (12):1303–1309, discussion 1310

[30] Takegami K, Thonar EJ, An HS, Kamada H, Masuda K. Osteogenic protein-1 enhances matrix replenishment by intervertebral disc cells previously exposed to interleukin-1. Spine. 2002; 27(12):1318–1325

[31] An HS, Takegami K, Kamada H, et al. Intradiscal administration of osteogenic protein-1 increases intervertebral disc height and proteoglycan content in the nucleus pulposus in normal adolescent rabbits. Spine. 2005; 30(1):25–31, discussion 31–32

[32] Masuda K, Imai Y, Okuma M, et al. Osteogenic protein-1 injection into a degenerated disc induces the restoration of disc height and structural changes in the rabbit anular puncture model. Spine. 2006; 31(7):742–754

[33] Miyamoto K, Masuda K, Kim JG, et al. Intradiscal injections of osteogenic protein-1 restore the viscoelastic properties of degenerated intervertebral discs. Spine J. 2006; 6(6):692–703

[34] Imai Y, An H, Thonar E, et al. Co-injected recombinant human osteogenic protein-1 minimizes chondroitinase ABC-induced intervertebral disc degeneration: an in vivo study using a rabbit model [poster]. Trans Orthop Res Soc. 2003:1143

[35] Imai Y, Okuma M, An HS, et al. Restoration of disc height loss by recombinant human osteogenic protein-1 injection into intervertebral discs undergoing degeneration induced by an intradiscal injection of chondroitinase ABC. Spine. 2007; 32(11):1197–1205

[36] Storm EE, Huynh TV, Copeland NG, Jenkins NA, Kingsley DM, Lee SJ. Limb alterations in brachypodism mice due to mutations in a new member of the TGF beta-superfamily. Nature. 1994; 368(6472):639–643

[37] Polinkovsky A, Robin NH, Thomas JT, et al. Mutations in CDMP1 cause autosomal dominant brachydactyly type C. Nat Genet. 1997; 17(1):18–19

[38] Thomas JT, Lin K, Nandedkar M, Camargo M, Cervenka J, Luyten FP. A human chondrodysplasia due to a mutation in a TGF-beta superfamily member. Nat Genet. 1996; 12(3):315–317

[39] Li X, Leo BM, Beck G, Balian G, Anderson GD. Collagen and proteoglycan abnormalities in the GDF-5-deficient mice and molecular changes when treating disk cells with recombinant growth factor. Spine. 2004; 29 (20):2229–2234

[40] Wang H, Kroeber M, Hanke M, et al. Release of active and depot GDF-5 after adenovirus-mediated overexpression stimulates rabbit and human intervertebral disc cells. J Mol Med (Berl). 2004; 82(2):126–134

[41] Chujo T, An HS, Akeda K, et al. Effects of growth differentiation factor-5 on the intervertebral disc—in vitro bovine study and in vivo rabbit disc degeneration model study. Spine. 2006; 31(25):2909–2917

[42] Yan J, Yang S, Sun H, et al. Effects of releasing recombinant human growth and differentiation factor-5 from poly(lactic-co-glycolic acid) microspheres for repair of the rat degenerated intervertebral disc. J Biomater Appl. 2014; 29(1):72–80

[43] Formica M, Cavagnaro L, Formica C, Mastrogiacomo M, Basso M, Di Martino A. What is the preclinical evidence on platelet rich plasma and intervertebral disc degeneration? Eur Spine J. 2015; 24(11):2377–2386

[44] Akeda K, An HS, Pichika R, et al. Platelet-rich plasma (PRP) stimulates the extracellular matrix metabolism of porcine nucleus pulposus and anulus fibrosus cells cultured in alginate beads. Spine. 2006; 31(9):959–966

[45] Kim HJ, Yeom JS, Koh YG, et al. Anti-inflammatory effect of platelet-rich plasma on nucleus pulposus cells with response of TNF-α and IL-1. J Orthop Res. 2014; 32(4):551–556

[46] Liu MC, Chen WH, Wu LC, et al. Establishment of a promising human nucleus pulposus cell line for intervertebral disc tissue engineering. Tissue Eng Part C Methods. 2014; 20(1):1–10

[47] Cho H, Holt DC, III, Smith R, Kim SJ, Gardocki RJ, Hasty KA. The effects of platelet-rich plasma on halting the progression in porcine intervertebral disc degeneration. Artif Organs. 2016; 40(2):190–195

[48] Nagae M, Ikeda T, Mikami Y, et al. Intervertebral disc regeneration using platelet-rich plasma and biodegradable gelatin hydrogel microspheres. Tissue Eng. 2007; 13(1):147–158

[49] Sawamura K, Ikeda T, Nagae M, et al. Characterization of in vivo effects of platelet-rich plasma and biodegradable gelatin hydrogel microspheres on degenerated intervertebral discs. Tissue Eng Part A. 2009; 15(12):3719–3727

[50] Chen WH, Liu HY, Lo WC, et al. Intervertebral disc regeneration in an ex vivo culture system using mesenchymal stem cells and platelet-rich plasma. Biomaterials. 2009; 30(29):5523–5533

[51] Gullung GB, Woodall JW, Tucci MA, James J, Black DA, McGuire RA. Platelet-rich plasma effects on degenerative disc disease: analysis of histology and imaging in an animal model. Evid Based Spine Care J. 2011; 2(4):13–18

[52] Obata S, Akeda K, Imanishi T, et al. Effect of autologous platelet-rich plasma-releasedon intervertebral disc degeneration in the rabbit anular puncture model: a preclinical study. Arthritis Res Ther. 2012; 14(6):R241

[53] Gui K, Ren W, Yu Y, Li X, Dong J, Yin W. Inhibitory effects of platelet-rich plasma on intervertebral disc degeneration: a preclinical study in a rabbit model. Med SciMonit. 2015; 21:1368–1375

[54] Tuakli-Wosornu YA, Terry A, Boachie-Adjei K, et al. Lumbar intradiskal platelet-rich plasma (PRP) injections: a prospective, double-blind, randomized controlled study. PM R. 2016; 8(1):1–10, quiz 10

[55] Tassabehji M, Fang ZM, Hilton EN, et al. Mutations in GDF6 are associated with vertebral segmentation defects in Klippel-Feil syndrome. Hum Mutat. 2008; 29(8):1017–1027

[56] Le Maitre CL, Freemont AJ, Hoyland JA. Expression of cartilage-derived morphogenetic protein in human intervertebral discs and its effect on matrix synthesis in degenerate human nucleus pulposus cells. Arthritis Res Ther. 2009; 11(5):R137

[57] Wei A, Williams LA, Bhargav D, et al. BMP13 prevents the effects of annular injury in an ovine model. Int J BiolSci. 2009; 5(5):388–396

[58] Huang KY, Yan JJ, Hsieh CC, Chang MS, Lin RM. The in vivo biological effects of intradiscal recombinant human bone morphogenetic protein-2 on the injured intervertebral disc: an animal experiment. Spine. 2007; 32(11):1174–1180

[59] Peeters M, Detiger SE, Karfeld-Sulzer LS, et al. BMP-2 and BMP-2/7 heterodimers conjugated to a fibrin/hyaluronic acid hydrogel in a large animal model of mild intervertebral disc degeneration. Biores Open Access. 2015; 4 (1):398–406

[60] Zou F, Jiang J, Lu F, et al. Efficacy of intradiscal hepatocyte growth factor injection for the treatment of intervertebral disc degeneration. Mol Med Rep. 2013; 8(1):118–122

[61] Mwale F, Demers CN, Petit A, et al. A synthetic peptide of link protein stimulates the biosynthesis of collagens II, IX and proteoglycan by cells of the intervertebral disc. J Cell Biochem. 2003; 88(6):1202–1213

[62] Mwale F, Masuda K, Pichika R, et al. The efficacy of Link N as a mediator of repair in a rabbit model of intervertebral disc degeneration. Arthritis Res Ther. 2011; 13(4):R120

[63] Than KD, Rahman SU, Wang L, et al. Intradiscal injection of simvastatin results in radiologic, histologic, and genetic evidence of disc regeneration in a rat model of degenerative disc disease. Spine J. 2014; 14(6):1017–1028

[64] Zhang H, Wang L, Park JB, et al. Intradiscal injection of simvastatin retards progression of intervertebral disc degeneration induced by stab injury. Arthritis Res Ther. 2009; 11(6):R172

[65] Hu MH, Yang KC, Chen YJ, Sun YH, Yang SH. Lovastatin prevents discography-associated degeneration and maintains the functional morphology of intervertebral discs. Spine J. 2014; 14(10):2459–2466

[66] Larson JW , III, Levicoff EA, Gilbertson LG, Kang JD. Biologic modification of animal models of intervertebral disc degeneration. J Bone Joint Surg Am. 2006; 88 Suppl 2:83–87

[67] Pierce A, Feng M, Masuda K, et al. Distribution, pharmacokinetics and excretion of 125-Iodine labeled BMP-7 (OP-1) following a single dose administration in lumbar IVD or knee joint of NZW rabbits. The Sixth International Conference on Bone Morphogenetic protein. Cavtat, Croatia 2006

[68] Reddi AH. Morphogenetic messages are in the extracellular matrix: biotechnology from bench to bedside. BiochemSoc Trans. 2000; 28(4):345–349

[69] Gruber HE, Hanley EN , Jr. Analysis of aging and degeneration of the human intervertebral disc. Comparison of surgical specimens with normal controls. Spine. 1998; 23(7):751–757

[70] Le Maitre CL, Frain J, Fotheringham AP, Freemont AJ, Hoyland JA. Human cells derived from degenerate intervertebral discs respond differently to those derived from non-degenerate intervertebral discs following application of dynamic hydrostatic pressure. Biorheology. 2008; 45(5):563–575

[71] Urban JP, Smith S, Fairbank JC. Nutrition of the intervertebral disc. Spine. 2004; 29(23):2700–2709

[72] Roberts S, Menage J, Urban JP. Biochemical and structural properties of the cartilage end-plate and its relation to the intervertebral disc. Spine. 1989; 14 (2):166–174

[73] Bae WC, Statum S, Zhang Z, et al. Morphology of the cartilaginous endplates in human intervertebral disks with ultrashort echo time MR imaging. Radiology. 2013; 266(2):564–574

[74] Rajasekaran S, Venkatadass K, Naresh Babu J, Ganesh K, Shetty AP. Pharmacological enhancement of disc diffusion and differentiation of healthy, ageing and degenerated discs: Results from in-vivo serial post-contrast MRI studies in 365 human lumbar discs. Eur Spine J. 2008; 17(5):626–643

[75] Rajasekaran S, Babu JN, Arun R, Armstrong BR, Shetty AP, Murugan S. ISSLS prize winner: A study of diffusion in human lumbar discs: a serial magnetic resonance imaging study documenting the influence of the endplate on diffusion in normal and degenerate discs. Spine. 2004; 29(23):2654–2667

[76] Carragee EJ, Don AS, Hurwitz EL, Cuellar JM, Carrino JA, Herzog R. 2009 ISSLS Prize Winner: does discography cause accelerated progression of degeneration changes in the lumbar disc: a ten-year matched cohort study. Spine. 2009; 34(21):2338–2345

[77] Gruber HE, Rhyne AL , III, Hansen KJ, et al. Deleterious effects of discography radiocontrast solution on human annulus cell in vitro: changes in cell

viability, proliferation, and apoptosis in exposed cells. Spine J. 2012; 12 (4):329–335

[78] Chee AV, Ren J, Lenart BA, Chen EY, Zhang Y, An HS. Cytotoxicity of local anesthetics and nonionic contrast agents on bovine intervertebral disc cells cultured in a three-dimensional culture system. Spine J. 2014; 14(3):491–498

[79] Kim KH, Park JY, Park HS, et al. Which iodinated contrast media is the least cytotoxic to human disc cells? Spine J. 2015; 15(5):1021–1027

[80] Eder C, Pinsger A, Schildboeck S, Falkner E, Becker P, Ogon M. Influence of intradiscal medication on nucleus pulposus cells. Spine J. 2013; 13 (11):1556–1562

[81] Quero L, Klawitter M, Nerlich AG, Leonardi M, Boos N, Wuertz K. Bupivacaine —the deadly friend of intervertebral disc cells? Spine J. 2011; 11(1):46–53

[82] Alini M, Eisenstein SM, Ito K, et al. Are animal models useful for studying human disc disorders/degeneration? Eur Spine J. 2008; 17(1):2–19

[83] Kawakami M, Matsumoto T, Hashizume H, Kuribayashi K, Chubinskaya S, Yoshida M. Osteogenic protein-1 (osteogenic protein-1/bone morphogenetic protein-7) inhibits degeneration and pain-related behavior induced by chronically compressed nucleus pulposus in the rat. Spine. 2005; 30 (17):1933–1939

[84] Olmarker K. Puncture of a lumbar intervertebral disc induces changes in spontaneous pain behavior: an experimental study in rats. Spine. 2008; 33 (8):850–855

[85] Yin W, Pauza K, Olan WJ, Doerzbacher JF, Thorne KJ. Intradiscal injection of fibrin sealant for the treatment of symptomatic lumbar internal disc disruption: results of a prospective multicenter pilot study with 24-month follow-up. Pain Med. 2014; 15(1):16–31

13 Treatment of Degenerative Disc Disease/Disc Regeneration: Stem Cells, Chondrocytes or Other Cells, and Tissue Engineering

Steven Presciutti and Howard An

Abstract

Intervertebral disc (IVD) degeneration remains a significant treatment challenge, but the use of stem cells has emerged as one of the most promising and exciting techniques to restore the degenerated disc. Many challenges remain. The use of stem cells in treating disc disease as well as the obstacles that remain are reviewed in this chapter in an evidence-based manner.

Keywords: intervertebral disc degeneration, mesenchymal stem cell, MSC, stem cells, tissue engineering

13.1 Historical Perspective

The intervertebral disc (IVD) is composed of the nucleus pulposus (NP), the annulus fibrosus (AF), and the two end plates of adjacent vertebral bodies. Adult NP primarily contains chondrocyte-like cells capable of synthesizing proteoglycans (PGs) and type II collagen and is contained within the AF, which principally contains fibroblast-like cells capable of synthesizing type I collagen.[1,2] Intervertebral disc degeneration (IDD) affecting the NP is characterized by attenuation of PG synthesis, development of NP dehydration, and an increase in waste products.[3,4,5,6] Alterations in the cell population of the IVD have been particularly implicated in the pathogenesis of IDD.[7] Loss of chondrogenic NP cells and their replacement by fibroblast-like cells has also been implicated in the later stages of IDD.[8] Over time, an imbalance in the production and degradation of extracellular matrix (ECM) components can lead to a perturbed mechanical balance between the NP and the AF, leading to structural compromise of the disc. This can ultimately result in a variety of clinically significant spinal disorders including radiculopathy and spinal stenosis. IDD has also been linked to low back pain itself; however, the exact relationship between the two remains unclear.[9,10]

Conventional treatment options include multiple nonoperative modalities (i.e., physical therapy, medication, epidural steroid injections) as well as eventually surgical options including spinal fusion or artificial disc replacement if nonoperative treatment fails.[11] Although short-term pain relief with these treatment modalities has been reported, long-term outcomes have been plagued with high rates of recurrent pain.[12] In addition, none of the aforementioned treatment strategies focus on halting or reversing the underlying disc degeneration process. In this regard, regenerative cellular therapy has attracted significant attention because of its potential to directly address the degenerative process. Cell-based therapies are particularly attractive in treatment of more advanced IDD, such as Pfirrmann grades IV or V (► Fig. 13.1).

Substantial progress has occurred in the fields of regenerative medicine, tissue engineering, and stem cell therapies with the aim of treating and reversing IDD as well as augmenting and enhancing current treatments. A stem cell can renew itself through cell division and can exert beneficial effects on other cell types through a variety of mechanisms (i.e., paracrine effects, cell–cell interactions). These characteristics make stem cells worthy of further investigation as a source of cells for treating IDD. Although not currently routinely employed in the management of IDD, these therapeutic characteristics of mesenchymal stem cells (MSCs) have led to an increasing number of preclinical and clinical studies attempting to demonstrate the efficacy and safety of progenitor cells for the treatment of IDD. The first reported use of cell-based therapies to treat IDD in humans was in 2005 by Haufe et al[13] and those initial positive results brought about intense interest among researchers and have resulted in many more preclinical and clinical studies investigating the role of cell-based therapies to treat IDD.

This chapter reviews the biology of stem cells, the clinical evidence concerning the use of MSCs, the hindrances to clinical use, and the potential risks associated with the application of MSCs for the treatment of IDD. Due to the fact that this specific subject matter uses terminology that can often times be confusing, a list of definitions is provided to the reader in ► Table 13.1.

13.2 Determining the Ideal Cell Type

Although considerable research has been dedicated to strategies that boost the ability of native disc cells to synthesize and maintain the ECM, the introduction of exogenous cells such as stem cells is gaining popularity as a potential treatment for IDD.[7] The goal of stem cell therapy is to replace or replenish diseased tissue through the localized differentiation of transplanted stem cells into native cells, which advance the healing process or directly restore the tissue physically. In addition, therapeutic stem cells also release trophic factors that have been shown to stimulate the metabolism of IVD cells as well as suppress inflammatory reactions.[14] Choosing the appropriate cell source, however, is vital for the successful outcome of cell therapy.[15] The choice of cells is based on their abundance, ease to obtain, and the capacity to differentiate into a desired cell type. The cells of choice also need to be viable in the hypoxic and the hypoglycemic environment found within the disc, with minimal or no immune response. They should have low or no risk for tumor growth.

Adult stem cells, like all stem cells, share at least two characteristics. First, they can make identical copies of themselves for long periods of time; this ability to proliferate is referred to as long-term self-renewal. Second, they can give rise to mature cell types that have characteristic morphologies (shapes) and specialized functions. The product of a stem cell undergoing division is at least one additional stem cell that has the same capabilities of the originating cell. Typically, stem cells generate an

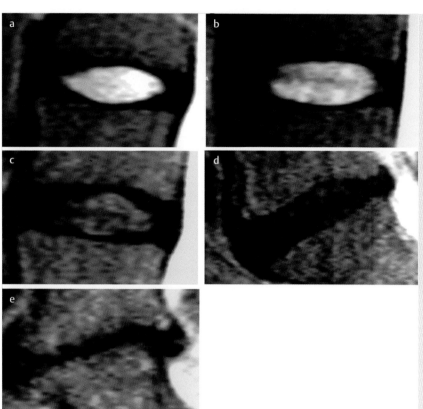

Fig. 13.1 Grading system for the assessment of lumbar disc degeneration. **(a)** Grade I: The structure of the disc is homogeneous, with a bright hyperintense white signal intensity and a normal disc height. **(b)** Grade II: The structure of the disc is inhomogeneous, with a hyperintense white signal. **(c)** Grade III: The structure of the disc is inhomogeneous, with an intermediate gray signal intensity. **(d)** Grade IV: The structure of the disc is inhomogeneous, with a hypointense dark gray signal intensity. **(e)** Grade V: The structure of the disc is inhomogeneous, with a hypointense black signal intensity. Grading is performed on T2-weighted mid-sagittal images. (Reprinted with permission from Pfirrmann et al. Magnetic resonance classification of lumbar intervertebral disc degeneration. Spine 2001;26 (17):1873–1878.)

Table 13.1 Cell-based therapy terminology

Adult stem cell	An undifferentiated cell found in a differentiated tissue that can renew itself and (with certain limitations) differentiate to yield all the specialized cell types of the tissue from which it originated		Ectoderm	The upper, outermost of the three primitive germ layers of the embryo; it gives rise to skin, nerves, and brain.
Allogenic	Two or more individuals (or cell lines) are stated to be allogenic to one another when the genes at one or more loci are not identical in sequence in each organism.		Embryonic stem (ES) cells	Primitive (undifferentiated) cells from the embryo that have the potential to become a wide variety of specialized cell types
Autologous transplant	Transplanted tissue derived from the intended recipient of the transplant. Such a transplant helps avoid complications of immune rejection.		Endoderm	Lower layer of a group of cells derived from the inner cell mass of the blastocyst; it later becomes the lungs and digestive organs.
Bone marrow	The soft, living tissue that fills most bone cavities and contains hematopoietic stem cells, from which all red and white blood cells evolve. The bone marrow also contains mesenchymal stem cells that a number of cell types come from, including chondrocytes, which produce cartilage.		Hematopoietic stem cell (HSC)	A stem cell from which all red and white blood cells evolve
			Mesenchymal stem cells (MSCs)	Cells from the immature embryonic connective tissue. A number of cell types come from mesenchymal stem cells, including chondrocytes, which produce cartilage.
Bone marrow stem cell (BMSC)	One of at least two types of multipotent stem cells: hematopoietic stem cell and mesenchymal stem cell		Mesoderm	The middle layer of the embryonic disk, which consists of a group of cells derived from the inner cell mass of the blastocyst. This middle germ layer is known as gastrulation and is the precursor to bone, muscle, and connective tissue.
Chondrocytes	Cartilage cells		Multipotent stem cells	Stem cells that have the capability of developing cells of multiple germ layers
Differentiation	The process whereby an unspecialized early embryonic cell acquires the features of a specialized cell such as a heart, liver, or muscle cell		Pluripotent stem cell (PSC)	A single stem cell that has the capability of developing cells of all germ layers (endoderm, ectoderm, and mesoderm)
			Precursor cells	In fetal or adult tissues, these are partly differentiated cells that divide and give rise to differentiated cells. Also known as progenitor cells.

Primary germ layers	The three initial embryonic germ layers—endoderm, mesoderm, and ectoderm—from which all other somatic tissue-types develop
Somatic cell	Any cell of a plant or animal other than a germ cell or germ cell precursor
Stem cell	A cell that has the ability to divide for indefinite periods in culture and to give rise to specialized cells
Totipotent	Having unlimited capability. The totipotent cells of the very early embryo have the capacity to differentiate into extra embryonic membranes and tissues, the embryo, and all postembryonic tissues and organs.

intermediate cell type or types before they achieve their fully differentiated state. The intermediate cell is called a precursor or progenitor cell. Progenitor or precursor cells are partly differentiated cells that divide and give rise to differentiated cells. Such cells are usually regarded as "committed" to differentiating along a particular cellular development pathway (▶ Fig. 13.2).

Most scientists use the term *pluripotent* to describe stem cells that can give rise to cells derived from all three embryonic germ layers—mesoderm, endoderm, and ectoderm. These three germ layers are the embryonic source of all cells of the body. All of the many different kinds of specialized cells that make up the body are derived from one of these germ layers (▶ Table 13.2). Pluripotent cells have the potential to give rise to any type of cell, a property observed in the natural course of embryonic development and under certain laboratory conditions.

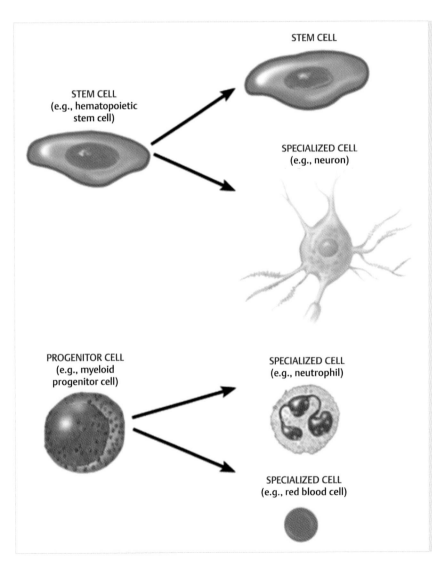

STEM CELL

STEM CELL
(e.g., hematopoietic stem cell)

SPECIALIZED CELL
(e.g., neuron)

PROGENITOR CELL
(e.g., myeloid progenitor cell)

SPECIALIZED CELL
(e.g., neutrophil)

SPECIALIZED CELL
(e.g., red blood cell)

Fig. 13.2 Distinguishing features of progenitor/precursor cells and stem cells. The product of a stem cell undergoing division is at least one additional stem cell that has the same capabilities of the originating cell. Shown here is an example of a hematopoietic stem cell (HSC) producing a second generation stem cell and a neuron. This is in contrast to a progenitor cell, which can yield two specialized cells upon cell division. Shown here is an example of a myeloid progenitor undergoing cell division to yield two specialized cells (a neutrophil and a red blood cell).

Table 13.2 Embryonic germ layers from which differentiated tissues develop

Embryonic germ layer	Differentiated tissue
Endoderm	Thymus
	Thyroid, parathyroid glands
	Larynx, trachea, lung
	Urinary bladder, vagina, urethra
	Gastrointestinal (GI) organs
	Lining of GI tract
	Lining of respiratory tract
Mesoderm	Bone marrow (blood)
	Adrenal cortex
	Lymphatic tissue
	Skeletal, smooth, and cardiac muscle
	Connective tissues (including bone, cartilage)
	Urogenital system
	Heart and blood vessels
Ectoderm	Skin
	Neural tissue (neuroectoderm)
	Adrenal medulla
	Pituitary gland
	Connective tissue of the head and face
	Eyes, ears

Because NP cells share similarities with chondrocytes in both phenotype and molecular markers, cells with the capacity of differentiating toward chondrocytes have largely been considered ideal in the treatment of IDD. Given this, autologous chondrocyte implantation has been attempted as a treatment strategy for IDD. Articular chondrocytes, such as NP cells, produce aggrecan and type II collagen and can be surgically obtained from the non–weight-bearing parts of the knee. In a study by Gorensek and colleagues,[16] the NP of rabbit IVDs was removed and autologous chondrocytes were transferred to the defect site. Discs injected with chondrocytes produced a hyaline-like cartilage in the center without any elastic fibers, but with a higher collagen to aggrecan ratio than in NP ECM. In a porcine denucleation model, autologous chondrocytes injected with a fibrin carrier showed dense cartilage formation by 3 months and cell viability up to 12 months after transplantation.[17] In vitro co-culture experiments have also suggested cartilage tissue stimulates NP cell anabolism through moderation of inflammation.[18] However, chondrocytes produce a lower PG to collagen ratio than NP cells,[19] so further work needs to be done to establish restoration of disc biochemical and biomechanical properties. Chondrocyte transplantation also suffers from some of the same limitations as NP cells (invasive second surgery and low supply of donor tissue), so chondrocytes themselves may not be an ideal source for cell therapy.

Given this, multiple sources of stem cells that have the ability to become chrondrocyte-like cells (i.e., NP cells) have also been explored as potential candidates and are discussed below. A list of the completed human clinical trials using cell-based therapies to treat IDD is provided in ▶ Table 13.3.[13,20,21,22,23,24] Similarly, ▶ Table 13.4 provides a list of the current ongoing clinical trials.[25,26,27,28,29,30]

13.2.1 Embryonic Stem Cells and Induced Pluripotent Stem Cells

Embryonic stem (ES cells) are pluripotent stem cells derived from discarded early-stage frozen embryos.[31] One major drawback is that there are only a limited number of cell lines available at present for study. ES cells are able to differentiate toward all derivatives of the three primary germ layers, including chondrocytelike cells.[32] Sheikh et al were able to show that the subsequent transplantation of these cells into the IVD of rabbits resulted in maintenance of the native cell's viability as well as their appropriate morphology.

Induced pluripotent stem cells (iPSCs) are similar to ES cells in both phenotype and potential for differentiation, and have also been reported to have the capacity of differentiating

Table 13.3 Clinical studies of cell therapy for intervertebral disc degeneration[a]

Location	Mode	Cell type	Indication	N	Outcome
United States[13]	Allogenic	Juvenile chondrocytes	IDD with low back pain	10	No improvement
Germany[20,21]	Allogenic	Adult mesenchymal precursor cells	IDD with low back pain	112	Improvement of low back pain and on radiograph
Japan[22]	Allogenic	Bone marrow MSCs	IDD with low back pain	2	Improvement on radiograph and on MRI
Spain[23]	Autologous	IVD cells	IVD herniation with back and / or leg pain	10	Improvement of low back pain and on MRI
United States[24]	Autologous	Adipose MSCs	IDD with low back pain	15	Improvement of low back pain and on MRI

Abbreviations: IDD, intervertebral disc degeneration; IVD, intervertebral disc; MRI, magnetic resonance imaging; MSCs, mesenchymal stem cells.

[a]Published as of December 2015.

Table 13.4 ongoing clinical trials of cell therapy for intervertebral disc degeneration

Location	Mode	Cell type	Indication	ClinicalTrials.gov identifier	Status
United States[25]	Allogenic	Juvenile chondrocytes	IDD with low back pain	NC-T01771471	Active, but not recruiting
United States[26]	Allogenic	Adult mesenchymal precursor cells	IDD with low back pain	NC-T01290367	Active, but not recruiting
Spain[27]	Allogenic	Bone marrow MSCs	IDD with low back pain	NC-T01860417	Active, but not recruiting
Austria, Germany[28]	Autologous	IVD cells	IVD herniation with back and / or leg pain	NC-T01640457	Recruiting
Korea[29]	Autologous	Adipose MSCs	IDD with low back pain	NC-T01643681	Recruiting
United States[30]	Autologous	Adipose MSCs	IDD with low back pain	NC-T02097862	Recruiting

Abbreviations: IDD, intervertebral disc degeneration; IVD, intervertebral disc; MSCs, mesenchymal stem cells.

toward chondrocytelike cells.[33]iPSCs are derived from somatic cells by inducing the expression of ectopic reprogramming transcriptional factors. Unfortunately, some of these factors are known oncogenes. Although some studies showed that these transcriptional factors can be replaced by small molecules,[34] tumorigenesis is still a major concern that limits the clinical utility of both ES cells and iPSCs.[35,36]

13.2.2 Mesenchymal Stem Cells

MSCs are multipotent cells derived from mesodermal tissues and they have the capacity to differentiate toward some or all of the specialized cell types of that original tissue. MSCs are reported to be nonimmunogenic and, in contrast to ES cells, do not as easily undergo malignant transformation.[37,38] Moreover, MSCs have the capacity for self-renewal, enabling maintenance of an undifferentiated phenotype in multiple subcultures.[39] However, in the appropriate environment, MSCs are capable of differentiating into multiple cell types including osteoblasts, adipocytes, chondrocytes, and neuronal cells.[40,41] The differentiation of MSCs toward chondrocytelike cells has been documented both in vitro and in vivo.[42,43,44,45] Although MSCs can be differentiated into chondrocytelike cells similar to those found in the NP, whether those cells are truly NP cells remains to be seen.[7] We next review the various tissues that have been explored as a source for MSCs.

Bone Marrow Stromal Cells

Bone marrow is an excellent source of MSCs for most orthopaedic applications including chondrogenic differentiation for the diseased IVD. Yamamoto and colleagues[46] investigated bone marrow–derived stromal cells in a direct contact co-culture system with native NP cells. The authors found significantly increased cell proliferation, deoxyribonucleic acid (DNA) synthesis, and PG synthesis in the NP cells. This was most pronounced in the NP cells that had direct cell-to-cell contact with the bone marrow MSCs. These in vitro findings have also been extended to an in vivo rat model by Allon and colleagues.[47] After injecting bone marrow–derived MSCs into the discs or rabbits, the authors were able to demonstrate an increase in PG content as well as partial restoration of both disc height and disc hydration.[48,49] Similarly in the ovine model, the injection of MSCs directly into the IVD has been shown to restore disc ECM, increase disc height, and reduce both radiological and histological grading scores 6 months following injection.[50,51]

Early clinical research has also been promising. Yoshikawa et al[22] reported two cases of autologous MSC implantation in markedly degenerative IVDs. Symptomatic and radiological improvement was demonstrated without significant adverse effects. In addition, a larger pilot study was subsequently conducted in which 10 patients suffering from low back pain associated with IDD were injected with autologous bone marrow–derived MSCs.[23]The authors found that improvements in patient-reported outcomes were similar to those observed following spinal fusion. These small human studies, along with numerous animal studies, suggest that MSC implantation could indeed be a useful tool for the treatment of IDD.

Adipose-Derived Stem Cells

Given the larger number of MSCs that can be obtained compared with bone marrow or other sources as well as the relative ease of procurement, adipose-derived stem cells (ADSCs) have gained significant attention in recent years. Multiple in vitro studies have been conducted that have found these MSCs to be a viable option for IVD regeneration.[52,53] Choi and colleagues[40] reported that chondrogenic differentiation of ADSCs was possible by co-culturing them with normal, healthy NP cells in monolayer. ADSCs cultured alone or with NP cells from degenerative discs were shown to have inferior results.

More recent studies have focused on fine-tuning the chondrogenic differentiation of these ADSCs in order to be more similar to actual NP cells. Lu and colleagues[54] reported that co-culture of human ADSCs and NP cells in a three-dimensional (3D) micromass culture resulted in differentiation of ADSCs into an NP cell–like phenotype. Likewise, Gaetani et al[55] showed that a 3D culture technique resulted in significantly increased matrix production and a 3D cell organization similar to IVD.

Other Mesenchymal Stem Cell Sources

Other stem cell sources have also been investigated for the treatment of IDD, although most of these other cell types are just beginning to be explored. Their true translational promise for the treatment of IDD remains to be seen. Vadala et al[56] investigated the use of adult muscle tissue as a stem cell source.

They used a co-culture in vitro model with NP cells and were able to show increased matrix production and DNA synthesis of the NP cells. Recent in vitro studies have also revealed the potential for human AF cells[57] and NP cells[58] to serve as a source of MSCs. The morbidity of harvesting one's own disc cells is a concern for the induction of further degeneration, however. Others studies have recently investigated the use of synovial cells as a stem cell source for IVD tissue engineering.[59,60,61]

Sakai and colleagues[62] demonstrated a population of progenitor cells within the actual NP itself. Although they were able to indentify such cells, the proportion of these cells within the disc was markedly reduced with age and degeneration. Other studies have also found highly proliferative cells expressing stem cell markers (i.e., Notch1, Delta4, Jagged1, C-KIT) within the disc.[63,64] These cells have been successfully isolated and have been shown to be capable of differentiating down the osteogenic, chondrogenic, and adipogenic lineage.[65] Although these endogenous stem cells offer huge potential, it remains to be seen whether they can be harnessed for regenerative purposes.

Human umbilical cord MSCs are multipotent and have been reported to differentiate into chondrogenic, adipogenic, and osteogenic lineages.[66]But the safety of allogenic transplantation in MSCs has not yet been established. Until further studies establish the immunologic safety of allogenic human umbilical cord MSC transplantation in humans, the utility of human umbilical cord MSCs is limited for the purpose of IDD treatment.

13.3 Understanding the Target Tissue

13.3.1 Influence of the Intervertebral Disc Microenvironment

To produce matrix, disc cells require an extracellular environment with sufficient oxygen (> 3%) and glucose (1 mM) and the pH must preferably not be acidic (optimally, ~7.0–7.2). In addition, the osmolarity must be high enough to stimulate matrix production as well as retain it locally (ideally, 350 mOsm).

These conditions are present in a normal, healthy disc[67] but in degenerative discs, osmolarity falls as aggrecan is lost, oxygen levels are variable, and the pH tends to become acidic.[68]These microenvironmental conditions are very specific, quite harsh, and differ from the native environments of the cells being considered as possible sources of MSCs (▶ Fig. 13.3). This could impair the functioning of any such implanted cells or even result in their death.[69]

For example, Wuertz and colleagues[70] reported that the acidic conditions often found in the degenerated disc caused an inhibition of aggrecan, collagen-1, and tissue inhibitor of metalloproteinase 3 (TIMP-3) expression. They also found a decrease in cell proliferation and viability as well as altered cell morphology of bone marrow–derived MSCs. Likewise, ADSCs were also shown to respond negatively to the environmental conditions found within degenerative IVDs.[52]

These difficult physiological conditions found in the healthy disc phenotype, let alone the degenerative one, poses a significant challenge. These conditions could theoretically be overcome with the use of growth factors as well as with the preconditioning of cultured cells prior to implantation to achieve better survival in the disc environment.[71]

13.3.2 The Target Cell

To successfully develop an MSC-based therapy for the treatment of IDD it is necessary to understand the phenotype of the target cell and ensure correct differentiation and synthesis of an appropriately functioning tissue. NP cells have routinely been described as chondrocytelike, with traditional chondrogenic gene markers (collagen type II alpha 1, aggrecan, SRY (sex determining region Y) box 9 [SOX9]) being used to assess MSC differentiation toward an NP cell phenotype.[72,73] However, whereas the NP and articular cartilage share a similar matrix composition, the ratio of PGs and collagens differs between the two tissues. In fact, the PG to collagen ratio in NP tissue is 27:1 as compared with only 2:1 in articular cartilage tissue.[74] Microarray studies have also identified differences in the phenotypic gene profile between NP and articular cartilage cells. Whereas

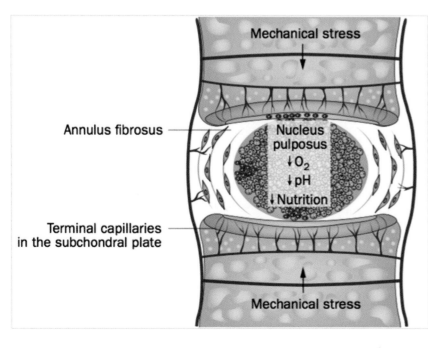

Fig. 13.3 The intravertebral disc (IVD)-specific niche is an obstacle to successful IVD regeneration using cell therapy. The specialized microenvironment of the IVD is characterized by low oxygen level, low pH, and poor nutrient supply, factors that present a major challenge to the survival and function of injected cells.

Mechanical stress

Annulus fibrosus

Nucleus pulposus
↓O_2
↓pH
↓Nutrition

Terminal capillaries in the subchondral plate

Mechanical stress

the functional significance of these molecules in the IVD is largely unknown, their use as phenotypic markers is vitally important to help define the NP cell phenotype.[75] Indeed, these markers (particularly CA12 and KRT-8, -18, and -19) are being used in more recent studies to better demonstrate MSC differentiation toward NP-like cells and not just toward more general chondrocytelike cells. This improvement in our understanding of the cells that are being generated from MSCs should provide better results moving forward.

13.4 Induction of Mesenchymal Stem Cell Discogenic Differentiation

13.4.1 Growth Factors

Disc cell metabolism is modulated by a variety of growth factors acting in both paracrine and autocrine roles.[5,76] These factors function to modulate the precise homeostasis of ECM production versus breakdown. In addition, growth factors have been shown to be very important in coaxing MSCs to differentiate into the desired cell line. In a 2005 study, Steck et al[77] demonstrated the ability of adult bone marrow–derived MSCs to differentiate toward the molecular phenotype of human IVD cells with the use of transforming growth factor (TGF)-β. This was further expanded upon by Tapp and colleagues.[78] In their study, they revealed that the treatment of TGF- β could significantly stimulate expression of PG and type I collagen in 3D-cultured sand rat ADSCs.

McCanless and colleagues[79] investigated the effects of bone morphogenetic protein (BMP)-2 and synthetic peptide B2A on cell proliferation and ECM synthesis by NP-like differentiated bone marrow–derived MSCs. The authors found that B2A induced proliferation, aggrecan synthesis, and stabilized collagen accumulation consistent with cells of the young, healthy NP.

Stoyanov and colleagues[71] also compared standard chondrogenic differentiation protocols using TGF- β with a novel technique utilizing hypoxia, growth and differentiation factor (GDF)-5, and co-culture with NP cells. The authors found that both hypoxia and GDF-5 were suitable for directing bone marrow–derived MSCs toward an NP-like phenotype. Feng et al[80] also examined the effects of GDF-5 on ADSCs. The authors found GDF-5 to be a potent inducer of chondrogenesis in ADSCs, and that ADSCs can be genetically engineered to express prochondrogenic growth factors as a promising therapeutic cell source for IVD tissue engineering.

In another example of genetic engineering, Yang and colleagues[81] engineered ADSCs to continuously express SOX9. The authors reported improved chondrogenic differentiation in the engineered cells, indicating a potential application in the treatment of IDD.

13.4.2 Scaffolds

Simply implanting a large number of stem cells into a target tissue can lead to a substantial amount of cell death rather than cell differentiation and matrix production. Additionally, after the removal of degenerated disc tissue, the implanted cells may need too much time to differentiate and generate new disc tissue and a more probable scenario might be that undesired scar tissue is formed instead.[82] The goal then is to improve the viability of the cells and to accelerate the process of matrix production, which has been shown to be achieved with the use of extracellular scaffolds. These scaffolds aid in cell delivery and provide a suitable microenvironment while the implanted cells generate new tissue.

The choice of scaffold is critical because it can directly affect the type of cell line that forms from MSCs. Scaffold fiber diameter and stiffness can influence cell function, proliferation, and orientation. They act as a cellular attachment site and can provide a privileged mechanical advantage for cell growth.[15] A good scaffold should also aid in the introduction of chemical stimuli by immobilizing growth factors and keeping them at a higher local concentration than in the surrounding liquid phase. The scaffold is also an important tool for tissue engineers because it can function as a delivery vehicle, not only allowing the implantation of cells into the intended site but also increasing their level of local retention thereafter. Numerous biomaterials have been described as scaffolds in the setting of stem cell delivery including polyactic glycolic acid (PLGA), poly-d-lactide, chitosan, alginate, collagens, gels, calcium polyphosphate, and demineralized bone matrix.[83]

Bertoloet al[84] compared the performance of four commercially available matrixes in supporting cell differentiation into NP-like cells. Bone marrow–derived human MSCs were seeded in these scaffolds or embedded in alginate as a 3D control for 5 weeks. MSCs in collagen matrices and gelatin produced more messenger ribonucleic acid (mRNA) and proteins of chondrogenic markers when compared with cells embedded in alginate or chitosan. PG accumulation and cell survival were also higher. Gene expression studies have shown that the phenotype of the differentiated MSCs was similar but not completely equivalent to that of NP cells, however.

Gruber and colleagues[85] developed a small animal model for autologous disc cell implantation. Cells were either placed onto a bioresorbable carrier or injected into the recipient disc of the sand rat alone. Immunocytologic identification of the engrafted cells showed that they integrated into the disc and were surrounded by normal matrix at time points up to 8 months after being placed. Another study has shown the ability of hyaluronan-based hydrogels to drive differentiation of MSCs when implanted into a nucleated bovine caudal disc.[86] The authors found that predifferentiation of the MSCs within the hydrogel prior to implantation was not necessary and in fact led to inferior results when compared with direct implantation.

Sato and colleagues[87] also investigated the regeneration of IVDs in a rabbit model. MSCs that had been cultured in a scaffold for 7 days were allografted into the IVDs of the rabbits whose NP had been vaporized with the use of a laser. The allografted cells not only survived but also produced hyalinelike cartilage, and narrowing of the disc spaces of the cell-containing scaffold group were found to be significantly inhibited after 12 weeks.

13.5 Challenges and Potential Risks

The cell density in the human disc is extremely low with between 2,000 and 5,000 cells/mm^3 in the adult human NP.[88] Nevertheless, despite the low cell densities required for replacement of 1 mL of tissue, about 2 to 5×10^6 of cells are needed. Therefore, due to the scarcity of MSCs in bone marrow or adipose tissue, cell proliferation and population expansion are still required to obtain sufficient cells for implantation.[89] This presents a significant challenge in not only harvesting but also successfully expanding these cells. In addition, the optimal number of cells for transplantation has not been established for cell survival or for therapeutic effect.

All cells normally perform a limited number of cell doublings when cultured in vitro, after which they become "senescent."[90] Senescent cells not only cease to have the ability to proliferate but also exhibit a distinct gene expression profile. These cells overexpress matrix metalloproteinases (MMPs), catabolic factors, and inflammatory molecules, which has been shown to affect tissue homeostasis.[91] This issue is an important aspect to be considered in culture expansion of MSCs for cell therapy. As discussed above, MSCs require extensive proliferation for use in cell replacement therapies if millions of them are to be implanted. Several studies have indicated that, even though MSCs are more resistant to senescence, repeated proliferation can lead to a decreased differentiation capacity.[92,93]

One method of obtaining sufficient cell numbers of MSCs for clinical application is by density gradient centrifugation followed by ex vivo expansion. This process may cause a selection for rapidly dividing cells, however, thereby increasing the risk of genetic and epigenetic mutations. This can potentially lead to the spontaneous transformation of MSCs, which has been suggested to be associated with tumor promotion.[89]

Moreover, Miura and colleagues[94] also found that murine bone marrow MSCs accumulated chromosomal abnormalities and were associated with both increased telomerase activity and c-myc expression during long-term culturing. Similarly, when the murine bone marrow–derived MSCs were delivered systemically to immunocompromised mice they generated fibrosarcomas in multiple organs. In contrast, the authors found a different behavior in human MSCs. They discovered that human bone marrow–derived MSCs demonstrated no signs of immortalization with continuous culture passages during expansion but did exhibit cell senescence. In a similar study in which human MSCs were populated to greater than 30 doublings, no karyotype abnormalities were noted nor was telomerase activity present.[95] The authors then transplanted the long-term cultured human MSCs into mice and were able to continue to demonstrate the absence of tumorigenesis.

However, other studies demonstrating in vitro malignant transformation of cultured human MSCs have challenged these findings. One study noted that cultured human MSCs exhibited a transformed phenotype and demonstrated chromosomal translocation and aneuploidy with increased telomerase activity. Moreover, when transplanted into immunocompromised mice, the cultured human MSCs grew solid tumors in multiple organs.[96] These findings have not been limited to bone marrow MSCs. ADSCs have also been shown to exhibit spontaneous transformation and cell immortalization.[97] When these cells were infused into immunocompromised mice, tumor formation occurred in almost all organs. However, in later experiments, the authors were unable to confirm the in vitro transformation of these ADSCs stem cells.[89,98]

Conversely, Bernardo and colleagues found that bone marrow MSCs can be safely expanded in vitro and are not susceptible to malignant transformation.[38] The authors investigated the susceptibility of bone marrow MSC transformation at different in vitro culture points. The study included 10 healthy bone marrow donors. The isolated MSCs were propagated in vitro until senescence, and the investigators found no chromosomal abnormalities as well as no telomerase activity.

A further potential risk associated with MSCs is the promotion of growth of established subclinical tumors within the transplant patient. Bian et al showed that human MSCs in vivo targeted established osteosarcomas and promoted tumor growth as well as pulmonary metastasis.[99] In animal studies, cotransplantation of cancer cells with MSCs promoted accelerated growth of the cancer cells.[100] However, the authors note that the studies that demonstrated the promotion of tumor growth by the addition of MSCs utilized either immortalized or modified MSC lines. In addition, 700 human subjects who received autologous or third-party MSCs showed no major side effects nor developed hematopoietic or solid tumors.[89] However, the follow-up period of most of the clinical trials was relatively short (1 month to 6.8 years). The clinical manifestation and occurrence of a tumor may certainly require longer surveillance.

13.6 Conclusion

Although animal and human data on the regenerative potential of cell-based therapy for IDD are promising, questions remain regarding the timing of treatment, optimal cell source, cell pretreatment, and cell carrier. A main hurdle is the limited understanding of IVD cell phenotypes and their modulation during disc development, homeostasis, and disease. Current knowledge indicates cellular injection therapy is safe, although long-term results are unknown. With the increasing number of clinical trials, cell therapy for IVD regeneration could bridge the gap between symptomatic care and aggressive surgical interventions in some patients with IDD.

The solution to overcoming the obstacles that exist in developing cell therapies for IVD regeneration is to address each concern through focused research, both in the laboratory and in the clinic. Well-controlled preclinical testing is needed to address the long-term efficacy in using committed cells compared with adverse effects and concerns about the use of stem cells. Consequently, the accumulation of well-designed and case-controlled clinical trials for each question, in a stepwise manner in concert with expert discussions and regulatory institutions, such as the US Food and Drug Administration (FDA), will be crucial to surmounting the obstacles to stem cell therapy in the treatment of IDD.

13.7 References

[1] Bibby SR, Urban JP. Effect of nutrient deprivation on the viability of intervertebral disc cells. Eur Spine J. 2004; 13(8):695–701

[2] Horner HA, Roberts S, Bielby RC, Menage J, Evans H, Urban JP. Cells from different regions of the intervertebral disc: effect of culture system on matrix expression and cell phenotype. Spine. 2002; 27(10):1018–1028

[3] Anderson DG, Li X, Balian G. A fibronectin fragment alters the metabolism by rabbit intervertebral disc cells in vitro. Spine. 2005; 30(11):1242–1246

[4] Freemont AJ. The cellular pathobiology of the degenerate intervertebral disc and discogenic back pain. Rheumatology (Oxford). 2009; 48(1):5–10

[5] Paesold G, Nerlich AG, Boos N. Biological treatment strategies for disc degeneration: potentials and shortcomings. Eur Spine J. 2007; 16(4):447–468

[6] Séguin CA, Pilliar RM, Roughley PJ, Kandel RA. Tumor necrosis factor-alpha modulates matrix production and catabolism in nucleus pulposus tissue. Spine. 2005; 30(17):1940–1948

[7] Sobajima S, Vadala G, Shimer A, Kim JS, Gilbertson LG, Kang JD. Feasibility of a stem cell therapy for intervertebral disc degeneration. Spine J. 2008; 8(6):888–896

[8] Kim KW, Lim TH, Kim JG, Jeong ST, Masuda K, An HS. The origin of chondrocytes in the nucleus pulposus and histologic findings associated with the transition of a notochordal nucleus pulposus to a fibrocartilaginous nucleus pulposus in intact rabbit intervertebral discs. Spine. 2003; 28(10):982–990

[9] Yang KH, King AI. Mechanism of facet load transmission as a hypothesis for low-back pain. Spine. 1984; 9(6):557–565

[10] Vanharanta H, Sachs BL, Spivey MA, et al. The relationship of pain provocation to lumbar disc deterioration as seen by CT/discography. Spine. 1987; 12(3):295–298

[11] Lewis G. Nucleus pulposus replacement and regeneration/repair technologies: present status and future prospects. J Biomed Mater Res B Appl Biomater. 2012; 100(6):1702–1720

[12] Karppinen J, Shen FH, Luk KD, Andersson GB, Cheung KM, Samartzis D. Management of degenerative disk disease and chronic low back pain. Orthop Clin North Am. 2011; 42(4):513–528, viii

[13] Haufe SM, Mork AR. Intradiscal injection of hematopoietic stem cells in an attempt to rejuvenate the intervertebral discs. Stem Cells Dev. 2006; 15(1):136–137

[14] Wang YT, Wu XT, Wang F. Regeneration potential and mechanism of bone marrow mesenchymal stem cell transplantation for treating intervertebral disc degeneration. J OrthopSci. 2010; 15(6):707–719

[15] Kandel R, Roberts S, Urban JPG. Tissue engineering and the intervertebral disc: the challenges. Eur Spine J. 2008; 17 Suppl 4:480–491

[16] Gorensek M, Jaksimović C, Kregar-Velikonja N, et al. Nucleus pulposus repair with cultured autologous elastic cartilage derived chondrocytes. Cell Mol Biol Lett. 2004; 9(2):363–373

[17] Acosta FL , Jr, Metz L, Adkisson HD, et al. Porcine intervertebral disc repair using allogeneic juvenile articular chondrocytes or mesenchymal stem cells. Tissue Eng Part A. 2011; 17(23–24):3045–3055

[18] Arana CJ, Diamandis EP, Kandel RA. Cartilage tissue enhances proteoglycan retention by nucleus pulposus cells in vitro. Arthritis Rheum. 2010; 62(11):3395–3403

[19] Mwale F, Roughley P, Antoniou J. Distinction between the extracellular matrix of the nucleus pulposus and hyaline cartilage: a requisite for tissue engineering of intervertebral disc. Eur Cell Mater. 2004; 8:58–63, discussion 63–64

[20] Meisel HJ, Ganey T, Hutton WC, Libera J, Minkus Y, Alasevic O. Clinical experience in cell-based therapeutics: intervention and outcome. Eur Spine J. 2006; 15 Suppl 3:S397–S405

[21] Meisel HJ, Siodla V, Ganey T, Minkus Y, Hutton WC, Alasevic OJ. Clinical experience in cell-based therapeutics: disc chondrocyte transplantation A treatment for degenerated or damaged intervertebral disc. BiomolEng. 2007; 24(1):5–21

[22] Yoshikawa T, Ueda Y, Miyazaki K, Koizumi M, Takakura Y. Disc regeneration therapy using marrow mesenchymal cell transplantation: a report of two case studies. Spine. 2010; 35(11):E475–E480

[23] Orozco L, Soler R, Morera C, Alberca M, Sánchez A, García-Sancho J. Intervertebral disc repair by autologous mesenchymal bone marrow cells: a pilot study. Transplantation. 2011; 92(7):822–828

[24] Coric D, Pettine K, Sumich A, Boltes MO. Prospective study of disc repair with allogeneic chondrocytes presented at the 2012 Joint Spine Section Meeting. J Neurosurg Spine. 2013; 18(1):85–95

[25] US National Library of Medicine. ClinicalTrials.gov. NCT01771471. https://clinicaltrials.gov/ct2/show/. 2014

[26] US National Library of Medicine. ClinicalTrials.gov. NCT01290367. https://clinicaltrials.gov/ct2/show/. 2014

[27] US National Library of Medicine. ClinicalTrials.gov. NCT01860417. https://clinicaltrials.gov/ct2/show/. 2014

[28] US National Library of Medicine. ClinicalTrials.gov. NCT01640457. https://clinicaltrials.gov/ct2/show/. 2014

[29] US National Library of Medicine. ClinicalTrials.gov. NCT01643681. https://clinicaltrials.gov/ct2/show/. 2014

[30] US National Library of Medicine. ClinicalTrials.gov. NCT02097862. https://clinicaltrials.gov/ct2/show/. 2014

[31] Thomson JA, Itskovitz-Eldor J, Shapiro SS, et al. Embryonic stem cell lines derived from human blastocysts. Science. 1998; 282(5391):1145–1147

[32] Sheikh H, Zakharian K, De La Torre RP, et al. In vivo intervertebral disc regeneration using stem cell-derived chondroprogenitors. J Neurosurg Spine. 2009; 10(3):265–272

[33] Chen J, Lee EJ, Jing L, Christoforou N, Leong KW, Setton LA. Differentiation of mouse induced pluripotent stem cells (iPSCs) into nucleus pulposus-like cells in vitro. PLoS One. 2013; 8(9):e75548

[34] Ichida JK, Blanchard J, Lam K, et al. A small-molecule inhibitor of tgf-Beta signaling replaces sox2 in reprogramming by inducing nanog. Cell Stem Cell. 2009; 5(5):491–503

[35] Knoepfler PS. Deconstructing stem cell tumorigenicity: a roadmap to safe regenerative medicine. Stem Cells. 2009; 27(5):1050–1056

[36] Gutierrez-Aranda I, Ramos-Mejia V, Bueno C, et al. Human induced pluripotent stem cells develop teratoma more efficiently and faster than human embryonic stem cells regardless the site of injection. Stem Cells. 2010; 28(9):1568–1570

[37] Le Blanc K, Frassoni F, Ball L, et al. Developmental Committee of the European Group for Blood and Marrow Transplantation. Mesenchymal stem cells for treatment of steroid-resistant, severe, acute graft-versus-host disease: a phase II study. Lancet. 2008; 371(9624):1579–1586

[38] Bernardo ME, Zaffaroni N, Novara F, et al. Human bone marrow derived mesenchymal stem cells do not undergo transformation after long-term in vitro culture and do not exhibit telomere maintenance mechanisms. Cancer Res. 2007; 67(19):9142–9149

[39] Oehme D, Ghosh P, Shimmon S, et al. Mesenchymal progenitor cells combined with pentosan polysulfate mediating disc regeneration at the time of microdiscectomy: a preliminary study in an ovine model. J Neurosurg Spine. 2014; 20(6):657–669

[40] Moroni L, Fornasari PM. Human mesenchymal stem cells: a bank perspective on the isolation, characterization and potential of alternative sources for the regeneration of musculoskeletal tissues. J Cell Physiol. 2013; 228(4):680–687

[41] Sensébé L, Krampera M, Schrezenmeier H, Bourin P, Giordano R. Mesenchymal stem cells for clinical application. Vox Sang. 2010; 98(2):93–107

[42] Shen B, Wei A, Tao H, Diwan AD, Ma DD. BMP-2 enhances TGF-beta3-mediated chondrogenic differentiation of human bone marrow multipotent mesenchymal stromal cells in alginate bead culture. Tissue Eng Part A. 2009; 15(6):1311–1320

[43] Umeda M, Kushida T, Sasai K, et al. Activation of rat nucleus pulposus cells by coculture with whole bone marrow cells collected by the perfusion method. J Orthop Res. 2009; 27(2):222–228

[44] Hee HT, Ismail HD, Lim CT, Goh JC, Wong HK. Effects of implantation of bone marrow mesenchymal stem cells, disc distraction and combined therapy on reversing degeneration of the intervertebral disc. J Bone Joint Surg Br. 2010; 92(5):726–736

[45] Abbah SA, Lam CX, Ramruttun KA, Goh JC, Wong HK. Autogenous bone marrow stromal cell sheets-loaded mPCL/TCP scaffolds induced osteogenesis in a porcine model of spinal interbody fusion. Tissue Eng Part A. 2011; 17(5–6):809–817

[46] Yamamoto Y, Mochida J, Sakai D, et al. Upregulation of the viability of nucleus pulposus cells by bone marrow-derived stromal cells: significance of direct cell-to-cell contact in coculture system. Spine. 2004; 29(14):1508–1514

[47] Allon AA, Aurouer N, Yoo BB, Liebenberg EC, Buser Z, Lotz JC. Structured coculture of stem cells and disc cells prevent disc degeneration in a rat model. Spine J. 2010; 10(12):1089–1097

[48] Zhang YG, Guo X, Xu P, Kang LL, Li J. Bone mesenchymal stem cells transplanted into rabbit intervertebral discs can increase proteoglycans. Clin OrthopRelat Res. 2005(430):219–226

[49] Sakai D, Mochida J, Iwashina T, et al. Regenerative effects of transplanting mesenchymal stem cells embedded in atelocollagen to the degenerated intervertebral disc. Biomaterials. 2006; 27(3):335–345

[50] Ghosh P, Moore R, Vernon-Roberts B, et al. Immunoselected STRO-3 + mesenchymal precursor cells and restoration of the extracellular matrix of degenerate intervertebral discs. J Neurosurg Spine. 2012; 16(5):479–488

[51] Ghosh P. STRO-3 Immunoselected allogeneic mesenchymal precursor cells injected into degenerate intervertebral discs reconstitute the proteoglycans of the nucleus pulposus—an experimental study in sheep. Orthopaedic Research Society Annual Scientific Meeting. Long Beach, California 2011

[52] Liang C, Li H, Tao Y, et al. Responses of human adipose-derived mesenchymal stem cells to chemical microenvironment of the intervertebral disc. J Transl Med. 2012; 10:49

[53] Choi EH, Park H, Park KS, et al. Effect of nucleus pulposus cells having different phenotypes on chondrogenic differentiation of adipose-derived stromal cells in a coculture system using porous membranes. Tissue Eng Part A. 2011; 17(19–20):2445–2451

[54] Lu ZF, Doulabi BZ, Wuisman PI, Bank RA, Helder MN. Influence of collagen type II and nucleus pulposus cells on aggregation and differentiation of adipose tissue-derived stem cells. J Cell Mol Med. 2008; 12 6B:2812–2822

[55] Gaetani P, Torre ML, Klinger M, et al. Adipose-derived stem cell therapy for intervertebral disc regeneration: an in vitro reconstructed tissue in alginate capsules. Tissue Eng Part A. 2008; 14(8):1415–1423

[56] Vadalà G, Sobajima S, Lee JY, et al. In vitro interaction between muscle-derived stem cells and nucleus pulposus cells. Spine J. 2008; 8(5):804–809

[57] Feng G, Yang X, Shang H, et al. Multipotential differentiation of human anulus fibrosus cells: an in vitro study. J Bone Joint Surg Am. 2010; 92 (3):675–685

[58] Erwin, WM, Islam, D, Eftekarpour, E, Inman, RD, Karim, MZ, Fehlings, MG. Intervertebral disc-derived stem cells: implications for regenerative medicine and neural repair. Spine. 2013; 38(3):211–216

[59] Chen S, Emery SE, Pei M. Coculture of synovium-derived stem cells and nucleus pulposus cells in serum-free defined medium with supplementation of transforming growth factor-beta1: a potential application of tissue-specific stem cells in disc regeneration. Spine. 2009; 34(12):1272–1280

[60] He F, Pei M. Rejuvenation of nucleus pulposus cells using extracellular matrix deposited by synovium-derived stem cells. Spine. 2012; 37(6):459–469

[61] Miyamoto T, Muneta T, Tabuchi T, et al. Intradiscal transplantation of synovial mesenchymal stem cells prevents intervertebral disc degeneration through suppression of matrix metalloproteinase-related genes in nucleus pulposus cells in rabbits. Arthritis Res Ther. 2010; 12(6):R206

[62] Sakai D, Nakamura Y, Nakai T, et al. Exhaustion of nucleus pulposus progenitor cells with ageing and degeneration of the intervertebral disc. Nat Commun. 2012; 3:1264

[63] Henriksson H, Thornemo M, Karlsson C, et al. Identification of cell proliferation zones, progenitor cells and a potential stem cell niche in the intervertebral disc region: a study in four species. Spine. 2009; 34(21):2278–2287

[64] Brisby H, Papadimitriou N, Brantsing C, Bergh P, Lindahl A, BarretoHenriksson H. The presence of local mesenchymal progenitor cells in human degenerated intervertebral discs and possibilities to influence these in vitro: a descriptive study in humans. Stem Cells Dev. 2013; 22(5):804–814

[65] Risbud MV, Guttapalli A, Tsai TT, et al. Evidence for skeletal progenitor cells in the degenerate human intervertebral disc. Spine. 2007; 32(23):2537–2544

[66] Li T, Xia M, Gao Y, Chen Y, Xu Y. Human umbilical cord mesenchymal stem cells: an overview of their potential in cell-based therapy. Expert Opin Biol Ther. 2015; 15(9):1293–1306

[67] Urban JP, McMullin JF. Swelling pressure of the lumbar intervertebral discs: influence of age, spinal level, composition, and degeneration. Spine. 1988; 13(2):179–187

[68] Bartels EM, Fairbank JCT, Winlove CP, Urban JP. Oxygen and lactate concentrations measured in vivo in the intervertebral discs of patients with scoliosis and back pain. Spine. 1998; 23(1):1–7, discussion 8

[69] Wuertz K, Godburn K, Neidlinger-Wilke C, Urban J, Iatridis JC. Behavior of mesenchymal stem cells in the chemical microenvironment of the intervertebral disc. Spine. 2008; 33(17):1843–1849

[70] Wuertz K, Godburn K, Iatridis JC. MSC response to pH levels found in degenerating intervertebral discs. Biochem Biophys Res Commun. 2009; 379 (4):824–829

[71] Stoyanov JV, Gantenbein-Ritter B, Bertolo A, et al. Role of hypoxia and growth and differentiation factor-5 on differentiation of human

mesenchymal stem cells towards intervertebral nucleus pulposus-like cells. Eur Cell Mater. 2011; 21:533–547

[72] Richardson SM, Hughes N, Hunt JA, Freemont AJ, Hoyland JA. Human mesenchymal stem cell differentiation to NP-like cells in chitosan-glycerophosphate hydrogels. Biomaterials. 2008; 29(1):85–93

[73] Henriksson HB, Svanvik T, Jonsson M, et al. Transplantation of human mesenchymal stems cells into intervertebral discs in a xenogeneic porcine model. Spine. 2009; 34(2):141–148

[74] Mwale F, Roughley P, Antoniou J. Distinction between the extracellular matrix of the nucleus pulposus and hyaline cartilage: a requisite for tissue engineering of intervertebral disc. Eur Cell Mater. 2004; 8:58–63, discussion 63–64

[75] Minogue BM, Richardson SM, Zeef L A, Freemont AJ, Hoyland JA. Characterization of the human nucleus pulposus cell phenotype and evaluation of novel marker gene expression to define adult stem cell differentiation. Arthritis Rheum. 2010; 62(12):3695–3705

[76] Yang SH, Wu CC, Shih TT, Sun YH, Lin FH. In vitro study on interaction between human nucleus pulposus cells and mesenchymal stem cells through paracrine stimulation. Spine. 2008; 33(18):1951–1957

[77] Steck E, Bertram H, Abel R, Chen B, Winter A, Richter W. Induction of intervertebral disc-like cells from adult mesenchymal stem cells. Stem Cells. 2005; 23(3):403–411

[78] Tapp H, Deepe R, Ingram JA, Kuremsky M, Hanley EN , Jr, Gruber HE. Adipose-derived mesenchymal stem cells from the sand rat: transforming growth factor beta and 3D co-culture with human disc cells stimulate proteoglycan and collagen type I rich extracellular matrix. Arthritis Res Ther. 2008; 10(4):R89

[79] McCanless JD, Cole JA, Slack SM, Bumgardner JD, Zamora PO, Haggard WO. Modeling nucleus pulposus regeneration in vitro: mesenchymal stem cells, alginate beads, hypoxia, bone morphogenetic protein-2, and synthetic peptide B2A. Spine. 2011; 36(26):2275–2285

[80] Feng G, Wan Y, Balian G, Laurencin CT, Li X. Adenovirus-mediated expression of growth and differentiation factor-5 promotes chondrogenesis of adipose stem cells. Growth Factors. 2008; 26(3):132–142

[81] Yang Z, Huang CY, Candiotti KA, et al. Sox-9 facilitates differentiation of adipose tissue-derived stem cells into a chondrocyte-like phenotype in vitro. J Orthop Res. 2011; 29(8):1291–1297

[82] van den Bogaerdt AJ, van der Veen VC, van Zuijlen PP, et al. Collagen cross-linking by adipose-derived mesenchymal stromal cells and scar-derived mesenchymal cells: Are mesenchymal stromal cells involved in scar formation? Wound Repair Regen. 2009; 17(4):548–558

[83] O'Halloran DM, Pandit AS. Tissue-engineering approach to regenerating the intervertebral disc. Tissue Eng. 2007; 13(8):1927–1954

[84] Bertolo A, Mehr M, Aebli N, Baur M, Ferguson SJ, Stoyanov JV. Influence of different commercial scaffolds on the in vitro differentiation of human mesenchymal stem cells to nucleus pulposus-like cells. Eur Spine J. 2012; 21 Suppl 6:S826–S838

[85] Gruber HE, Johnson TL, Leslie K, et al. Autologous intervertebral disc cell implantation: a model using Psammomysobesus, the sand rat. Spine. 2002; 27(15):1626–1633

[86] Peroglio M, Eglin D, Benneker LM, Alini M, Grad S. Thermoreversible hyaluronan-based hydrogel supports in vitro and ex vivo disc-like differentiation of human mesenchymal stem cells. Spine J. 2013; 13(11):1627–1639

[87] Sato M, Kikuchi M, Ishihara M, et al. Tissue engineering of the intervertebral disc with cultured annulus fibrosus cells using atelocollagen honeycomb-shaped scaffold with a membrane seal (ACHMS scaffold). Med BiolEngComput. 2003; 41(3):365–371

[88] Liebscher T, Haefeli M, Wuertz K, Nerlich AG, Boos N. Age-related variation in cell density of human lumbar intervertebral disc. Spine. 2011; 36(2):153–159

[89] Casiraghi F, Remuzzi G, Abbate M, Perico N. Multipotent mesenchymal stromal cell therapy and risk of malignancies. Stem Cell Rev. 2013; 9(1):65–79

[90] Hayflick L. The limited in vitro lifetime of human diploid cell strains. Exp Cell Res. 1965; 37:614–636

[91] Campisi J, d'Adda di Fagagna F. Cellular senescence: when bad things happen to good cells. Nat Rev Mol Cell Biol. 2007; 8(9):729–740

[92] Schellenberg A, Stiehl T, Horn P, et al. Population dynamics of mesenchymal stromal cells during culture expansion. Cytotherapy. 2012; 14(4):401–411

[93] Li J, Pei M. Cell senescence: a challenge in cartilage engineering and regeneration. Tissue Eng Part B Rev. 2012; 18(4):270–287

[94] Miura M, Miura Y, Padilla-Nash HM, et al. Accumulated chromosomal instability in murine bone marrow mesenchymal stem cells leads to malignant transformation. Stem Cells. 2006; 24(4):1095–1103

[95] Kim J, Kang JW, Park JH, et al. Biological characterization of long-term cultured human mesenchymal stem cells. Arch Pharm Res. 2009; 32(1):117–126

[96] Wang Y, Huso DL, Harrington J, et al. Outgrowth of a transformed cell population derived from normal human BM mesenchymal stem cell culture. Cytotherapy. 2005; 7(6):509–519

[97] Rubio D, Garcia-Castro J, Martín MC, et al. Spontaneous human adult stem cell transformation. Cancer Res. 2005; 65(8):3035–3039

[98] de la Fuente R, Bernad A, Garcia-Castro J, Martin MC, Cigudosa JC. Cancer Res. 2010; 70(16):6682

[99] Bian ZY, Fan QM, Li G, Xu WT, Tang TT. Human mesenchymal stem cells promote growth of osteosarcoma: involvement of interleukin-6 in the interaction between human mesenchymal stem cells and Saos-2. Cancer Sci. 2010; 101(12):2554–2560

[100] Meier RP, Müller YD, Morel P, Gonelle-Gispert C, Bühler LH. Transplantation of mesenchymal stem cells for the treatment of liver diseases, is there enough evidence? Stem Cell Res (Amst). 2013; 11(3):1348–1364

14 Nucleus Replacement and Repair: Autologous Disc Chondrocyte Transplantation

Christian Hohaus, Timothy Ganey, and Hans Jörg Meisel

Abstract

Intervertebral disc (IVD) degeneration is in 40% of younger individuals and in more than 90% of individuals older than 50 years of age, a common disorder with a negative impact on life quality. Available treatment options, conservative as well as operative procedures, are limited and don't treat the underlying biological reason, IVD degeneration. Total regeneration of the degenerated IVD is not currently considered a therapeutic assurance. The goals of regenerative medicine at this time are to prevent further progression of disc degeneration and its associated symptoms.

What has been shown to date, and therefore available in limited geographies and jurisdictions, is that expanded and transplanted autologous cells are safe and appear to arrest if not reverse degenerative disc disease (DDD) following treatment for sequestrectomy. In our clinical trial with more than 140 patients, the largest number of patients with degenerated IVD disease treated with cell transplantation under defined study conditions, all patients have benefited from transplantation in reduced back pain as one measure of an enhanced quality of life and were able to return to work after transplantation. Moreover, the reduction in reherniation rate was more than 50% better than the control group.

The use of autologous chondrocytes requires the ex vivo expansion of cells, adding burdens of cost, time, and regulation that add to the intricacy of the procedure beyond the medical interface. This limitation of the procedure could be avoided by the use of a one-step procedure, using stem cells obtained from autologous adipose tissue, with shows promising results in preclinical studies.

Cell transplantation appears to present an effective treatment option in DDD. The transplantation of autologous disc cells is currently the only biological treatment option with good clinical results under defined study conditions.

Keywords: autologous disc cell transplantation, cell therapy, clinical study, degenerative disc disease, intervertebral disc, low back pain

14.1 Introduction

Low back pain is extremely common, affecting nearly three quarters of the population sometime in their life. More than 80% of the population will suffer from lumbar back pain once in their lifetime.[1,2,3,4] Although most people recover within 3 months, in some patients chronic back or leg pain leads to long-term physical disability, and the reduced quality of life that it imposes.

Disc anatomy would be expected to play a pivotal role and correlate with the underlying pain, yet abnormal spine and disc morphology including disc herniation has been described as a normal component of an asymptomatic population.[5,6]

IVD degeneration is influenced by multiple factors such as age and genetic loading,[7] biomechanical forces,[8] and environmental factors such as immobilization, trauma, and application of nicotine.[9] Age-related diseases such as diabetes, arterial hypertension, and complications attendant to vascular diseases have been defined as relevant factors as well.[10]

Accepting the vast prevalence of asymptomatic disc degeneration as noted, "normal" IVDs present an optimal balance between anabolic and catabolic processes that are regulated by anabolic growth factors, catabolic enzymes, and pro-inflammatory cytokines.[11] Among the key anabolic growth factors that have been noted are insulin-like growth factor (IGF)-1, transforming growth factor (TGF)-β, and bone morphogenetic proteins (BMPs).[12] Interleukin (IL)-1 and TGF-α clearly are involved in catabolic activities in the healthy IVD.[13] Catabolic processes contribute to changing disc morphology and variations in matrix composition that initially alters biochemical composition, and ultimately result in the loss of proteoglycans and type II collagen. Following a restructuring of the matrix, an increase in cell death and decreasing nutrition further impose conditions and predisposition to mechanobiological consequence and precipitate a self-imposing insult that furthers the degenerative process.[14,15,16,7,18]

Therapeutic options for treating degenerative disc disease (DDD) resulting from this knowledge have informed strategies including the substitution of growth factors, gene therapy tissue engineering, and cell transplantation. Some of these efforts have met with suggestive success to the extent that proteoglycan synthesis has been shown to increase in a canine model after direct injection of recombinant TGF-β in combination with epidermal growth factor.[19] Similarly, the direct stimulation of cells with BMP-7 in rabbit IVDs resulted in an increase in proteoglycan synthesis as well as restoration of disc height.[20,21,22] The intradiscal application of BMP-7 for regeneration of IVD degeneration in a natural canine model, however, did not promote disc regeneration but instead resulted in the formation of extradiscal bone.[23] A pilot clinical study combining matrix components and growth factors that was directly injected into degenerated discs stimulated IVD regeneration that was durable over the course of a 12-month follow-up.[24] Despite the success achieved, the concern for therapeutic support for such techniques seemed severely limited by the availability of viable cells and the limitation in application only in early stages of disc degeneration.[25] Transplantation of mesenchymal stem cells (MSCs) has also gained increasing attention,[26,27,28,29] although critics of that strategy have weighed in on limitations of cell viability as concerning.[25]

Given that disc herniation is thought to be an extension of progressive disc degeneration that attends the normal aging process, seeking an effective therapy that staves disc degeneration has been considered a logical attempt to reduce back pain. Disc herniation is the most common reason for radicular symptoms in the lumbar spine leading to an operative treatment. Herniated material from the degenerated disc has been considered a potential donor for nucleus pulposus (NP) cells and chondrocytes because of their extended viability.[30] Culturing and expanding these cells is not simple but is possible, and following successful transplantation cells produce both type-II collagen as well as appropriate proteoglycans.[31] Transplantation of these expanded cultured cells would create an option to enlarge the viable cell content in the degenerated disc and to increase the necessary extracellular matrix (ECM).

14.2 Preclinical Study Using Autologous Disc Cell Transplantation for Nucleus Regeneration in the Dog

This study[31] was performed to test the hypothesis that restoration of IVD morphology could be achieved by transplantation of cultured autologous chondrocytes into the NP. The study addressed the question of whether the introduction of cultured autologous disc–derived cells would repair a damaged disc and inhibit degenerative changes. The dogs were divided into two basic groups; 4 animals receiving autologous cells containing bromodeoxyuridine (BrdU) as a nuclear marker, the other 14 receiving autologous cells without a nuclear marker. Animals were radiographed to establish a baseline for preexisting spine pathology.

Lumbar IVDs at three levels (L1–2, L2–3, and L3–4) were identified as study levels for the procedure and disc tissue was collected. The sampled disc cells were expanded in culture through several passages, producing approximately 6 million cells with the goal of establishing a population of disc cells capable of producing matrix and sustaining an expanded volume within the damaged disc. In this study, the L1–2 IVD had tissue removed but did not receive chondrocyte transplantation, the L2–3 disc was approached but not violated and served as a surgical control, and the L3–4 level had disc material removed and received chondrocyte transplantation 12 weeks later via left-side minimally invasive puncture of the IVD under fluoroscopic imaging.

An important criterion for evaluating the success of cell transplantation in the disc repair procedure was identifying that matrix regeneration was attributable to transplanted, cultured, expanded disc cells rather than a result of inherent disc capacity for self-repair. BrdU, an analog nucleotide of thymidine, was incorporated into the nucleus during deoxyribonucleic acid (DNA) synthesis and could later be identified by immunohistochemical techniques. As such, it was possible to analyze morphology in situ after repair, and delineate cells that were transplanted from those already present in the host tissue.

The animals were humanely euthanized 3, 6, 9, and 12 months following the cell transplantation. Immediately after the dogs were killed, their lumbar spines were removed and the tissue analyzed (▶ Fig. 14.1). Magnetic resonance imaging (MRI) and X-ray analysis with coronal slices of the spinal column were performed to interpret disc height. Tissue analyses

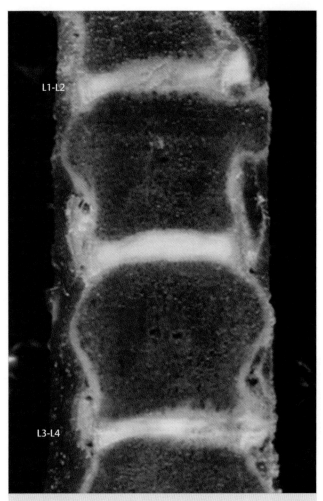

Fig. 14.1 Gross pathology at 12-month follow-up after autologous chondrocyte transplantation in the canine model. Level L3–4 was transplanted, level L1–2 received no treatment and displayed more scar tissue, and level L2–3 was the control level with a normal intervertebral disc.

included light microscopy and immunohistochemistry for assessing BrdU content (▶ Fig. 14.2) and collagen expression.

The results of this animal study were extremely promising for further clinical applications: Autologous disc cells were expanded in culture and returned to the disc by a minimally invasive procedure after 12 weeks. Under defined conditions, it was possible to assure phenotype and assess metabolic capacity of the cells prior to transplantation. These transplanted disc cells remained viable after transplantation as shown by BrdU incorporation and maintained a capacity for proliferation after transplantation as depicted by histology. They produced an ECM that contained components similar to normal IVD tissue. Both type I and type II collagens were demonstrated in the regenerated IVD matrix by immunohistochemistry following chondrocyte transplantation. And there was a statistically significant correlation between transplanting cells and retention of disc height that was demonstrated at longer intervals following transplantation.[31]

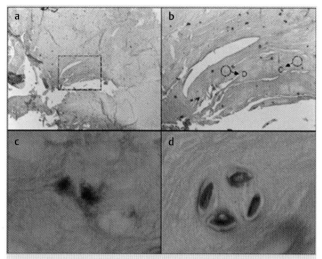

Fig. 14.2 Staining of paraffin sections of the regenerated intervertebral disc 6 months following cell transplantation. Bromodeoxyuridine (BrdU)-containing chondrocytes were detected and stained by immunohistochemical procedures using 3,3'-diaminobenzidine (DAB) as the chromogen. Sections were counterstained by eosin. BrdU-positive cells are colored black. **(a)** Nucleus regenerate overview (25 ×). **(b)** BrdU-stained transplanted cells (200 ×), **(c,d)** single BrdU-stained transplanted chondrocytes, pericellular de novo synthesis of nucleus matrix (1,000 ×).

14.3 Clinical Application of Autologous Disc Chondrocyte Transplantation in Degenerative Disc Disease

After these positive and promising results demonstrating both safety and efficacy, a randomized controlled study (the Euro Disc Randomized Trial) was designed to embrace a representative patient group, examining not only the traumatic, less degenerative disc, but also to include patients with persistent symptoms that had not responded to conservative treatment where an indication for surgical treatment was given. Between 2002 and 2006 a total number of 148 patients were included in this clinical trial from seven German spine centers.[32][33]

14.3.1 Patient Selection

Eligibility to participate in the study was limited to patients having exclusively one level requiring surgical intervention. Criteria for surgical therapy were progressive sciatic pain with futile conservative treatment or neurological deficits caused by root nerve compression. Magnetic resonance imaging (MRI) of the lumbar spine was mandatory. The trial was limited to patients between 18 and 60 years of age, with a body mass index (BMI) below 28.

Exclusion criteria to participating in the study included sclerotic changes, edema, Modic changes of type 2 or 3 in preoperative MRI, and spondylolisthesis. Patients with generalized diseases or progressive neurological deficits were excluded, as well as pregnancy.

14.3.2 Operative Treatment

Each patient participating in the clinical trial underwent surgical treatment for prolapsed disc. This was done as a minimally invasive open sequestrectomy using a tubular retractor system for minimal affection of the lumbar muscles. The use of an operative microscope after opening the yellow ligament was mandatory. This procedure was performed by an experienced neurosurgeon with the patient under general anesthesia. Randomization was done after closure of the fascia thoracolumbalis, directly from the operating room to prevent surgical bias in the evaluation of patients. The harvested cells from the sequestered disc material were cultured by co.Don AG (Teltow, Germany) under Good Manufacturing Practice (GMP) conditions. Patients were not blinded to their treatment.

14.3.3 Transplantation

Cell implantation was performed 3 months after the primary operative procedure to assure that the anulus had healed and would contain the cells. Prior to intervention with the cells, an MRI was used to detect possible early recurrent sequestration or progressive degeneration. In the prepared solution for the transplantation were more than 5 million living disc cells.

Under fluoroscopic control the affected disc was punctured with a minimal caliber cannula opposite the side of the previous disc herniation procedure (▶ Fig. 14.3). Using a pressure-volume test[34] prior to the delivery of any chondrocytes, surgeons were able to place the cells with confidence that they would be retained at the site of delivery.

Following cell transplantation, patients were placed for 24 hours in a lying position. After that time they were mobilized. They were urged to wear a lumbar orthesis for the next 3 weeks to provide an additional external stabilization to the treated segments.

14.3.4 Follow-up

The primary clinical evaluation criterion used to evaluate patient recovery was the Oswestry Low Back Pain Disability Questionnaire (OPDQ). Secondary criteria included the 36-item Short Form Health Survey (SF-36), Prolo Score,[35] Quebec Back Pain Disability Scale (QBPD), MRI, and X-ray evaluation.

All patients were scheduled for preoperative evaluation as well as seen 3 months following sequestrectomy as the time point for the transplantation in the treatment group. Additional examinations were conducted 3, 6, 12, and 24 months after transplantation. A long-term follow-up to evaluate durability of treatment is planned for 10 years after transplantation.

14.3.5 Results

An interim analysis with 28 patients was published in 2007 and showed a clear benefit for the patients transplanted with autologous disc–derived cells.[32] A final analysis of the Euro Disc Randomized Trial was not possible due to a lot of inconstancy in the data collection between the centers.

In 2014 an evaluation of the data from 78 patients with a mean age of 33.5 years (19–57 years) who were included between 2002 and 2006 in the Euro Disc Trial through the

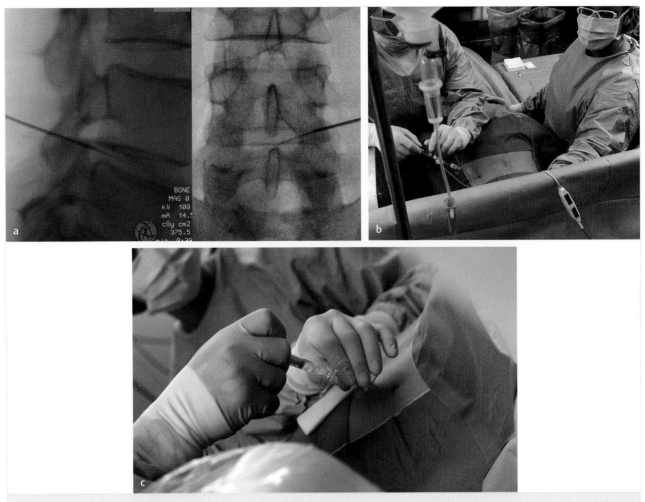

Fig. 14.3 Intraoperative picture of the fluoroscopically guided minimally invasive puncture of the intervertebral disc. **(a)** Fluoroscopic view after puncture of the disc. **(b)** Pressure-volume test. **(c)** Transplantation.

Department of Neurosurgery at the BG Klinikum Bergmann-strost in Halle, Germany, was begun. Of the 36 patients randomized into the treatment group, 3 patients dropped out for personal reasons. From the remaining 33 patients, 21 were successfully transplanted at the L5–S1 level and 12 at the L4–5 level following pressure-volume–test assurance in all patients with annulus fibrous (AF) containment before transplantation. The control group comprised 35 patients with disc herniation at the L5–S1 level and 7 patients at the L4–5 level.

For descriptive analysis of efficacy, the total sum score as well as the disability index of the OPDQ and the total sum score of the QBPD were taken into account from the initial presurgical presentation through the 2-year follow-up. Based on the mean total sum score as well as the disability index of the OPDQ, differences in initial presentations between the control group and those receiving autologous cells were not seen.

Surgery as an intervention was a positive experience, and as expected, substantially reduced the patient's disability and pain. The trend in reduction of the total sum score continued to decrease in the patients whose treatment was supplemented by cell transplantation over the 2-year follow-up. The patients in the control group did not sustain continual improvement. At the 2-year follow-up we noticed in the control group an increase in all measured clinical parameters. The difference was not statistically significant but showed a clear benefit for the treatment group (▶ Fig. 14.4).

A statistically significant difference was shown between the groups by measure of the rate of reherniation of disc material. The rate of recurrent herniation was 6.1% (2/33) in the autologous disc chondrocyte transplantation (ADCT) group. In the control group we detected 16.7% (7/42) recurrent herniations. From each group one patient had to be operated on again due to development of neurological deficits from the recurrent herniation.

14.4 Discussion

Cell transplantation in DDD is possible and the results of the clinical study offer some optimism for the future treatment of patients with intervertebral DDD. Autologous disc cell transplantation after sequestrectomy proved to be a safe and technically feasible procedure in the hands of skilled and select surgeons. Transplanted chondrocytes were shown to be viable in situ and to create a functional matrix in preclinical work, and

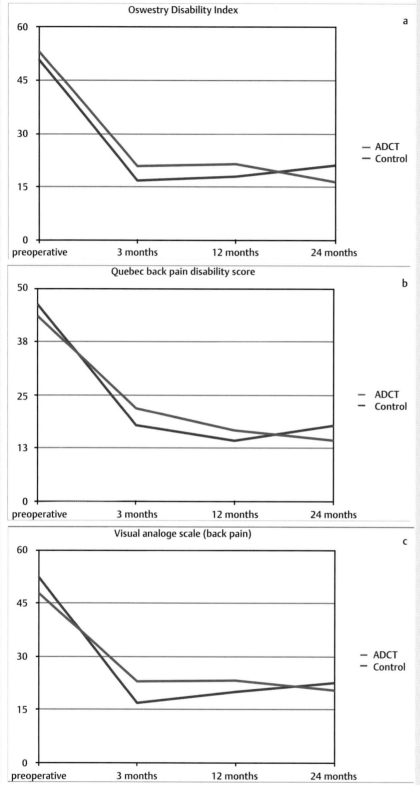

Fig. 14.4 Description analysis of efficacy after 24 months. (a) Oswestry Disability Index. (b) Quebec Back Pain Disability Scale score. (c) Visual Analog Scale (back pain). Abbreviations: ADCT, autologous disc chondrocyte transplantation.

the assumption of translation of cell viability as one of the accenting potentials of the clinical outcome seems likely.

The results for patients in the Euro Disc Randomized Trial from the Department of Neurosurgery at the BG Klinikum Bergmannstrost provide strong evidence for both the safety and efficiency of the disc-derived cell transplantation applied following sequestrectomy to delay or inhibit ongoing processes of disc degeneration. After transplantation a clear decrease in scores for the OPDQ, QBPD, and Visual Analog Scale (VAS) in ADCT-treated patients for disability and pain were measured.

Assigning an ideal group of patients who might profit most from the autologous disc cell transplantation needs additional work in larger populations of patients as well in a broader scope of clinical practice.

The technique of autologous disc cell transplantation is only possible for patients who underwent a sequestrectomy. There may be merit in transplanting disc cells at earlier stages of degeneration prior to significant loss of matrix from the IVD, but for autologous considerations this unfortunately requires an operation. Surgery to harvest cell material in the early stages of disc degeneration introduces the risk of infection to the disc and the bone, plus the risk of nerve root injury and other potential complications, and therefore the larger medical community has not been able to establish an ethical or medical foundation for this consideration.

For patients with MRI findings graded according to the Pfirrmann classification[36] between Grade I and Grade III with accompanying symptomatic nerve root compression in concert with a sequestered NP prolapse planning to undergo a minimally invasive operative procedure, the possibility of autologous disc cell transplantation might be an intervention that could be entertained. For other patients with intervertebral DDD who do not need to undergo operative treatment with sequestrectomy, a therapeutic option could be the transplantation of adipose-derived stem cells, and regenerative cells that are specifically expanded but allogenically derived. Our previous work in the animal model demonstrated that these cells can be transplanted at surgery using fluoroscopic guidance, and that these cells can be injected directly into the IVD with the expectation that they will remain viable and produce appropriate, tissue-specific matrix.[33,37]

If future results of adipose-derived and regenerative cell studies present promising outcomes, cell therapy might be accepted as a safe and easy technique for producing cells for minimally invasive transplantation into a symptomatic degenerative IVD without open operative intervention. Among the first clinical studies using stem cells for treatment of intervertebral DDD, that by Orozco et al illustrates the technical feasibility and safety of therapeutic intervention with stem cells.[38] Ten patients with chronic back pain diagnosed with lumbar disc degeneration with intact AF were treated with autologous expanded bone marrow MSCs injected into the NP area. The follow-up time was one year and there was no control group. Treated patients exhibited rapid improvement of pain and disability. The authors compare this favorably with the results of other procedures such as spinal fusion or total disc replacement. Critics of this study suggest that the lack of correlation of disc degeneration, a failure to adequately measure disc height and water content, and a variety of etiologies confound the outcome assessment. Those criticisms aside for what might constitute an ideal study, the positive effects should be studied further and could transfer to a controlled randomized study to include more specificity in the inclusion criteria. To that challenge, sources of cells also harbor choice. A particular option for patients could be the transplantation of juvenile allogeneic chondrocyte cells. Coric et al demonstrated in a small group of patients the technical feasibility and safety of this procedure by using juvenile allogenic chondrocyte cells harvested from the articular surface of cadaveric donor tissue.[39] These cells were transplanted using a fibrin glue–like carrier, which has been shown in a separate pilot study to be sufficient on its own account.[40]

14.5 Conclusion

Total regeneration of the degenerated IVD is not currently considered a therapeutic assurance. The goals of regenerative medicine at this time are to prevent further progression of disc degeneration and its associated symptoms. What has been shown to date, and therefore been available in limited geographies and jurisdictions, is that expanded and transplanted autologous cells are safe and appear to arrest if not reverse DDD following treatment for sequestrectomy.[37]

Our own experience embraces more than 140 patients treated with autologous disc cell transplantation over the last 10 years. This is the largest number of patients with degenerated IVD disease treated with cell transplantation under defined study conditions. All patients have benefited from transplantation with reduced back pain as one measure of an enhanced quality of life. All of the patients treated were able to return to work after transplantation. There was no postoperative back pain after cell transplantation, nor was there any inflammatory complication such as spondylodiscitis or local reaction after the cell transplantation in these patients. Moreover, a stable disc height was reconciled in the MR images, and a reduction in reherniation rate was more than 50% better than that in the control group.

The principal limitation, however, comes from the fact that the use of autologous chondrocytes requires the ex vivo expansion of cells, adding burdens of cost, time, and regulation that add to the intricacy of the procedure beyond the medical interface. One way to circumvent these disadvantages is the use of a one-step procedure, using stem cells obtained from autologous adipose tissue. Ongoing studies will yield more information about the possibility of using stem cells for regenerative therapies in intervertebral DDD.

Cell transplantation appears to present an effective treatment option in DDD. A graft-versus-host reaction as a common problem after cell transplantation is reduced by the avascular nature of the NP.[41] The effect of the transplantation is limited by the survival of the transplanted cells in the hostile environment of the degenerated disc.[42] The development of specialized carriers that preserve the acidic environment of the IVD such as injectable hydrogels and atelocollagen as well as hyaluronic acid (HA) are other factors that could facilitate the survival of transplanted cells and induce matrix production.[43,44] Once confidence in the outcomes of the cell interventions for disc treatment has been accepted in the medical lexicon, then it will be possible for refinement and reimbursement within the regenerative framework to achieve an equilibrium of medical intention balanced in both economic and health ergonomics.

14.6 References

[1] Stewart WF, Ricci JA, Chee E, Morganstein D, Lipton R. Lost productive time and cost due to common pain conditions in the US workforce. JAMA. 2003; 290(18):2443–2454

[2] Ricci JA, Stewart WF, Chee E, Leotta C, Foley K, Hochberg MC. Back pain exacerbations and lost productive time costs in United States workers. Spine. 2006; 31(26):3052–3060

[3] Walker BF. The prevalence of low back pain: a systematic review of the literature from 1966 to 1998. J Spinal Disord. 2000; 13(3):205–217

[4] Wadell G. A new clinical model for treatment of low back pain. Spine. 1987; 12:632–644

[5] Boden SDMP, McCowin PR, Davis DO, Dina TS, Mark AS, Wiesel S. Abnormal magnetic-resonance scans of the cervical spine in asymptomatic subjects. A prospective investigation. J Bone Joint Surg Am. 1990; 72(8):1178–1184

[6] Brinjikji W, Luetmer PH, Comstock B, et al. Systematic literature review of imaging features of spinal degeneration in asymptomatic populations. AJNR Am J Neuroradiol. 2015; 36(4):811–816

[7] Battié MC, Videman T, Gibbons LE, Fisher LD, Manninen H, Gill K. 1995 Volvo Award in clinical sciences. Determinants of lumbar disc degeneration.A study relating lifetime exposures and magnetic resonance imaging findings in identical twins. Spine. 1995; 20(24):2601–2612

[8] Lotz JC, Staples A, Walsh A, Hsieh AH. Mechanobiology in intervertebral disc degeneration and regeneration. Conference proceedings: Annual International Conference of the IEEE Engineering in Medicine and Biology Society 2004;7:5459

[9] Pye SR, Reid DM, Adams JE, Silman AJ, O'Neill TW. Influence of weight, body mass index and lifestyle factors on radiographic features of lumbar disc degeneration. Ann Rheum Dis. 2007; 66(3):426–427

[10] Anderson DG, Tannoury C. Molecular pathogenic factors in symptomatic disc degeneration. Spine J. 2005; 5(6) Suppl:260S–266S

[11] Freimark D, Czermak P. Cell-based regeneration of intervertebral disc defects: review and concepts. Int J Artif Organs. 2009; 32(4):197–203

[12] Masuda K, Oegema TR , Jr, An HS. Growth factors and treatment of intervertebral disc degeneration. Spine. 2004; 29(23):2757–2769

[13] Zhang Y, An HS, Toofanfard M, Li Z, Andersson GB, Thonar EJ. Low-dose interleukin-1 partially counteracts osteogenic protein-1-induced proteoglycan synthesis by adult bovine intervertebral disk cells. Am J Phys Med Rehabil. 2005; 84(5):322–329

[14] Buckwalter JA. Aging and degeneration of the human intervertebral disc. Spine. 1995; 20(11):1307–1314

[15] Jandial R, Aryan HE, Park J, Taylor WT, Snyder EY. Stem cell-mediated regeneration of the intervertebral disc: cellular and molecular challenge. Neurosurg Focus. 2008; 24(3–4):E21

[16] Gruber HE, Hanley EN , Jr. Analysis of aging and degeneration of the human intervertebral disc. Comparison of surgical specimens with normal controls. Spine. 1998; 23(7):751–757

[17] Nachemson A, Lewin T, Maroudas A, Freeman MA. In vitro diffusion of dye through the end-plates and the annulus fibrosus of human lumbar inter-vertebral discs. Acta OrthopScand. 1970; 41(6):589–607

[18] Roughley PJ. Biology of intervertebral disc aging and degeneration: involvement of the extracellular matrix. Spine. 2004; 29(23):2691–2699

[19] Thompson JP, Oegema TR , Jr, Bradford DS. Stimulation of mature canine intervertebral disc by growth factors. Spine. 1991; 16(3):253–260

[20] An HS, Takegami K, Kamada H, et al. Intradiscal administration of osteogenic protein-1 increases intervertebral disc height and proteoglycan content in the nucleus pulposus in normal adolescent rabbits. Spine. 2005; 30(1):25–31, discussion 31–32

[21] Chaofeng W, Chao Z, Deli W, et al. Nucleus pulposus cells expressing hBMP7 can prevent the degeneration of allogenic IVD in a canine transplantation model. J Orthop Res. 2013; 31(9):1366–1373

[22] Masuda K, Imai Y, Okuma M, et al. Osteogenic protein-1 injection into a degenerated disc induces the restoration of disc height and structural changes in the rabbit anular puncture model. Spine. 2006; 31(7):742–754

[23] Willems N, Bach FC, Plomp SG, et al. Intradiscal application of rhBMP-7 does not induce regeneration in a canine model of spontaneous intervertebral disc degeneration. Arthritis Res Ther. 2015; 17:137

[24] Klein RG, Eek BC, O'Neill CW, Elin C, Mooney V, Derby RR. Biochemical injection treatment for discogenic low back pain: a pilot study. Spine J. 2003; 3 (3):220–226

[25] Sakai D, Mochida J, Iwashina T, et al. Differentiation of mesenchymal stem cells transplanted to a rabbit degenerative disc model: potential and limitations for stem cell therapy in disc regeneration. Spine. 2005; 30(21):2379–2387

[26] Sakai D, Mochida J, Iwashina T, et al. Regenerative effects of transplanting mesenchymal stem cells embedded in atelocollagen to the degenerated intervertebral disc. Biomaterials. 2006; 27(3):335–345

[27] Feng G, Zhao X, Liu H, et al. Transplantation of mesenchymal stem cells and nucleus pulposus cells in a degenerative disc model in rabbits: a comparison of 2 cell types as potential candidates for disc regeneration. J Neurosurg Spine. 2011; 14(3):322–329

[28] Rodrigues-Pinto R, Richardson SM, Hoyland JA. Identification of novel nucleus pulposus markers: Interspecies variations and implications for cell-based therapiesfor intervertebral disc degeneration. Bone Joint Res. 2013; 2 (8):169–178

[29] Clarke LE, McConnell JC, Sherratt MJ, Derby B, Richardson SM, Hoyland JA. Growth differentiation factor 6 and transforming growth factor-beta differentially mediate mesenchymal stem cell differentiation, composition, and micromechanical properties of nucleus pulposus constructs. Arthritis Res Ther. 2014; 16(2):R67

[30] Gorensek M, Jaksimović C, Kregar-Velikonja N, et al. Nucleus pulposus repair with cultured autologous elastic cartilage derived chondrocytes. Cell Mol Biol Lett. 2004; 9(2):363–373

[31] Ganey T, Libera J, Moos V, et al. Disc chondrocyte transplantation in a canine model: a treatment for degenerated or damaged intervertebral disc. Spine. 2003; 28(23):2609–2620

[32] Meisel HJ, Siodla V, Ganey T, Minkus Y, Hutton WC, Alasevic OJ. Clinical experience in cell-based therapeutics: disc chondrocyte transplantation. A treatment for degenerated or damaged intervertebral disc. Biomol Eng. 2007; 24 (1):5–21

[33] Hohaus C, Ganey TM, Minkus Y, Meisel HJ. Cell transplantation in lumbar spine disc degeneration disease. Eur Spine J. 2008; 17 Suppl 4:492–503

[34] Brock M, Görge HH, Curio G. Intradiscal pressure-volume response: a methodological contribution to chemonucleolysis. Preliminary results. J Neurosurg. 1984; 60(5):1029–1032

[35] Prolo DJ, Oklund SA, Butcher M. Toward uniformity in evaluating results of lumbar spine operations. A paradigm applied to posterior lumbar interbody fusions. Spine. 1986; 11(6):601–606

[36] Pfirrmann CW, Metzdorf A, Zanetti M, Hodler J, Boos N. Magnetic resonance classification of lumbar intervertebral disc degeneration. Spine. 2001; 26 (17):1873–1878

[37] Ganey T, Hutton WC, Moseley T, Hedrick M, Meisel HJ. Intervertebral disc repair using adipose tissue-derived stem and regenerative cells: experiments in a canine model. Spine. 2009; 34(21):2297–2304

[38] Orozco L, Soler R, Morera C, Alberca M, Sánchez A, García-Sancho J. Intervertebral disc repair by autologous mesenchymal bone marrow cells: a pilot study. Transplantation. 2011; 92(7):822–828

[39] Coric D, Pettine K, Sumich A, Boltes MO. Prospective study of disc repair with allogeneic chondrocytes presented at the 2012 Joint Spine Section Meeting. J Neurosurg Spine. 2013; 18(1):85–95

[40] Yin W, Pauza K, Olan WJ, Doerzbacher JF, Thorne KJ. Intradiscal injection of fibrin sealant for the treatment of symptomatic lumbar internal disc disruption: results of a prospective multicenter pilot study with 24-month follow-up. Pain Med. 2014; 15(1):16–31

[41] Sheikh H, Zakharian K, De La Torre RP, et al. In vivo intervertebral disc regeneration using stem cell-derived chondroprogenitors. J Neurosurg Spine. 2009; 10(3):265–272

[42] Sakai D. Future perspectives of cell-based therapy for intervertebral disc disease. Eur Spine J. 2008; 17 Suppl 4:452–458

[43] Li H, Liang C, Tao Y, et al. Acidic pH conditions mimicking degenerative intervertebral discs impair the survival and biological behavior of human adipose-derived mesenchymal stem cells. ExpBiol Med (Maywood). 2012; 237 (7):845–852

[44] Henriksson H, Hagman M, Horn M, Lindahl A, Brisby H. Investigation of different cell types and gel carriers for cell-based intervertebral disc therapy, in vitro and in vivo studies. J Tissue Eng Regen Med. 2012; 6(9):738:747

15 Annulus Fibrosus Repair

Olivia M. Torre, Michelle A. Cruz, Andrew C. Hecht, and James C. Iatridis

Abstract

This chapter describes the clinical need for annulus fibrosus (AF) repair as well as the state of the art in AF repair procedures and next-generation AF repair strategies that aim to improve upon currently available treatments. AF injury from herniation and degeneration can result in complications such as accelerated degeneration and prolonged chronic pain. Discectomy is the standard treatment for painful conditions associated with the ruptured AF from herniation, and is highly effective at reducing acute radicular pain; however, it does not promote repair and there is a risk of reherniation. AF closure devices can augment discectomy procedures by reducing the reherniation risk, but they do not promote tissue repair. AF repair research is broad and involves technologies including experimental biomaterials, drug and cellular-based therapies, and combination treatments. A key challenge is to design AF repair strategies that withstand complex loads on the spine while promoting integration and regeneration with the native tissue. Natural and synthetic biomaterials have been developed to mimic certain AF properties, and some show substantial promise for sealing AF defects. The most promising strategies to promote AF repair involve combinations of biological factors, cell delivery, and biomaterials. However, regulatory considerations hinder the translation of such complex strategies to clinical use. Several promising experimental strategies exist and require further material development and validation.

Keywords: annulus fibrosus, biomaterials, cell delivery, intervertebral disc, regeneration, repair

15.1 Historical and Clinical Perspective

The annulus fibrosus (AF) contains the highly pressurized nucleus pulposus (NP) in order to maintain intervertebral disc (IVD) height under the large spinal loads and deformations that occur during activities of daily life. Degenerative changes or traumatic injury can lead to herniation of NP tissue through defects in the AF. Unrepaired AF defects can directly result in debilitating painful conditions by leading to compression of adjacent nerve roots by herniated tissue,[1,2] and can indirectly result in painful conditions by leading to accelerated IVD degeneration, which can predispose to biomechanical instability, chronic inflammation, and increased nociception.[3,4] AF repair following herniation is challenging due to the limited self-healing capacity of the IVD and the need to withstand complex repetitive loading.[5]

Walter E. Dandy provided the first report of a lumbar IVD herniation in 1929, in which he observed the detachment of an IVD fragment and described the associated painful conditions related to the herniated material bulging into the spinal canal.[6] Pain and disability from herniation was long-believed to be associated with extent of mechanical compression of the herniated tissue on the nerve root.[7] However, clinical and scientific observations that nerve root–related pain gradually resolved without any change in the mechanical deformation implicated neural inflammation due to contact of the nerve with autologous NP tissue.[8,9] Mixter and Barr described a procedure to relieve the painful conditions associated with IVD herniation in 1934, giving rise to the field of lumbar discectomy in which extruded NP tissue is removed.[10] Since Mixter and Barr's report, discectomy procedures have vastly improved to become less invasive with faster recovery times and improved patient outcomes. Discectomy is now the most commonly performed surgical procedure to alleviate low back and leg pain with 300,000 procedures performed yearly in the United States.[11,12,13,14] However, discectomy procedures do not involve repairing the existing AF injury resulting from the herniation, and can enlarge the defect size in the process of removing herniated tissue (▶ Fig. 15.1). Sealing such large iatrogenic defects from discectomy poses distinct biological and mechanical challenges involving larger defects in a specific area. In contrast, defects resulting from degenerative changes with age may be smaller in size and in more locations. Furthermore, adjacent AF tissue quality impacts repair potential and ranges from high-quality tissue with good mechanical integrity (e.g., in younger patients with defects associated with injuries) to degenerated tissue of poorer mechanical integrity (e.g., in patients with herniation due to chronic degenerative conditions).

AF repair strategies include devices (sutures and implants), experimental biomaterials (sealants and scaffolds), biologics and cell-based therapies, and combinatorial strategies (▶ Fig. 15.2). The objectives of this chapter are to provide a summary of the current state of the art in AF repair techniques for defects resulting from herniation and subsequent discectomy procedures, and an overview of experimental biomaterial, biological, and cell-based strategies aiming to improve upon current treatment options.

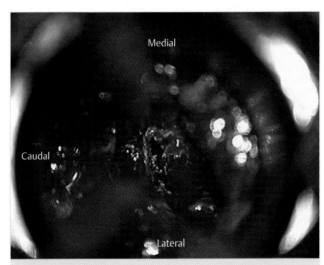

Fig. 15.1 Intraoperative image of large annular defect after discectomy.

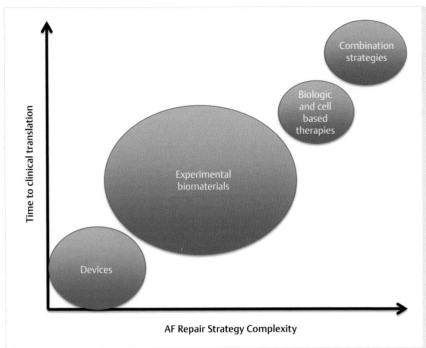

Fig. 15.2 Annulus fibrosus (AF) repair strategies currently used and under investigation in the context of time to clinical translation and complexity of the repair strategy. The relative sizes of each category indicate the prevalence of their use or investigational interest.

15.2 Current Procedures for Annulus Fibrosus Repair

Discectomy procedures can afford superior clinical outcomes after a failure of nonoperative treatments for lumbar IVD herniation.[14] However, the challenge of a microdiscectomy is to determine how much disc material needs to be removed. Typically, the loose or herniated pieces are removed and an annular defect remains. The more disc that is removed by the surgeon the greater the risk of degeneration, and if too little is removed the risk of reherniation is greater. Consequently, there is a balance between removing sufficient amounts of NP tissue to prevent reherniation and removing so much NP tissue that the remaining IVD is at risk for further injury to the end plates, faster rates of degeneration, IVD height loss, and subsequent pain at the same spinal level.[15] The rate of reherniation, postsurgical pain, and recurrent pain at the same level of the discectomy is 5 to 25%,[16,17,18,19,20] demonstrating an important clinical need to develop AF repair strategies. An ideal AF repair strategy would prevent reherniation, seal the remaining defects, and restore the mechanical behavior of the AF to a healthy level.[5] However, current surgical treatment options for radicular pain associated with herniation do not offer effective repair strategies, and developing AF repair strategies remains an unmet clinical challenge.

15.2.1 Causes of Annulus Fibrosus Injury

The AF undergoes structural changes with degeneration, age, and pathological loading, and these changes include tears, fissures, and defects to the lamellar layers and can result in AF rupture and herniation.[5,21] AF punctures, defects, and simulated discectomy procedures in healthy IVDs are known to accelerate IVD degeneration in animal models and organ culture.[22,23,24,25,26,27] Although some clinical data suggest discectomy procedures result in accelerated IVD degeneration,[28] it is difficult to separate effects of discectomy from degeneration that might have occurred at that spinal level due to existing herniation and AF damage.[28]

15.2.2 Currently Available Annulus Fibrosus Repair Strategies

Currently available AF repair strategies include suturing and implants, which focus on AF closure or prevention of reherniation (▶ Fig. 15.3), and several have been used in clinical trials (▶ Table 15.1). Suturing AF defects was a promising solution due to its simplicity; however, it was ineffective in restoring intradiscal pressure in animal models[29] and suturing procedures are very challenging in the posterior AF region due to surrounding nerve roots. An improved suturing system is commercially available in Europe, and has offered slightly lower, but not significantly decreased, reherniation rates and no additional risk (Xclose, Anulex Technologies Inc., Minnetonka, MN).[30] However, this technology was removed from the U.S. market. The PushLock knotless suture anchor, approved for rotator cuff repair, has been studied as a potential AF closure device[31] however, this approach is suitable only for patients with sufficient tissue integrity of the ruptured AF and vertebral end plate, and is therefore only feasible for a small subset of patients. Barbed polyethylene annular closure device implants tested in goats in vivo demonstrated material deformation, end plate damage, and device expulsion after 6 weeks, presumably due to a mismatch in mechanical properties.[32] The Barricaid (Intrinsic Therapeutics, Woburn, MA), is an implant for AF closure consisting of a titanium bone anchor and polymer mesh positioned in the annular defect, and shows promise for preventing reherniation and retaining IVD height.[33,34,35]

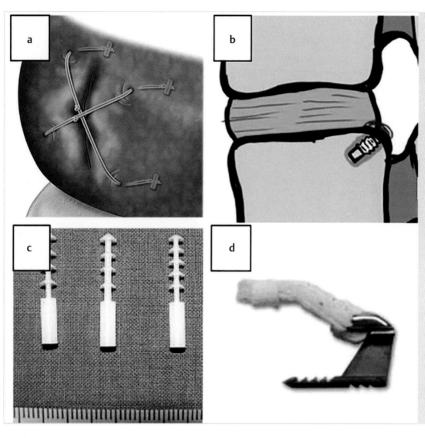

Fig. 15.3 Devices for annulus fibrosus repair. **(a)** The Xclose (Anulex Technologies; Minnetonka, MN) modified suture system is approved for use in Europe.[30] **(b)** The PushLock knotless suture anchor (Arthrex; Naples, FL), approved for rotator cuff repair, has been studied as an annular closure device.[31] **(c)** Annular closure device implants have been tested in in vivo goat models.[32] **(d)** The Barricaid annular closure device (Intrinsic Therapeutics; Woburn, MA) is approved for use in Europe.[35]

Table 15.1 Summary of AF repair devices that are approved, in clinical trials, or under investigation

Device	Company	Countries where approved	Function	Reference
Xclose	Anulex Technologies; Minnetonka, MN	Europe, USA (510k)	Modified sutures with anchors	32
PushLock	Arthrex; Naples, FL	USA (rotator cuff repair), under investigation	Knotless suture anchor	33
Annular closure device	-	Under investigation	Barbed polyethylene implants for AF defect closure	34
Barricaid	Intrinsic Therapeutics Inc.; Woburn, MA	Europe	Large annular defect closure in region of herniation consisting of woven mesh and titanium bone anchor	35,36,37

Abbreviations: AF, annulus fibrosus.

Currently available devices and treatments do not seal defects in the AF or promote tissue regeneration, and have not demonstrated a capacity to restore biomechanical function. Next-generation AF repair techniques are under development using experimental biomaterials with greater biomimicry and with cell delivery that are likely to be important for long-term clinical success, yet many challenges exist.

15.2.3 Clinical Challenges of Annulus Fibrosus Repair

Designing a regenerative AF repair technique is highly challenging due to the clinical, biological, and mechanical demands and generally good success of current discectomy procedures.[5] Pure biomimicry of the AF is challenging due to the complex hierarchical, multilamellar structure of the AF, whose structure and material properties depend on location in the IVD. The IVD is avascular with low cellularity, providing a limited innate healing response. Innate repair of the IVD is poorly understood and efforts to promote repair activity through cell delivery, protein delivery, and gene therapy require extensive further investigation. Furthermore, there is limited information on the native AF cell phenotype, making it more challenging to design cell therapies. Nevertheless, several biomaterials and cell-based therapies exist that show promise to address at least some of these challenges and improve AF repair.

15.3 Experimental Biomaterials

Next-generation AF repair strategies include experimental biomaterials for AF repair that are formed as hydrogels to serve as AF sealants or in fibrous forms to better mimic AF structure (▶ Fig. 15.4). Design criteria for AF sealants were previous proposed to be[36] (1) strongly adhesive, (2) biocompatible, (3) able to withstand immediate repetitive loading, and (4) injectable for easy delivery at the time of surgery.

Biomaterials for AF replacement further aim to match native AF biomechanical and/or biological properties. Although a biomaterial possessing all these design criteria has yet to be been identified, this active field of research has produced many promising candidates. Various experimental biomaterials show promise as parts of tissue-engineered AF repair strategies and include natural, synthetic, combined, and electrospun materials (▶ Table 15.2).

15.3.1 Natural Biomaterials

Natural biomaterials such as fibrin,[36,44,45,46] collagen,[37,47,48,49,50] alginate,[39,51,52] and silk[53] have been investigated for their use as injectable AF sealants with the goal of preventing reherniation following discectomy and providing mechanical stabilization. The primary advantages of natural biomaterials are high biocompatibility and ability to maintain highly viable cellular populations and ability to be formed as injectable hydrogels. Natural biomaterials have been modified to improve their adhesion to native tissue, biocompatibility, mechanical properties, and injectability with varied success.

Fibrin is a natural protein involved in blood clotting that has been commercially available for use as glue in many orthopaedic surgeries. Fibrin was used for IVD repair with some success in a porcine model[54] and early clinical trials.[55] However, Phase III clinical trials of fibrin injection in patients with low back pain showed no significant differences in outcomes compared with saline injections[44] (Clinical Trial ID: NCT01011816), suggesting fibrin alone is not a useful material for AF repair. Adding genipin, a natural compound extracted from gardenia fruit, cross-links fibrin (FibGen) and resulted in increased shear mechanical properties to match AF tissues, slower degradation times compared with fibrin, and high cell viability in vitro.[45,46]FibGen was able to withstand over 14,000 cycles of repetitive compression loading, restore IVD height, and restore compressive mechanical properties in injured bovine IVDs ex vivo.[36] FibGen matches many of the criteria for design of an AF repair material and remains a promising candidate as an AF sealant.

High-density collagen, a major extracellular matrix (ECM) component of the AF, cross-linked with riboflavin has shown cell infiltration from native tissue and promising short-term mechanical properties matching the undamaged IVD in an in vivo rat model.[37,47]Atelocollagen honeycomb-shaped scaffolds seeded with mature rabbit AF cells and implanted in a rabbit IVD degeneration model promoted short-term maintenance of cell viability, IVD height, and proteoglycan production[48,49,50]; however, mechanical properties of the implants were not evaluated. Modified collagen biomaterials show promise as AF sealants due to their injectability and biocompatibility; however, they require further mechanical testing and validation in the long term in vivo.

Shape-memory porous alginate is capable of recovering its original geometry once rehydrated and has the potential for minimally invasive delivery; however, it has material behaviors substantially lower than native AF.[39] Alginate composites with collagen and chitosan have demonstrated enhanced cell compatibility and proliferation capacity when compared with alginate alone, and also tunable porosity to promote tissue integration and biocompatibility.[39,51,52] Whereas alginate-based biomaterials have promising adhesion, biocompatibility, and injectability, further mechanical testing is required to validate these materials as candidates for AF repair.

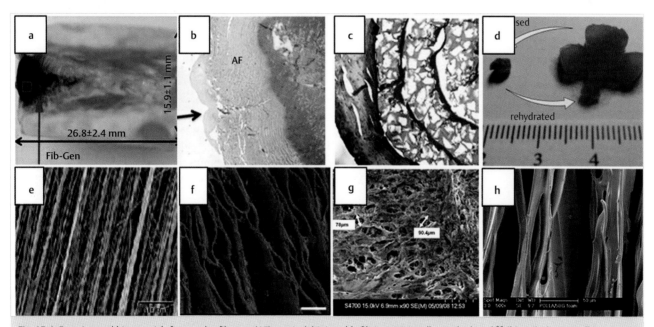

Fig. 15.4 Experimental biomaterials for annulus fibrosus (AF) repair. (a) Injectable fibrin-genipin adhesive hydrogel.[36] (b) High-density collagen cross-linked with riboflavin.[37] (c) Composite BBG-poly(polycaprolactone-triol-malate) (PPCLM) construct seeded with rat chondrocytes.[38] (d) Shape-memory porous alginate scaffolds for AF regeneration.[39] (e) Electrospun polyurethane.[40] (f) Lamellar silk.[41] (g) Type II collagen–hyaluronic acid hydrogel.[42] (h) PDLLA/Bioglass composite foam scaffold.[43]

Table 15.2 Summary of natural, synthetic, and electrospun materials designed for AF repair

	Material	Model	AF repair design criteria				References
			Adhesive	*Biocompatible*	*Withstands Repetitive Loading*	*Injectable*	
Natural	Fibrin-genipin	In vitro (human AF) Ex vivo (bovine) In vivo (rat)	Yes	21 d High viability in vitro 16 wk Cell infiltration in vivo	Withstood 14,000 compression cycles	Yes	37,39,40
	High-density collagen	In vivo Rat	Yes	6 mo High viability Cell infiltration	-	Yes	41,42
	Atelocollagen	In vitro Rabbit AF cells	-	21 d High viability Collagen II, GAG	-	Yes	43
	Shape-memory alginate	In vitro Porcine AF cells	-	21 d Total collagen, GAG	-	Yes	47
	Alginate-collagen	Ex vivo Porcine organ culture	-	5 wk High viability	-	Yes	46
	Alginate-chitosan	In vitro Canine AF cells	-	4 wk Collagen I, collagen II, aggrecan	-	No	54
	Porous silk	In vitro Bovine AF cells	-	4 wk High viability Total collagen, GAG	-	No	49
Synthetic	Malic acid	In vitro Rat AF cells	-	4 d High viability GAG, aggrecan, collagen II	Withstood 500 press load/release cycles, 30% max strain	Yes	55
	PTMC-PU	Ex vivo Bovine organ culture with human MSCs	Yes	14 d Collagen V	Withstood 3-h sinusoidal load cycles for 7 d	No	56
	PDLLA/45S5 Bioglass	In vitro Bovine AF cells	-	4 wk Actin fiber formation sGAG, collagen	-	No	57
Combined Natural and Synthetic	Collagen type I-alginate-polyethylene	In vitro Sheep AF cells	-	3 d High viability	-	No	58
	Bone matrix gelatin-PPCLM	In vitro Rabbit chondrocytes	-	4 wk High viability Collagen II, proteoglycan	-	No	59
Electrospun	PCL	In vitro Porcine AF cells Bovine MSCs	-	6 wk High viability Total collagen, GAG	-	No	60,61,62
	PU-PCL	In vitro Bovine AF cells	-	21 d Proliferation Total collagen, GAG	-	No	63

Abbreviations: AF, annulus fibrosus; GAG, glycosaminoglycan; MSCs, mesenchymal stem cells; PCL, poly-ε-caprolactone; PDLLA, poly(d,l-lactide); PPCLM, poly(polycaprolactone-triol-malate); PTMC-PU, poly(trimethylene-carbonate)-polyurethane; PU-PCL, polyurethane-poly-ε-caprolactone; sGAG, sulfated glycosaminoglycan.

Validation in large animal models for AF repair is required for these natural biomaterials, yet many variations of these materials have already undergone regulatory approval for other applications, which may provide a relatively fast track for clinical translation. Many natural biomaterials are inherently weak and require extensive optimization to enhance mechanical properties and cell and drug delivery capabilities. Natural biomaterials also have chemistry that is more complex and commonly less flexibility for chemical modification than synthetic biomaterials.

15.3.2 Synthetic Biomaterials

Synthetic polymeric materials have been extensively investigated for AF repair, and are particularly useful due to their predicable properties, consistent synthesis between batches, and the ability to tune chemical, mechanical, and structural properties based on specific design criteria. Synthetic materials do not easily adhere to the native AF and require modifications to improve biocompatibility and AF tissue integration. Most synthetic scaffolds are used in full tissue-engineering applications with cell or drug delivery (see Section 15.4, Biological Therapies), yet a few are used for structural repair alone.

A malic acid–based scaffold supported growth of rat AF cells and had supported high gene and protein expression of ECM molecules as well as little immune or foreign body response in vivo upon implantation.[56] However, the stiffest formulation had a compressive modulus tensile strength several orders of magnitude lower than AF tissues, so it is likely to be unfeasible for AF repair.

Different combinations of synthetic biomaterials have been investigated together to enhance their capacity to mimic the complex structure of inner and outer components of the AF, to combine different mechanical or biological properties into a more favorable composite, and to provide an additional barrier or membrane to further reduce the chances of reherniation. A combination of poly(trimethylene-carbonate) (PTMC) and polyurethane membrane was injected into injured bovine IVDs and tested in a dynamically loaded organ culture bioreactor.[57] Improved IVD height and decreased herniation were observed in IVDs treated with both the scaffold and membrane, suggesting that the combined approach using the polyurethane membrane was an effective repair strategy. A composite poly(d,l-lactide)(PDLLA)/45S5-Bioglass scaffold was seeded with bovine AF cells and promoted actin fiber formation after 4 weeks, glycoaminoglycan (GAG), type I collagen, and type II collagen production.[43] Combinations of synthetic materials have increased design complexity, and membrane fixation is technically difficult. Multiple biomaterials have more potential for complications and higher regulatory challenges, therefore simpler biomaterial design solutions are more attractive.

15.3.3 Combined Natural and Synthetic Biomaterials

Self-assembling type I collagen and polyethylene hydrogels with circumferentially aligned fibrils have been fabricated using contraction of AF cell–seeded collagen around an inner polyethylene disc and showed the ability to maintain high cell viability in vitro.[58] Mimicking the circumferential alignment of native AF tissue may help confer similar shear and tensile properties, and self-assembling collagen is a promising technique to achieve this; however, long-term validation and mechanical testing and characterization of adhesive properties are still required for this material.

The combination of poly(polycaprolactone-triol-malate) (PPCLM) and demineralized bone matrix gelatin resulted in matched compressive and tensile AF properties and collagen and GAG production by seeded adult rabbit chondrocytes in vitro, and tissue ingrowth after 2 weeks in mice in vivo with limited inflammatory response.[38] However, integration between the PPCLM and bone matrix gelatin would require further optimization to withstand the high loads and complex strain patterns known to be present in the AF in vivo.

15.3.4 Electrospun Biomaterials

Electrospinning is a fabrication method particularly useful for AF repair materials because of the ability to create ordered, aligned fibers using various natural and synthetic materials, and to incorporate biological components. The aligned lamellar layers of the AF confer its unique mechanical properties and tissue structure and function. Therefore, mimicking this architecture using electrospinning has great potential for an effective repair strategy. Poly-ε-caprolactone (PCL) fibers electrospun to create a multilayered structure consisting of fibers of alternating angles has demonstrated mechanical properties comparable to native tissue as well as the ability to maintain cell viability and produce ECM in culture.[59,60,61] Electrospun polyurethane supports bovine AF cell growth and ECM production in vitro with high yield strain.[62] Electrospun scaffolds show the greatest promise for replicating the native AF fiber and lamellar structure and material behaviors. However, these materials integrate poorly, do not withstand high loads, and substantial further development is required for application to humans.

15.4 Biological Therapies

Biomaterials used as scaffolds have the potential to restore biomechanical behaviors while simultaneously delivering biological components such as growth factors, proteins, small molecules, and cells. Scaffolds have the capacity to deliver drugs locally at high doses that would be impossible to achieve with systemic delivery. Biological functionalization of scaffolds has the greatest potential for promoting AF tissue repair or regeneration, which is likely to be important for long-term success over the many cycles of loading occurring over decades of life. AF regeneration is an ambitious goal; however, bioactive repairs of the IVD may prove successful if they can slow, halt, or reverse degeneration processes, promote tissue proliferation and growth, prevent pain, and/or restore IVD function.[63,64,65] Various biologics, drugs, and cells have potential to be used for AF repair strategies (▶ Table 15.3); however, there are several obstacles to achieving AF repair through biological delivery. Clinical studies determining the effective dosages and kinetics of promising biological compounds are required. Optimal delivery strategies will likely include biomaterial scaffolds; however, regulatory approval of repair strategies consisting of multiple components is more challenging because of strict regulations for combinatorial strategies involving biological compounds.

Table 15.3 Summary of growth factors, chemokines, peptides, drugs, and cellular therapies that show potential for AF repair

	Biologic	Model	Carrier	Dose	Test duration	Significant effects	References
Growth Factors	Platelet rich plasma	In vitro Bovine AF cells	Media	25%	4 d	Increased DNA proliferation, production of GAG, collagen I, collagen II, aggrecan, decorin, versican	69
		In vivo Rabbit	None	0.1 mL	4 wk	Improved IVD height and MRI signal intensity	70
	Osteogenic protein-1	In vivo Rabbit	5% lactose	100 µg /10 µL	24 wk	Improved IVD height and MRI signal intensity, increased proteoglycan content, decreased degenerative grade	75
Chemokines and Peptides	CCL5	Ex vivo Bovine IVD	None	-	7 d	CCL5 observed in conditioned media of degenerated IVDs in organ culture, increased mRNA expression, increased stem cell recruitment	77
	CXCL10	In vitro Human AF cells	None	1,000 nM	20 h	Cell migration was stimulated by presence of chemokine	81
	Link N	In vivo Rabbit	Saline	100 µg /10 µL	12 wk	Increased aggrecan and decreased proteinase	83
	Substance P receptor antagonist	In vitro Human AF cells	Media	1–50 µM	7 d	Decreased pro-inflammatory cytokine expression	84
Drugs	Simvastatin	In vivo Rat	PEG	5–15 mg/ mL	2–4 wk	Improved MRI signal intensity, and increased BMP-2, aggrecan, collagen II	86,87
	Infliximab	In vitro Human AF cells	Fibrin-genipin	10–30 mg/ mL	20 d	Decreased inflammatory cytokine expression	88
Cell Delivery	Human juvenile chondrocytes	In vivo Rat	Fibrin	4×10^5 cells	12 wk	Maintained MRI signal intensity, increased GAG production	90
	Rabbit MSCs	In vivo Rabbit	Saline	1×10^5 cells	3–9 wk	MSCs leaked from IVD after injection	91
	Canine ADRCs	In vivo Canine	Hyaluronic acid	2×10^6 cells	12 wk	Maintained MRI signal intensity, increased collagen II and aggrecan	92
	Human AF cells	In vivo Mouse	Fibrin + collagen	6×10^5 cells	28 d	Increased collagen I and collagen II, GAG content	93

Abbreviations: ADRC, adipose-derived regenerative cells; AF, annulus fibrosus; BMP, bone morphogenetic protein; DNA, deoxyribonucleic acid; ECM, extracellular matrix; GAG, glycosaminoglycan; IVD, intervertebral disc; MRI, magnetic resonance imaging; mRNA, messenger ribonucleic acid; MSCs, mesenchymal stem cells.

15.4.1 Growth Factors

Growth factors such as platelet rich plasma (PRP) and osteogenic protein-1 (OP-1) can stimulate tissue repair and protein synthesis in the IVD. PRP consists of a variety of concentrated growth factors such as platelet-derived growth factor, transforming growth factor, and vascular endothelial growth factor (VEGF). These factors are delivered in a small volume of plasma and are already commonly used to treat muscle, ligament, and tendon injuries.[66,67] PRP-treated bovine AF cells demonstrated increased proliferation, collagen content, and GAG content. Similarly, treatment of whole IVDs with PRP increased ECM synthesis ex vivo.[68] In a preclinical rabbit AF puncture study, animals with PRP injection retained 90% of IVD height 6 weeks after injection as compared with 70% in control groups, and maintained GAG production, magnetic resonance imaging (MRI) signal intensity, and cellular morphology that was similar to uninjured controls.[69] When injected, PRP has natural gelation properties, which is beneficial for local delivery and retention of growth factors at the injury site. It is currently unclear which of the factors is the most important for these effects, or if the combination of factors is necessary for repair.[70] Clinical studies in humans have been performed using PRP injections to treat degenerated IVDs with improved outcomes[71] however, use of PRP to help regenerate the AF specifically requires further investigation.

OP-1, also known as bone morphogenetic protein (BMP)-7, is used surgically to promote bone growth.[72] It has also been shown to promotes the synthesis of proteoglycans and collagen of IVD cells in vitro.[73] OP-1 injection 4 weeks after IVD puncture in rabbits resulted in the recovery of the degenerated IVD visible on MRI and histology, demonstrating proteoglycan production as well as restoration of IVD height.[74] Direct injection of PRP and OP-1 has shown promising results in animal models and their current use in orthopaedic surgeries offers promise for human IVD repair.

15.4.2 Chemokines and Peptides

Delivery of chemokines, peptides, and proteins to the injured AF may be required to promote cell recruitment, stimulate ECM synthesis, and inhibit inflammatory responses as part of a strategy to regenerate the AF for long-term repair. These are important targets because degenerated IVDs have less cells, degraded ECM, and high levels of catabolism and inflammation when compared with healthy IVDs.[75] CCL5 is a chemotactic factor involved in tissue damage responses and increased stem cell migration, and messenger ribonucleic acid (mRNA) expression was observed in degenerated IVD cells in bovine organ culture[76] indicating this could be a potential therapy to induce migration of regenerative stem cells in the AF. CXCL10 is a chemokine with angiostatic properties stimulated by tumor necrosis factor (TNF)-α and expressed in herniated tissue, suggesting that it is important for prevention of vascularization and early inflammation in the injured IVD.[77,78,79] During in vitro migration assays, isolated human AF cells migrated when stimulated with CXCL10.[80] Delivering chemokines such as CCL5 or CXCL10 into injured areas of the AF has the potential to recruit endogenous progenitor stem cells,[81] which may be more

effective than recruiting mature AF cells for stimulating regenerative repair.

Synthetic peptides such as Link protein N-terminal peptide (Link N) and substance P receptor antagonist may provide more cost-effective therapeutics for AF repair strategies compared with growth factors. Link N is a peptide involved in proteoglycan aggregate stabilization that was shown in a rabbit in vivo model to partially restore loss of IVD height, downregulate metalloproteinase and proteolytic activity, and increase GAG and collagen content.[82] Substance P is a neuropeptide that stimulates production of pro-inflammatory cytokines in human IVD cells. Inhibiting substance P receptors using NK1 R antagonist was effective in blocking inflammatory effects on human IVD cells.[83] Injection of peptides may have the beneficial effect of promoting ECM production and anti-inflammatory properties, and because their low molecular weight allows more rapid transport than for larger proteins. However, further work is required to determine the kinetics of biological peptide delivery, optimal dosing, and long-term effects in humans.

15.4.3 Drugs

Drugs currently approved for other therapeutic applications are attractive candidates for AF repair because of simplified regulatory considerations. Statins, for example, have been repurposed for treatment of IVDs because they stimulate BMP-2 expression and maintain chondrogenic phenotypes of IVD cells.[84] Simvastatin treatment delivered in poly(ethylene glycol) (PEG)-based hydrogels after AF puncture injury in a rat model reversed or prevented degeneration in the IVD.[85,86] Infliximab, an anti-TNF-α drug, was delivered to AF cells in vitro and showed feasibility of using a FibGen scaffold for sustained drug release and sustained bioactivity for 20 days.[87] Small-molecule delivery also has the potential to augment scaffolds with bioactive characteristics by promoting ECM synthesis and reducing inflammation, so that combinations of small molecules and scaffolds for delivery warrant further investigation.

15.5 Cell Delivery

Cellular therapies can potentially improve IVD repair by addressing the low cellularity found in the ECM of degenerated human IVDs. Clinical studies that address low back pain with cell delivery have reported varied success. Delivery of bone marrow mesenchymal stem cells (MSCs) and juvenile articular chondrocytes has been observed to decrease low back pain,[88] although the mechanisms for decreased pain and any occurrence of IVD repair is unknown. A better understanding of cellular mechanisms in injury repair will help inform and optimize future cell-based repair strategies.

Injections of cells alone in preclinical studies have produced mixed results and it is currently unclear which cell type is optimal for AF repair. Delivery of juvenile chondrocytes from human knee cartilage to injured rat IVDs in vivo resulted in improved IVD height and GAG production as compared with untreated controls[89]; however, this is not a clinically relevant cell source to treat large numbers of patients with low back pain. Allogenic MSCs injected into injured rabbit IVDs in vivo resulted in the formation of anterolateral osteophytes; however, a scaffold was not used to deliver the cells and osteophyte formation could be attributed to cell leakage.[90] The most promising candidates for long-term AF repair are those that will promote long-term tissue regeneration in combination with restoration of mechanical properties using scaffolds.[63] Allogenic adipose-derived stem cell–seeded hyaluronic acid (HA) implanted in canines improved ECM production compared with acellular scaffolds.[91] Human AF cell–seeded fibrin and collagen scaffolds promoted GAG production and cell survival in mice in vivo.[92] Cellular delivery via a biomaterial scaffold may result in the best regenerative outcomes; however, complexity of designing these combinatorial strategies lengthens their time to clinical translation, and substantial work is still required to validate these in large animal models and humans.

Although one small clinical trial found no improvement in discogenic back pain, five other trials found improvements in both pain and on radiographic measures.[88] Between these trials, patients had different indications, and different cell types and numbers of cells injected were used, therefore it remains unclear which strategy will be the most effective.

15.6 Outlook

Although discectomy procedures are very effective at reducing acute radicular pain and disability, the unrepaired AF can result in complications including reherniation or degeneration-associated pain at the same level and long-term low back and/or leg pain. AF repair remains an important clinical priority. Current procedures and devices undergoing clinical trials show potential to reduce reherniation rates. Research on AF repair remains broad in scope with technologies that include experimental biomaterials with drug and/or cell delivery. Integration with the native tissue under immediate large spinal loading remains a key challenge for designing natural and synthetic biomaterials for AF repair. Many cell and drug delivery procedures also show promise for effect, although lack of mechanistic investigations makes it difficult to optimize treatment method and delivery. It is likely that the most effective treatments to promote regeneration and restoration of AF tissue structure and function following injury will require a combination of strategies.

15.7 References

[1] Rydevik B, Brown MD, Lundborg G. Pathoanatomy and pathophysiology of nerve root compression. Spine. 1984; 9(1):7–15

[2] Tarulli A W, Raynor EM. Lumbosacral radiculopathy. Neurol Clin. 2007; 25 (2):387–405

[3] Carragee EJ, Don AS, Hurwitz EL, Cuellar JM, Carrino JA, Herzog R. 2009 ISSLS Prize Winner: does discography cause accelerated progression of degeneration changes in the lumbar disc: a ten-year matched cohort study. Spine. 2009; 34(21):2338–2345

[4] Iatridis JC, Nicoll SB, Michalek AJ, Walter BA, Gupta MS. Role of biomechanics in intervertebral disc degeneration and regenerative therapies: what needs repairing in the disc and what are promising biomaterials for its repair? Spine J. 2013; 13(3):243–262

[5] Guterl CC, See EY, Blanquer SBG, et al. Challenges and strategies in the repair of ruptured annulus fibrosus. Eur Cell Mater. 2013; 25:1–21

[6] Dandy WE. Loose cartilage from intervertebral disk. Arch Surg. 1929; 19 (4):660–672

[7] Olmarker K, Holm S, Rosenqvist AL, Rydevik B. Experimental nerve root compression. A model of acute, graded compression of the porcine cauda equina and an analysis of neural and vascular anatomy. Spine. 1991; 16 (1):61–69

[8] Garfin SR, Rydevik BL, Brown RA. Compressive neuropathy of spinal nerve roots. A mechanical or biological problem? Spine. 1991; 16(2):162–166

[9] Olmarker K, Rydevik B, Nordborg C. Autologous nucleus pulposus induces neurophysiologic and histologic changes in porcine cauda equina nerve roots. Spine. 1993; 18(11):1425–1432

[10] Mixter WJ, Barr JS. Rupture of the intervertebral disc with involvement of the spinal canal*. J Neurosurg. 1934; 211:210–215

[11] Deyo RA, Mirza SK, Martin BI. Back pain prevalence and visit rates: estimates from U.S. national surveys, 2002. Spine. 2006; 31(23):2724–2727

[12] Deyo RA, Weinstein JN. Low back pain. N Engl J Med. 2001; 344(5):363–370

[13] Atlas SJ, Deyo RA, Patrick DL, Convery K, Keller RB, Singer DE. The Quebec Task Force classification for Spinal Disorders and the severity, treatment, and outcomes of sciatica and lumbar spinal stenosis. Spine. 1996; 21(24):2885–2892

[14] Weinstein, JN, Lurie, JD, Tosteson, TD, et al. Surgical vs nonoperative treatment for lumbar disk herniation: the Spine Patient Outcomes Research Trial (SPORT) observational cohort. JAMA. 2006; 296(20):2451–2459

[15] McGirt MJ, Ambrossi GL, Datoo G, et al. Recurrent disc herniation and long-term back pain after primary lumbar discectomy: review of outcomes reported for limited versus aggressive disc removal. Neurosurgery. 2009; 64 (2):338–344, discussion 344–345

[16] Carragee EJ, Han MY, Suen PW, Kim D. Clinical outcomes after lumbar discectomy for sciatica: the effects of fragment type and anular competence. J Bone Joint Surg Am. 2003; 85-A(1):102–108

[17] Carragee EJ, Spinnickie AO, Alamin TF, Paragioudakis S. A prospective controlled study of limited versus subtotal posterior discectomy: short-term outcomes in patients with herniated lumbar intervertebral discs and large posterior anular defect. Spine. 2006; 31(6):653–657

[18] Daneyemez M, Sali A, Kahraman S, Beduk A, Seber N. Outcome analyses in 1072 surgically treated lumbar disc herniations. Minim Invasive Neurosurg. 1999; 42(2):63–68

[19] Lebow RL, Adogwa O, Parker SL, Sharma A, Cheng J, McGirt MJ. Asymptomatic same-site recurrent disc herniation after lumbar discectomy: results of a prospective longitudinal study with 2-year serial imaging. Spine. 2011; 36 (25):2147–2151

[20] Henriksen L, Schmidt K, Eskesen V, Jantzen E. A controlled study of microsurgical versus standard lumbar discectomy. Br J Neurosurg. 1996; 10 (3):289–293

[21] Stokes IA, Iatridis JC. Mechanical conditions that accelerate intervertebral disc degeneration: overload versus immobilization. Spine. 2004; 29 (23):2724–2732

[22] Michalek AJ, Iatridis JC. Height and torsional stiffness are most sensitive to annular injury in large animal intervertebral discs. Spine J. 2012; 12(5):425–432

[23] Masuda K, Aota Y, Muehleman C, et al. A novel rabbit model of mild, reproducible disc degeneration by an anulus needle puncture: correlation between the degree of disc injury and radiological and histological appearances of disc degeneration. Spine. 2005; 30(1):5–14

[24] Sobajima S, Kompel JF, Kim JS, et al. A slowly progressive and reproducible animal model of intervertebral disc degeneration characterized by MRI, X-ray, and histology. Spine. 2005; 30(1):15–24

[25] Illien-Jünger S, Lu Y, Purmessur D, et al. Detrimental effects of discectomy on intervertebral disc biology can be decelerated by growth factor treatment during surgery: a large animal organ culture model. Spine J. 2014; 14 (11):2724–2732

[26] Melrose J, Smith SM, Little CB, Moore RJ, Vernon-Roberts B, Fraser RD. Recent advances in annular pathobiology provide insights into rim-lesion mediated intervertebral disc degeneration and potential new approaches to annular repair strategies. Eur Spine J. 2008; 17(9):1131–1148

[27] Osti OL, Vernon-Roberts B, Fraser RD. 1990 Volvo Award in experimental studies. Anulus tears and intervertebral disc degeneration. An experimental study using an animal model. Spine. 1990; 15(8):762–767

[28] Rahme R, Moussa R, Bou-Nassif R, et al. What happens to Modic changes following lumbar discectomy? Analysis of a cohort of 41 patients with a 3- to 5-year follow-up period. J Neurosurg Spine. 2010; 13(5):562–567

[29] Ahlgren BD, Lui W, Herkowitz HN, Panjabi MM, Guiboux JP. Effect of anular repair on the healing strength of the intervertebral disc: a sheep model. Spine. 2000; 25(17):2165–2170

[30] Bailey A, Araghi A, Blumenthal S, Huffmon GV, Anular Repair Clinical Study Group. Prospective, multicenter, randomized, controlled study of anular repair in lumbar discectomy: two-year follow-up. Spine. 2013; 38(14):1161–1169

[31] Suh BG, Uh JH, Park SH, Lee GW. Repair using conventional implant for ruptured annulus fibrosus after lumbar discectomy: surgical technique and case series. Asian Spine J. 2015; 9(1):14–21

[32] Bron JL, van der Veen AJ, Helder MN, van Royen BJ, Smit TH, Skeletal Tissue Engineering Group Amsterdam, Research Institute MOVE. Biomechanical and in vivo evaluation of experimental closure devices of the annulus fibrosus designed for a goat nucleus replacement model. Eur Spine J. 2010; 19 (8):1347–1355

[33] Lequin MB, Barth M, Thomé C, Bouma GJ. Primary limited lumbar discectomy with an annulus closure device: one-year clinical and radiographic results from a prospective, multi-center study. Korean J Spine. 2012; 9 (4):340–347

[34] Wilke H-J, Ressel L, Graf N, Heuer F. Can prevention of a reherniation be investigated? Establishment of a herniation model and experiments with an anular closure device. Spine J. 2013; 38(10):E587–E593

[35] Parker SL, Grahovac G, Vukas D, et al. Effect of an annular closure device (Barricaid) on same level recurrent disc herniation and disc height loss after primary lumbar discectomy: two-year results of a multi-center prospective cohort study. Clin Spine Surg. 2016:[Epub ahead of print]

[36] Likhitpanichkul M, Dreischarf M, Illien-Junger S, et al. Fibrin-genipin adhesive hydrogel for annulus fibrosus repair: performance evaluation with large animal organ culture, in situ biomechanics, and in vivo degradation tests. Eur Cell Mater. 2014; 28:25–37, discussion 37–38

[37] Borde B, Grunert P, Hartl R, Bonassar LJ. Injectable, high-density collagen gels for annulus fibrosus repair: an in vitro rat tail model. J Biomed Mater Res A. 2015; 103(8):2571–2581

[38] Wan Y, Feng G, Shen FH, Laurencin CT, Li X. Biphasic scaffold for annulus fibrosus tissue regeneration. Biomaterials. 2008; 29(6):643–652

[39] Guillaume O, Daly A, Lennon K, Gansau J, Buckley SF, Buckley CT. Shape-memory porous alginate scaffolds for regeneration of the annulus fibrosus: effect of TGF-β3 supplementation and oxygen culture conditions. Acta Biomater. 2014; 10(5):1985–1995

[40] Yeganegi M, Kandel RA, Santerre JP. Characterization of a biodegradable electrospun polyurethane nanofiber scaffold: mechanical properties and cytotoxicity. Acta Biomater. 2010; 6(10):3847–3855

[41] Park S-H, Gil ES, Mandal BB, et al. Annulus fibrosus tissue engineering using lamellar silk scaffolds. J Tissue Eng Regen Med. 2012; 6 Suppl 3:s24–s33

[42] Calderon L, Collin E, Velasco-Bayon D, Murphy M, O'Halloran D, Pandit A. Type II collagen-hyaluronan hydrogel–a step towards a scaffold for intervertebral disc tissue engineering. Eur Cell Mater. 2010; 20:134–148

[43] Helen W, Gough JE. Cell viability, proliferation and extracellular matrix production of human annulus fibrosus cells cultured within PDLLA/Bioglass composite foam scaffolds in vitro. Acta Biomater. 2008; 4(2):230–243

[44] Colombini A, Ceriani C, Banfi G, Brayda-Bruno M, Moretti M. Fibrin in intervertebral disc tissue engineering. Tissue Eng Part B Rev. 2014; 20 (6):713–721

[45] Guterl CC, Torre OM, Purmessur D, et al. Characterization of mechanics and cytocompatibility of fibrin-genipin annulus fibrosus sealant with the addition of cell adhesion molecules. Tissue Eng Part A. 2014; 20(17–18):2536–2545

[46] Schek RM, Michalek AJ, Iatridis JC. Genipin-crosslinked fibrin hydrogels as a potential adhesive to augment intervertebral disc annulus repair. Eur Cell Mater. 2011; 21:373–383

[47] Grunert P, Borde BH, Hudson KD, Macielak MR, Bonassar LJ, Härtl R. Annular repair using high-density collagen gel: a rat-tail in vivo model. Spine. 2014; 39(3):198–206

[48] Sato M, Asazuma T, Ishihara M, et al. An atelocollagen honeycomb-shaped scaffold with a membrane seal (ACHMS-scaffold) for the culture of annulus fibrosus cells from an intervertebral disc. J Biomed Mater Res A. 2003; 64 (2):248–256

[49] Sato M, Kikuchi M, Ishihara M, et al. Tissue engineering of the intervertebral disc with cultured annulus fibrosus cells using atelocollagen honeycomb-shaped scaffold with a membrane seal (ACHMS scaffold). Med BiolEngComput. 2003; 41(3):365–371

[50] Sato M, Asazuma T, Ishihara M, et al. An experimental study of the regeneration of the intervertebral disc with an allograft of cultured annulus fibrosus cells using a tissue-engineering method. Spine. 2003; 28(6):548–553

[51] Guillaume O, Naqvi SM, Lennon K, Buckley CT. Enhancing cell migration in shape-memory alginate-collagen composite scaffolds: In vitro and ex vivo assessment for intervertebral disc repair. J Biomater Appl. 2015; 29(9):1230–1246

[52] Shao X, Hunter CJ. Developing an alginate/chitosan hybrid fiber scaffold for annulus fibrosus cells. J Biomed Mater Res A. 2007; 82(3):701–710

[53] Chang G, Kim H-J, Kaplan D, Vunjak-Novakovic G, Kandel RA. Porous silk scaffolds can be used for tissue engineering annulus fibrosus. Eur Spine J. 2007; 16(11):1848–1857

[54] Buser Z, Kuelling F, Liu J, et al. Biological and biomechanical effects of fibrin injection into porcine intervertebral discs. Spine. 2011; 36(18):E1201–E1209

[55] Yin W, Pauza K, Olan WJ, Doerzbacher JF, Thorne KJ. Intradiscal injection of fibrin sealant for the treatment of symptomatic lumbar internal disc disruption: results of a prospective multicenter pilot study with 24-month follow-up. Pain Med. 2014; 15(1):16–31

[56] Wan Y, Feng G, Shen FH, Balian G, Laurencin CT, Li X. Novel biodegradable poly(1,8-octanediol malate) for annulus fibrosus regeneration. MacromolBiosci. 2007; 7(11):1217–1224

[57] Pirvu T, Blanquer SBG, Benneker LM, et al. A combined biomaterial and cellular approach for annulus fibrosus rupture repair. Biomaterials. 2015; 42:11–19

[58] Bowles RD, Williams RM, Zipfel WR, Bonassar LJ. Self-assembly of aligned tissue-engineered annulus fibrosus and intervertebral disc composite via collagen gel contraction. Tissue Eng Part A. 2010; 16(4):1339–1348

[59] Koepsell L, Zhang L, Neufeld D, Fong H, Deng Y. Electrospunnanofibrouspolycaprolactone scaffolds for tissue engineering of annulus fibrosus. MacromolBiosci. 2011; 11(3):391–399

[60] Nerurkar NL, Baker BM, Sen S, Wible EE, Elliott DM, Mauck RL. Nanofibrous biologic laminates replicate the form and function of the annulus fibrosus. Nat Mater. 2009; 8(12):986–992

[61] Nerurkar NL, Elliott DM, Mauck RL. Mechanics of oriented electrospun nanofibrous scaffolds for annulus fibrosus tissue engineering. J Orthop Res. 2007; 25(8):1018–1028

[62] Wismer N, Grad S, Fortunato G, Ferguson SJ, Alini M, Eglin D. Biodegradable electrospun scaffolds for annulus fibrosus tissue engineering: effect of scaffold structure and composition on annulus fibrosus cells in vitro. Tissue Eng Part A. 2014; 20(3–4):672–682

[63] Chan SCW, Gantenbein-Ritter B. Intervertebral disc regeneration or repair with biomaterials and stem cell therapy—feasible or fiction? Swiss Med Wkly. 2012; 142:w13598

[64] Benneker LM, Andersson G, Iatridis JC, et al. Cell therapy for intervertebral disc repair: advancing cell therapy from bench to clinics. Eur Cell Mater. 2014; 27 SUPPL:5–11

[65] Zhang Y, Chee A, Thonar EJ-MA, An HS. Intervertebral disk repair by protein, gene, or cell injection: a framework for rehabilitation-focused biologics in the spine. PM R. 2011; 3(6) Suppl 1:S88–S94

[66] Alsousou J, Thompson M, Hulley P, Noble A, Willett K. The biology of platelet-rich plasma and its application in trauma and orthopaedic surgery: a review of the literature. J Bone Joint Surg Br. 2009; 91(8):987–996

[67] Paoloni J, De Vos RJ, Hamilton B, Murrell GA, Orchard J. Platelet-rich plasma treatment for ligament and tendon injuries. Clin J Sport Med. 2011; 21 (1):37–45

[68] Pirvu, TN, Schroeder, JE, Peroglio, M, et al. Platelet-rich plasma induces annulus fibrosus cell proliferation and matrix production. Eur Spine J. 2014; 23(4):745–753

[69] Gui K, Ren W, Yu Y, Li X, Dong J, Yin W. Inhibitory effects of platelet-rich plasma on intervertebral disc degeneration: a preclinical study in a rabbit model. Med SciMonit. 2015; 21:1368–1375

[70] Lubkowska A, Dolegowska B, Banfi G. Growth factor content in PRP and their applicability in medicine. J Biol Regul Homeost Agents. 2012; 26(2) Suppl 1:3S–22S

[71] Tuakli-Wosornu YA, Terry A, Boachie-Adjei K, et al. Lumbar intradiskal platelet-rich plasma (PRP) injections: a prospective, double-blind, randomized controlled study. PM R. 2016; 8(1):1–10, quiz 10

[72] White AP, Vaccaro AR, Hall JA, Whang PG, Friel BC, McKee MD. Clinical applications of BMP-7/OP-1 in fractures, nonunions and spinal fusion. Int Orthop. 2007; 31(6):735–741

[73] Takegami K, An HS, Kumano F, et al. Osteogenic protein-1 is most effective in stimulating nucleus pulposus and annulus fibrosus cells to repair their matrix after chondroitinase ABC-induced in vitro chemonucleolysis. Spine J. 2005; 5(3):231–238

[74] Masuda K, Imai Y, Okuma M, et al. Osteogenic protein-1 injection into a degenerated disc induces the restoration of disc height and structural changes in the rabbit anular puncture model. Spine. 2006; 31(7):742–754

[75] Adams MA, Roughley PJ. What is intervertebral disc degeneration, and what causes it? Spine. 2006; 31(18):2151–2161

[76] Pattappa G, Peroglio M, Sakai D, et al. CCL5/RANTES is a key chemoattractant released by degenerative intervertebral discs in organ culture. Eur Cell Mater. 2014; 27:124–136, discussion 136

[77] Poleganov MA, Pfeilschifter J, Mühl H. Expanding extracellular zinc beyond levels reflecting the albumin-bound plasma zinc pool potentiates the capability of IL-1beta, IL-18, and IL-12 to Act as IFN-gamma-inducing factors on PBMC. J Interferon Cytokine Res. 2007; 27(12):997–1001

[78] Kalwitz G, Andreas K, Endres M, et al. Chemokine profile of human serum from whole blood: migratory effects of CXCL-10 and CXCL-11 on human mesenchymal stem cells. Connect Tissue Res. 2010; 51(2):113–122

[79] Romagnani P, Annunziato F, Lasagni L, et al. Cell cycle-dependent expression of CXC chemokine receptor 3 by endothelial cells mediates angiostatic activity. J Clin Invest. 2001; 107(1):53–63

[80] Hegewald, AA, Neumann, K, Kalwitz, G, et al. The chemokines CXCL10 and XCL1 recruit human annulus fibrosus cells. Spine. 2012; 37(2):101–107

[81] Henriksson HB, Svala E, Skioldebrand E, Lindahl A, Brisby H. Support of concept that migrating progenitor cells from stem cell niches contribute to normal regeneration of the adult mammal intervertebral disc: a descriptive study in the New Zealand white rabbit. Spine. 2012; 37(9):722–732

[82] Mwale F, Masuda K, Pichika R, et al. The efficacy of Link N as a mediator of repair in a rabbit model of intervertebral disc degeneration. Arthritis Res Ther. 2011; 13(4):R120

[83] Kepler CK, Markova DZ, Koerner JD, et al. Substance P receptor antagonist suppresses inflammatory cytokine expression in human disc cells. Spine. 2015; 40(16):1261–1269

[84] Zhang H, Lin C-Y. Simvastatin stimulates chondrogenic phenotype of intervertebral disc cells partially through BMP-2 pathway. Spine. 2008; 33(16): E525–E531

[85] Than, KD, Rahman, SU, Wang, L, et al. Intradiscal injection of simvastatin results in radiologic, histologic, and genetic evidence of disc regeneration in a rat model of degenerative disc disease. Spine J. 2014; 14(6):1017–1028

[86] Zhang, H, Wang, L, Park, JB, et al. Intradiscal injection of simvastatin retards progression of intervertebral disc degeneration induced by stab injury. Arthritis Res Ther. 2009; 11(6):R172

[87] Likhitpanichkul M, Kim Y, Torre OM, et al. Fibrin-genipin annulus fibrosus sealant as a delivery system for anti-TNFα drug. Spine J. 2015; 15(9):2045–2054

[88] Sakai D, Andersson GBJ. Stem cell therapy for intervertebral disc regeneration: obstacles and solutions. Nat Rev Rheumatol. 2015; 11(4):243–256

[89] Kim AJ, Adkisson DH, Wendland M, Seyedin M, Berven S, Lotz JC. Juvenile chondrocytes may facilitate disc repair. Open Tissue Eng Regen Med J. 2010; 3:28–35

[90] Vadalà, G, Sowa, G, Hubert, M, Gilbertson, LG, Denaro, V, Kang, JD. Mesenchymal stem cells injection in degenerated intervertebral disc: cell leakage may induce osteophyte formation. J Tissue Eng Regen Med. 2012; 6 (5):348–355

[91] Ganey T, Hutton WC, Moseley T, Hedrick M, Meisel H-J. Intervertebral disc repair using adipose tissue-derived stem and regenerative cells: experiments in a canine model. Spine. 2009; 34(21):2297–2304

[92] Colombini A, Lopa S, Ceriani C, et al. In vitro characterization and in vivo behavior of human nucleus pulposus and annulus fibrosus cells in clinical-grade fibrin and collagen-enriched fibrin gels. Tissue Eng Part A. 2015; 21(3–4):793–802

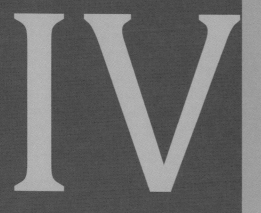

16 Summary of Clinical Trials with Biological Treatment Approaches for Spinal Disease

Gernot Lang, Ibrahim Hussain, Micaella Zubkov, Yu Moriguchi, Brenton Pennicooke, Rodrigo Navarro-Ramirez, and Roger Härtl

Abstract

Biological-based treatment approaches for cartilaginous and ligamentous parts of the body have laid the foundation for these strategies to be translated to spinal disease. Preclinical reports of different biomolecular, cell-based, and tissue-engineered therapies in animal models have shown promising results, with some of these therapies previously or currently being assessed in human clinical trials.

Although few, these clinical trials have been instrumental in determining how different stages of intervertebral disc (IVD) degeneration correlate with the efficacy of various treatments, as well as which therapies show short-term, but not long-term benefits. This robust topic within the spinal disease research landscape will continue to advance over the coming decades via more comprehensive understanding of the molecular interaction between host tissue, implanted biologics such as stem cells, and anti-inflammatory proteins. Furthermore, as these therapies gain traction, improvements in the surgeon's ability to deliver treatments safely will also become a major part of future clinical trials. In this chapter, we present an update on completed, aborted, and currently active clinical trials evaluating biological treatment approaches for spinal disease.

Keywords: annulus, biologics, intervertebral disc, nucleus, tissue engineering, regeneration

16.1 Historical Perspective

Current treatment options for degenerative disc disease (DDD), both conservative and surgical, fail to treat the underlying pathology, leading to symptomatlogy and complications. Biological treatment approaches have emerged as a feasible strategy for treating pathological intervertebral disc (IVD) segments without the adverse effects associated with conventional approaches. The aim of biological treatment strategies for DDD is to restore native biomechanics of the IVD and at the same time induce regeneration by promoting anabolism of IVD cells. Early-stage degenerated discs contain a sufficient amount of viable cells to replenish a healthy extracellular matrix (ECM) with assistance from engineered biomolecules, such as recombinant genes or proteins. Mid-stage degenerated discs are characterized by less active cells that are rapidly disappearing, at which point cell-based therapy is the most viable option. When the disc's structure and function are severely compromised, it has reached terminal-stage degeneration. At this point, it is necessary to replace the degenerated disc with a disclike composite impregnated with autologous tissues or tissues generated in vitro[1,2] (► Fig. 16.1).

The concept of using tissue engineering technology to treat musculoskeletal disorders is not new. One of the first biological treatment approaches for DDD was proposed by Wehling et al

in 1997, who described using gene therapy to engineer cells with the ability to regenerate ECM components.[3] In 2001, Orozco et al were the first to use autologous mesenchymal stem cells (MSCs) harvested from the patients' bone marrow for injection into the nucleus pulposus (NP) of a degenerated disc. Since then, many similar experiments have been conducted to explore cell therapy techniques to treat DDD, but almost all were pilot studies and contained very small study populations. To date, only a few clinical trials targeting IVD repair or regeneration have been published, and several ongoing clinical trials aimed at disc repair have yet to publish their findings (► Table 16.1).

Thus, the application of biological treatment strategies for the regeneration of IVDs remains a largely undiscovered field, especially with respect to clinical trials. Much work remains to be done before biomolecular- and cell-based therapies become prevalent treatment options for DDD, such as identifying and characterizing the roles of endogenous IVD stem cells, MSCs, platelet rich plasma (PRP), and cytokine inhibitors (► Fig. 16.2).

The following pages summarize and evaluate the literature on published and ongoing clinical trials that employ biological approaches for the treatment of DDD from the perspective of evidence-based medicine (EBM).

16.2 Growth Factors

A well-established compound in growth factor therapy applications is Growth and Differentiation Factor 5 (GDF-5), also known as Bone Morphogenetic Protein (BMP-14), a member of the BMP subfamily belonging to the transforming growth factor (TGF)-β superfamily. In vitro and in vivo experiments have shown that recombinant human GDF-5 (rhGDF-5) can stimulate gene expression and synthesis of collagen 2 (COL2) and aggrecan (ACAN) in bovine and human NP cells.[4,5] Phase I clinical trials of intradiscal rhGDF-5 showed no drastic adverse effects, and in 2016, a multicenter, randomized, double-blind, placebo-controlled Phase II clinical trial was completed that evaluated the safety, tolerability, and preliminary effectiveness of two different doses of intradiscal rhGDF-5 (single administration) for the treatment of early-stage lumbar disc degeneration.[6,7,8,9] Twenty-four participants were randomized into three groups, and administered a single injection of 1.0 mg rhGDF-5, 2.0 mg rhGDF-5, or sterile water (placebo control). The inclusion criteria were persistent low back pain (LBP) with at least 3 months of conservative therapy at one suspected symptomatic lumbar level, as confirmed by standardized provocative discography. Only 17 patients completed the entire study protocol. Clinical measurement scores (neurological assessment, Oswestry Disability Index [ODI], Visual Analog Scale [VAS], and quality-of-life Short Form Health Survey [SF-36]) did not reveal significant differences

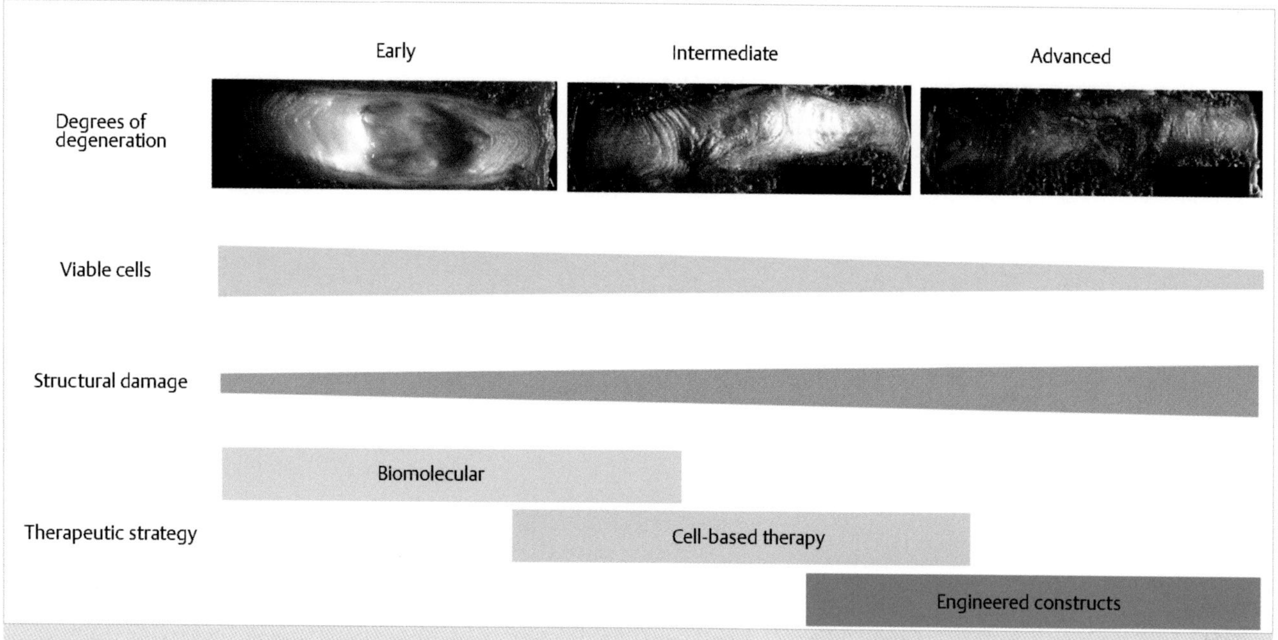

Fig. 16.1 Summary of biological approaches for intervertebral disc (IVD) repair based on the degree of degeneration.

Table 16.1 Published results of clinical trials targeting IVD repair or regeneration

Haufe et al[25] 2006	
Purpose	To analyze whether hematopoietic precursor stem cells (HSCs) prompt regeneration of disc tissue when injected into degenerated IVDs
Study type	Therapy (intervention), Phase I
Study design	Prospective study
Patient	Discogenic LBP; all patients had attempted endoscopic discectomy to eliminate pain ($N = 10$)
Intervention	Single intradiscal injection of 1 mL of HSCs harvested from patient's pelvic bone marrow
Comparison	None
Outcome	Follow-up at 6 and 12 mo: VAS
Status/Conclusion	Status: Complete No SAEs. No effect: no patients experienced relief of LBP 80% later underwent surgery
Meisel et al[24] 2007	
Purpose	To assess the long-term efficacy of autologous disc chondrocyte transplantation (ADCT) in DDD
Study type	Therapy (intervention), Phase I
Study design	Prospective, randomized, multicenter clinical; not blinded (EuroDisc)
Patient	Single-level DDD, Modic 1, failed conservative treatment ($N = 28$)
Intervention	Discectomy to harvest cells from index IVD, culture of disc cells and transplantation into index IVD 12 weeks following discectomy
Comparison	Discectomy only
Outcome	OPDQ, QBPD, MRI at 3, 6, 12, and 24 months postop; patients' experiences with surgery
Status/Conclusion	Status: Complete ADCT is a safe procedure ODI + OPDQ are slightly lower in the treatment group No statistical analysis No control group

Table 16.1 *(continued)*

Yoshikawa et al[30] 2010

Purpose	To analyze the regenerative ability of MSCs in degenerated IVDs
Study type	Therapy (intervention), Phase I
Study design	Clinical case report
Patient	DDD, failed conservative treatment (*N* = 2)
Intervention	Collagen sponge holding MSCs cultured from patient's bone marrow grafted to degenerated disc; collagen soaked in 10^5 cells/mL suspension
Comparison	None
Outcome	JOA, VAS, MRI, CT, and X-ray at 6 months and 2 years postop
Status/Conclusion	Status: Complete Low power (n = 2) No SAE Clinical outcome scores improved Morphological outcome questionable (MRI)

Orozco et al[32] 2011

Purpose	To assess the feasibility, safety, and efficacy of MSCs for degenerated IVDs
Study type	Therapy (intervention), Phase I
Study design	Prospective pilot study
Patient	DDD and LBP; failed conservative treatment for 6 months (*N* = 10)
Intervention	Injection of cultured MSCs into NP
Comparison	None
Outcome	MRI, SF-36, VAS, and ODI at 3, 6, and 12 months postop; 85% of improvement occurred within first 3 months
Status/Conclusion	Status: Complete No SAEs No control group Low power Clinical and radiographic outcomes showed improvement 85% of improvement occurred within the first 3 months

Coric et al[43] 2013

Purpose	US Investigational New Drug Application (IND) Phase I study to evaluate the safety of cell-based therapy with juvenile chondrocytes for the treatment of lumbar DDD with mechanical LBP
Study type	Therapy (intervention), Phase I
Study design	Prospective, U.S. FDA-regulated IND feasibility trial
Patient	LBP and single-level DDD (Pfirrmann III–IV) without annular rupture; failed ≥ 12 weeks conservative therapy (N = 15)
Intervention	1–2 mL intradiscal injection of juvenile chondrocytes (10^7 cells/mL) with fibrin carrier; cells harvested from articular surface of cadaveric donor tissue
Comparison	None
Outcome	Neurological examinations, serum liver and renal function, ODI, NRS, and SF-36 at 1, 3, 6, and 12 months post-treatment; MRI at 1, 6, and 12 months
Status/Conclusion	Status: Complete Improvements in ODI and NRS No control group Low power No SAE reported

Pettine et al[26] 2015

Purpose	To evaluate the use of autologous bone marrow–concentrated cells (BMCs) to treat discogenic LBP in an attempt to avoid or delay lumbar fusion or artificial disc replacement

Table 16.1 *(continued)*

Study type	Therapy (intervention), Phase I
Study design	Prospective, open-label, nonrandomized, two-arm study, single center
Patient	LBP: ODI ≥ 30, VAS ≥ 40 mm (100-mm scale), height loss < 30%, Modic II or less (N = 26)
Intervention	Intradiscal injection of 2–3 mL BMC (single or two adjacent levels), cell concentration varied between patients
Comparison	None
Outcome	ODI, VAS, MRI (Pfirrmann) at 12 months postop; bone marrow concentration analyses
Status/Conclusion	Status: Complete No SAEs Low power No control group Improvement in clinical measures Radiological measures inconclusive

Tuakli-Wosornu et al[13] 2015

Purpose	To determine whether single injections of PRPs into degenerative IVDs will improve pain and function
Study type	Therapy (intervention), Phase I
Study design	Prospective, double-blind, randomized controlled study
Patient	≥ 6 months LBP, failed conservative treatment, presence of a grade 3 or 4 annular fissure (N = 47)
Intervention	Intradiscal PRP injection (1–2 mL); (N = 29)
Comparison	Omnipaque 180, Amersham Health, Princeton, NJ
Outcome	NRS, FRI, physical SF-36, and NASS Outcome Questionnaire at 1, 4 and 8 weeks post-op
Status/Conclusion	Status: Complete Short follow up (2 months) Slight improvement in all clinical scores in experimental group compared to control No SAEs

DePuy Spine[6,7,8,9] 2016

Purpose	To evaluate safety and preliminary effectiveness of intradiscal rhGDF-5 in patients with early lumbar DDD
Study type	Therapy (intervention), Phase I/II
Study design	Open-label, single administration, dose finding
Patient	Single-level LBP (L3–4 to L5–S1) (L3/L4 to L5/S1) with ≥ 3 months of conservative therapy; ODI of ≥ 30; LBP score ≥ 4 cm (VAS) (N=32)
Intervention	Intradiscal injection of rhGDF-5, 0.25 mg (N=7) and 1.0 mg (N=25)
Comparison	None
Outcome	ODI, VAS, SF-36, neurological assessment
Status/Conclusion	Status: Complete 37.5% of patients were lost to follow-up No statistical analysis Clinical outcomes reveal minimal improvement No effect compared to placebo

Mesoblast Ltd.[41,42] 2016

Purpose	To determine safety of MPCs and carrier injection treatments, and its effectiveness in reducing chronic LBP
Study type	Therapy (intervention), Phase II
Study design	Prospective, double-blind, controlled, multicenter
Patient	Chronic LBP ≥ 6 months, single-level DDD L1–S1, failed 3 months of conservative treatment, ODI ≥ 30, (N = 100)
Intervention	Single intradiscal (NP) injection of MPCs in hyaluronic acid; volumes and concentrations not indicated

Table 16.1 (continued)

Comparison	Sham control: single injection of saline/hyaluronic acid solution
Outcome	VAS and safety evaluation at 1, 3, 6, 12, 24, and 36 months post-injection; MRI at 6,12, 24, and 36 months post-injection
Status/Conclusion	Ongoing study Results of this study are not yet available on ClinicalTrials.gov (as of time of publication)

Abbreviations: CT, computed tomography; DDD, degenerative disc disease; HSCs, hematopoietic stem cells; IND, investigational new drug; IVD, intervertebral disc; JOA, Japanese Orthopaedic Association; LBP, low back pain; MPCs, mesenchymal precursor cells; MRI, magnetic resonance imaging; MSCs, mesenchymal stem cells; NASS, North American Spine Society; NP, nucleus pulposus; ODI, Oswestry Disability Index; OPDQ, Oswestry Low Back Pain Disability Questionnaire; PRP, platelet rich plasma; QBPD, Quebec Back Pain Disability Scale; rhGDF-5, recombinant human growth and differentiation factor 5; SAE, serious adverse event; VAS, Visual Analog Scale.

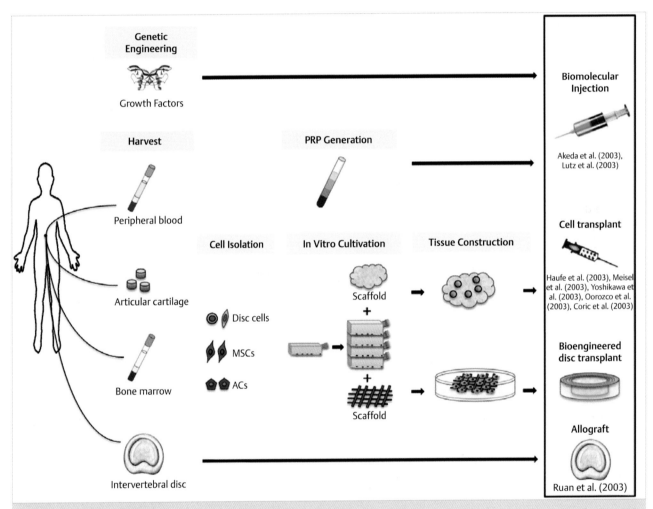

Fig. 16.2 Generation and application of biological repair strategies for intervertebral disc disease. Abbreviations: AC, autologous chrondrcytes; MSC, mesenchymal stem cell; PRP, platelet rich plasma.

between the groups at 12-month follow-up. Furthermore, the groups receiving the intradiscal rhGDF-5 saw higher rates of non–life-threatening adverse effects, including higher procedural pain. Although formal results have not been published yet, larger studies and longer follow-up will be required to assess the effectiveness of this treatment.

16.2.1 Platelet Rich Plasma

PRP is a fraction of plasma that can be obtained by centrifugal separation of whole blood. A platelet contains the vast majority of biologically active molecules required for blood coagulation, such as adhesive proteins, coagulation factors, and protease inhibitors.[10] More specifically, PRP includes growth factors such as TGF-β, platelet-derived growth factor (PDGF), epidermal growth factor (EGF), vascular endothelial growth factor (VEGF), and insulin-like growth factor (IGF)-1. These factors enhance cell viability, promote ECM metabolism, and stimulate proliferation of IVD cells.[11] Clinical studies in autologous injection models of degenerated discs have shown PRP to upregulate proteoglycan (PG) synthesis rate, which leads to a restoration in disc height corresponding to the increased number of PG molecules. The presence of these factors in PRP led to the proposal to use it as an intradiscal injection to stimulate regeneration or at least slow the degenerative process in diseased IVDs.

Akeda et al demonstrated the feasibility of intradiscal PRP-releasate injection for reducing LBP in patients with DDD at L4–5 and L5–S1.[12] Although this trial was just a pilot study, it provided an initial platform for intradiscal injections of PRP. The soluble releasate (2.0 mL), isolated from clotted PRP, was injected into the center of the NP under fluoroscopic guidance. Mean disc height, as assessed on T2-weighted axial magnetic resonance imaging (MRI), did not significantly change over the follow-up period, but VAS pain scores significantly decreased at 1 and 12 months after treatment despite no additional/further injections of PRP. More recently, a prospective, double-blind, randomized controlled trial (RCT) evaluated the efficacy of intradiscal PRP injections in 47 patients with discogenic LBP.[13] After 8 weeks, patients receiving PRP had significantly less pain, better functional results, and higher patient satisfaction compared with controls. However, this effect did not persist, and at 1 year post-procedure there were no differences between the groups based on these metrics. No adverse events of infection, neurological injury, or progressive herniation were reported. Although this study initially described promising results, the follow-up period of the control group was extremely short, lasting for only 8 weeks, which may compromise the impact and validity of the data. Longer follow-up and imaging analysis will help demonstrate the clinical impact of this therapy.

16.3 Anti–TNF-α Treatment

Inhibition of pro-inflammatory cytokines such as tumor necrosis factor (TNF)-α may protect the IVD from further degeneration. TNF-α inhibitors are currently used for the treatment of chronic inflammatory diseases such as Crohn's disease, ankylosing spondylitis, psoriasis, and rheumatoid arthritis. The most commonly used types of TNF-α inhibitors are the monoclonal antibodies adalimumab, infliximab, certolizumab, and the fusion protein etanercept. Several pilot studies and RCTs investigated the effects of etanercept, infliximab and adalimumab in patients with symptomatic lumbar DDD. The overall results demonstrated a significant reduction in leg and back pain in patients with sciatica compared with placebo groups.[14,15,16,17,18] Mechanistically, Olmarker et al supported these findings by showing that etanercept and infliximab prevent NP thrombus formation and intraneural edema, as well as a reduction in nerve conduction velocity.[19] Other studies have shown that a short course of adalimumab injections significantly reduces the risk for spine surgery by 61% for 3 years in patients with acute sciatica secondary to disc herniation.[20] Although promising, these therapies are limited by three major issues. First, it is unclear if the mechanism behind radicular pain

relief translates to early-stage discogenic pain prior to disc herniation. Second, IVDs that have reached terminal degeneration may not respond due to the lack of structure-building cells that have already been compromised by chronic inflammation. Third, the well-established side-effect profile of these medications may mitigate their utility in treating discogenic back pain. Their immuno-compromising nature may cause infection by opportunistic pathogens, including reactivation of latent tuberculosis. Furthermore, reports of rare white blood cell cancers (T-cell lymphomas) have been linked to these medications.[21]

16.4 Cell-based Therapy for Disc Regeneration

Biomolecular treatment of IVDs becomes less effective with progressively higher grades of degeneration due to a reduction in the number of responsive target cells.[22] Cell-based therapy can be an effective alternative biological treatment strategy for discs with mid-stage degeneration that are characterized by a decreased number of functional cells. Rather than injecting active biomolecules into the disc to increase metabolism, vital whole cells are delivered into the disc to help synthesize a de novo ECM or to further augment endogenous cell-mediated synthesis of the ECM.

16.4.1 Autologous Disc Chondrocytes

Autologous disc chondrocyte transplantation (ADCT) was initially performed within the EuroDisc Trial.[23,24] This multicenter RCT aimed to assess the safety, efficacy, and postoperative pain of patients undergoing ADCT after discectomy compared with patients undergoing discectomy only. Twenty-eight patients presenting with single-level disc disease were included in the study. Patients who received ADCT showed significant postoperative improvement according to their Oswestry Low Back Pain Disability Questionnaire (OPDQ) compared with controls; this difference between groups persisted for 2 years following treatment.[23] The efficiency of the treatment was assessed morphologically by evaluating the NP's signal intensity on T2-weighted MRI scans as well as the increase in disc height. The study revealed 16% higher fluid retention within the NP of patients treated with ADCT compared with controls, but no difference in mean disc height. ADCT systems are currently manufactured and marketed in Germany (co. don AG; Teltow, Germany), but have not yet been approved by the U.S. Food and Drug Administration (FDA).

16.4.2 Autologous Hematopoietic Stem Cells

The first stem cell–based clinical trial published in the field of disc regeneration investigated whether the intradiscal injection of hematopoietic precursor stem cells (HPSCs) obtained from pelvic bone marrow followed by 2 weeks of hyperbaric oxygen therapy provided rejuvenating effects.[25] None of the 10 patients enrolled in this study experienced any improvement in discogenic low back pain after one year, and 80% of patients underwent surgical treatment within one year of receiving the injection.

16.4.3 Autologous Bone Marrow Aspirate/Bone Marrow–Concentrated Cells

Biological treatment strategies containing autologous chondrocytes and MSCs require specialized methods for harvesting, culturing, and expanding cells. Furthermore, after expansion these cells are implanted in the IVD during a separate, delayed procedure. Bone marrow–concentrated cells (BMCs) for ADCT, which include multiple types of progenitor cells (▶ Fig. 16.2), provide a less cumbersome and invasive way to utilize autologous bone marrow. Pettine et al first reported using BMCs as a novel treatment for discogenic low back pain in 2015.[26] Twenty-six patients had BMCs harvested from the iliac crest, followed by immediate intradiscal injections to either one or two IVDs. Clinical outcome measures including ODI and VAS revealed a reduction of pain over one year postoperatively, and 40% of patients presented improved radiographic scores. Furthermore, patients who received more than 2,000 colony-forming unit fibroblasts (CFU-F) per milliliter of bone marrow aspirate had significantly improved pain scores over 3 and 6 months when compared with patients who received < 2,000 CFU-F/mL.

16.4.4 Allogenic Mesenchymal Precursor Cells/Mesenchymal Stem Cells

MSCs derived from bone marrow are extensively studied cells in regenerative medicine because of their accessibility via minimally invasive procedures and expansion capabilities in in vitro conditions. Furthermore, recent research has demonstrated anti-inflammatory effects of MSCs in various animal models and injury conditions, such as myocardial infarction, renal ischemia, burn wounds, and osteoarthritis.[27,28,29] Multiple attempts have been conducted over the past decade to apply mesenchymal precursor cells (MPCs) or MSCs to the intradiscal space to treat chronic low back pain (LBP). Please refer to Chapter 13 for additional background information on the properties of MSCs.

Yoshikawa et al investigated the effects of autologous MSCs as a supplemental treatment to improve disc regeneration in two patients undergoing surgical intervention for DDD.[30] Both patients had chronic LBP, radiculopathy, and paresthesias. First, MSCs were harvested from the patients' iliac crest and cultured in vitro. In a second procedure, a partial laminotomy was performed to decompress the stenotic spinal canal, followed by placement of several pieces of collagen sponge impregnated with autologous MSCs into the degenerated IVD (▶ Fig. 16.3). Two years after surgery, both patients had significant symptomatic relief and T2-weighted MR images illustrated high signal intensity within the treated IVDs, indicating high NP hydration without progression of degeneration. Due to the small number of patients and a lack of a control group, it remains uncertain to what extend the application of MSCs contributed to the improved MRI and clinical outcome. One year later, Orozco et al used a similar technique to evaluate intradiscal MSCs in 10 patients with LBP due to DDD[31] (▶ Fig. 16.3). All patients reported a rapid improvement in pain (up to 85% at 3-month follow-up), but the primary radiographic outcome of disc height was not seen.

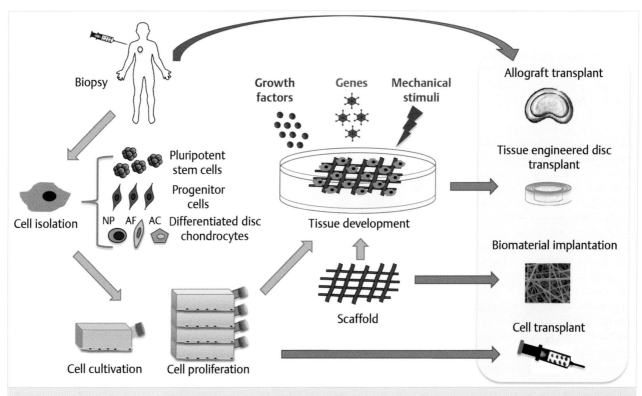

Fig. 16.3 Bone marrow–based cell therapies for degenerative disc disease. Abbreviations: AC, articular cartilage; AF, annulus fibrosus; NP, nucleus pulposus.

Although the changes in the patients' states were obvious, it remains unclear how the MSCs contributed to their improvement. Recent publications suggest that NP cells co-cultured with MSCs in direct contact are able to stimulate the MSCs to differentiate into NP-like cells with a chondrocyte-like phenotype.[32,33,34,35,36] Furthermore it has been shown that MSCs have the ability to stimulate NP cells to produce ECM components.[37,38] Lastly, MSCs' immunomodulatory effects reduce inflammation and thus may reduce symptomatic pain via this mechanism.[38,39] This study proved the feasibility and safety of using MSCs to treat DDD, and demonstrated the potential to provide significant pain relief for patients while preserving spinal biomechanics and avoiding the risks associated with major surgery.

Mesoblast Ltd. is an Australian-based company developing a commercially available cell line of MPCs expanded in vitro for discogenic LBP.[40] A Phase II clinical trial was recently completed, in which 100 patients with discogenic LBP received intradiscal injections of saline, hyaluronic acid (HA), or varying concentrations of MPCs. Whereas all experimental protocols were well-tolerated 24 months out, the higher concentrations of MPCs showed lower efficacy and higher adverse events. Nonetheless, of those receiving the intradiscal MPCs, 44% showed reduction in pain, improvement in function, and no need for further interventional procedures.[41] Mesoblast Ltd. is currently initiating Phase III clinical trials in a study enrolling 360 patients with an estimated completion date in February 2019. Patients meeting inclusion criteria include those with at least 6 months of LBP and radiographic evidence of DDD, and will undergo a double-blinded, placebo-controlled, clinical trial. Participants will be randomized into three groups, one of which will serve as the control group, receiving an intradiscal injection of saline. The two experimental arms will receive intradiscal injections of rexlemestrocel-L (MPCs) alone versus rexlemestrocel-L with HA. Another group in Spain has taken a similar approach and is currently conducting a Phase II trial using MSCs in an intradiscal injection for treatment of DDD. Results have not been published yet, but they will provide a relevant comparison to the Mesoblast trial.[42]

16.4.5 Allogeneic Juvenile Disc Chondrocytes

Allogeneic juvenile articular chondrocytes are another promising cell source for treating DDD via disc regeneration because they are immunoprivileged and have a similar biological profile to disc chondrocytes. In a prospective cohort study, Coric et al demonstrated that an injectable fibrin-based composite infused with juvenile chondrocytes called NuQu (ISTO Technologies, St. Louis, MO) attenuated symptoms in patients having refractory LBP that was unresponsive to conservative therapy ($n = 15$).[43] Phase I results showed significant reduction in ODI and significant improvement in quality of life (as assessed by SF-36) at 12 months following the procedure without any adverse events. Despite these results, a Phase II clinical trial was recently terminated early, due to questions concerning the safety and efficacy of this therapy. Published results are pending.

16.5 Allogenic IVD and Tissue-engineered IVD Implantation for DDD

Currently, both in vivo and in vitro experiments on tissue-engineered IVDs (TE-IVDs) are in their preliminary stages. Please refer to Chapter 7 for more information on these topics. At this point, no clinical trials are being implemented in humans. One promising clinical study conducted by Ruan et al demonstrated that whole allogenic IVDs could be implanted into humans.[44] This study included five patients between the ages of 41 and 56 years who suffered from a cervical disc herniation. These patients underwent a transplantation of fresh-frozen composite disc allografts plus end plates after en bloc resection. The disc allografts were harvested from 13 previously healthy young female donors, aged 20 to 30 years, who died from trauma. Within 2 hours of cardiac arrest and after other organs were harvested, the cervical spine was removed en bloc from vertebral levels C3 to T1 from the donors under sterile conditions. The harvested allografts were then implanted and the patients were followed with serial flexion-extension X-rays 2 months after surgery and every 3 months thereafter to monitor the status of the grafts and the sagittal stability and mobility of the segment.[44] Additionally, the patients received an MRI before and after the operation and at the last follow-up visit to assess the adequacy of cord decompression and the hydration of the transplanted disc. It is important to note that these patients did not receive any immunosuppressive agents, and were simply monitored with serial weekly measurements of erythrocyte sedimentation rate, C-reactive protein, and peripheral blood counts. The study demonstrated that at the 5-year follow-up, the motion and stability of the implanted spinal segments were preserved, but only 40% of the implanted grafts contained optimal levels of hydration on T2-weighted MRI. Still, union of the graft and host end plates was observed 3 months after surgery and there was improvement in neurological symptoms in all patients that persisted at 5 year follow-up. There were no immunoreactions reported.[44] These results are very promising, and introduce the possibility of transplanting cervical discs from donors set to undergo anterior cervical discectomies to subjects with severe DDD. Future experimentation may consider the viability of these human allografts when treated with growth factors or repopulated with living cells.

16.6 Future Perspective

Multiple approaches for the biological treatment of DDD are still in their infancy, and future studies will further elucidate the mechanisms and molecular pathophysiology of this disease. Biomolecular treatments have overall fallen out of favor, as it is unrealistic to assume that a one-time boost with these therapies would have a long-lasting effect. The results of the aforementioned clinical trials support this notion, although other compounds are still being considered for applications in DDD. Cell-based therapies appear to be more promising, as these cells are inherently regenerative, and may perpetuate positive clinical and radiographic findings with single-dose treatments. However, a major limiting factor for both approaches is that the injection of biomolecular and cell-based therapies into the disc is in and of itself destructive. The procedure in most cases is performed in degenerated discs that have an intact annulus fibrosus that have not succumbed to frank herniation at the time of treatment. It remains unclear what role an iatrogenic annular and NP injury may have in the natural progression of disc degeneration, and what interaction it has with the therapy being delivered.

Although tissue engineering is progressing in its development, using TE-IVDs for total disc replacement (TDR) still presents challenges in both implementation and functionality. Implanting biological constructs as functional disc substitutes requires substantially more invasive procedures, putting patients at increased operative morbidity, and presents technical complexities that must be accounted for before clinical trials can commence. Using minimally invasive spine (MIS) surgery techniques presents an attractive alternative for overcoming these hurdles. Additionally, implant displacement is a common complication associated with IVD implants that are positioned in a stand-alone fashion, predominantly due to axial loading forces the human spine is subjected to as evidenced by studies in prosthetic TDR implants.[45] This implies that experimental results obtained from studies testing IVD implants in quadrupedal animal models must be interpreted with caution before applying the intervention to humans, even when results are promising. Furthermore, manufacturing an implant that remains viable within a mechanically and trophically inhospitable environment remains technically difficult. However, the combined use of implants with either temporary axial distraction via a fixator[46] or prolonged mechanical support with rigid, but biodegradable materials[47] can enhance the in vivo performance of the IVD implant.

Gene therapy, discussed in detail in Chapter 11, was among the first biological therapies proposed, but has recently been abandoned. The procedure is conducted either by directly injecting the viral vector into the host tissue or by transfecting harvested cells in vitro followed by reimplantation of the cells back into the respective tissue. Adenovirus and retrovirus are the major vectors commonly used in clinical trials, particularly for the treatment of cystic fibrosis and human immunodeficiency virus (HIV). At present, there are no clinical trials utilizing gene therapy for the treatment of DDD. Major concerns regarding the safety of gene therapy limit its applicability for treating degenerative tissue disease, particularly the potential mutagenesis of transfected genes, which could present greater risks than benefits.[48,49,50] Over the past few years, numerous clinical trials using gene therapy in other fields have advanced this science and justified its safety profile,[51] paving the way for future Phase I studies in the repair of degenerated discs.

16.7 References

[1] An HS, Masuda K, Cs-Szabo G, et al. Biologic repair and regeneration of the intervertebral disk. J Am AcadOrthop Surg. 2011; 19(7):450–452

[2] Maidhof R, Alipui DO, Rafiuddin A, Levine M, Grande DA, Chahine NO. Emerging trends in biological therapy for intervertebral disc degeneration. Discov Med. 2012; 14(79):401–411

[3] Wehling P, Schulitz KP, Robbins PD, Evans CH, Reinecke JA. Transfer of genes to chondrocytic cells of the lumbar spine. Proposal for a treatment strategy of spinal disorders by local gene therapy. Spine. 1997; 22(10):1092–1097

[4] Chujo T, An HS, Akeda K, et al. Effects of growth differentiation factor-5 on the intervertebral disc—in vitro bovine study and in vivo rabbit disc degeneration model study. Spine. 2006; 31(25):2909–2917

[5] Stoyanov JV, Gantenbein-Ritter B, Bertolo A, et al. Role of hypoxia and growth and differentiation factor-5 on differentiation of human mesenchymal stem cells towards intervertebral nucleus pulposus-like cells. Eur Cell Mater. 2011; 21:533–547

[6] DePuy Spine, J-CPL. A Clinical Trial to Evaluate the Safety, Tolerability and Preliminary Effectiveness of Single Administration Intradiscal rhGDF-5 for the Treatment of Early Stage Lumbar Disc Degeneration. : ClinicalTrials.gov; 2010 [updated 01/26/2016]

[7] DePuySpine. A Clinical Trial to Evaluate the Safety, Tolerability and Preliminary Effectiveness of Single Administration Intradiscal rhGDF-5 for the Treatment of Early Stage Lumbar Disc Degeneration: ClinicalTrials.gov; 2010 [updated 01/26/2016]. https://clinicaltrials.gov/ct2/show/study?term=GDF-5+Disc&rank=3.

[8] DePuy Spine. A Multicenter, Randomized, Double-blind, Placebo Controlled, Clinical Trial to Evaluate the Safety, Tolerability and Preliminary Effectiveness of 2 Doses of Intradiscal rhGDF-5 (Single Administration) for the Treatment of Early Stage Lumbar Disc Degeneration. 2016. https://clinicaltrials.gov/ct2/show/NCT01124006?term=rhGDF-5+intervertebral+disc&rank=4. Accessed June 29, 2016

[9] DePuySpine. Intradiscal rhGDF-5 Phase I/II Clinical Trial: ClinicalTrials.gov; June 2008 [updated 01/26/2016]. https://clinicaltrials.gov/ct2/show/NCT00813813?term=rhGDF-5&rank=1&submit_fld_opt=

[10] Harrison P, Cramer EM. Platelet alpha-granules. Blood Rev. 1993; 7(1):52–62

[11] Gruber HE, Norton HJ, Hanley EN , Jr. Anti-apoptotic effects of IGF-1 and PDGF on human intervertebral disc cells in vitro. Spine. 2000; 25(17):2153–2157

[12] Akeda K, Imanisha T, Ohishi K, et al. Intradiscal injection of autologous platelet-rich-plasma for the treatment of lumbar disc degeneration preliminary prospective clinical trial for discogenic low back pain patients. Poster no. 2194 presented at ORS Annual Meeting 2012

[13] Tuakli-Wosornu YA, Terry A, Boachie-Adjei K, et al. Lumbar intradiskal platelet-rich plasma (PRP) injections: a prospective, double-blind, randomized controlled study. PM R. 2016; 8(1):1–10, quiz 10

[14] Freeman BJ, Ludbrook GL, Hall S, et al. Randomized, double-blind, placebo-controlled, trial of transforaminal epidural etanercept for the treatment of symptomatic lumbar disc herniation. Spine. 2013; 38(23):1986–1994

[15] Genevay S, Stingelin S, Gabay C. Efficacy of etanercept in the treatment of acute, severe sciatica: a pilot study. Ann Rheum Dis. 2004; 63(9):1120–1123

[16] Cohen SP, Bogduk N, Dragovich A, et al. Randomized, double-blind, placebo-controlled, dose-response, and preclinical safety study of transforaminal epidural etanercept for the treatment of sciatica. Anesthesiology. 2009; 110 (5):1116–1126

[17] Okoro T, Tafazal SI, Longworth S, Sell PJ. Tumor necrosis alpha-blocking agent (etanercept): a triple blind randomized controlled trial of its use in treatment of sciatica. J Spinal Disord Tech. 2010; 23(1):74–77

[18] Karppinen J, Korhonen T, Malmivaara A, et al. Tumor necrosis factor-alpha monoclonal antibody, infliximab, used to manage severe sciatica. Spine. 2003; 28(8):750–753, discussion 753–754

[19] Olmarker K, Rydevik B. Selective inhibition of tumor necrosis factor-alpha prevents nucleus pulposus-induced thrombus formation, intraneural edema, and reduction of nerve conduction velocity: possible implications for future pharmacologic treatment strategies of sciatica. Spine. 2001; 26 (8):863–869

[20] Genevay S, Finckh A, Zufferey P, Viatte S, Balagué F, Gabay C. Adalimumab in acute sciatica reduces the long-term need for surgery: a 3-year follow-up of a randomised double-blind placebo-controlled trial. Ann Rheum Dis. 2012; 71 (4):560–562

[21] Mariette X, Tubach F, Bagheri H, et al. Lymphoma in patients treated with anti-TNF: results of the 3-year prospective French RATIO registry. Ann Rheum Dis. 2010; 69(2):400–408

[22] Gruber HE, Ingram JA, Davis DE, Hanley EN , Jr. Increased cell senescence is associated with decreased cell proliferation in vivo in the degenerating human annulus. Spine J. 2009; 9(3):210–215

[23] Meisel HJ, Ganey T, Hutton WC, Libera J, Minkus Y, Alasevic O. Clinical experience in cell-based therapeutics: intervention and outcome. Eur Spine J. 2006; 15(3) Suppl 3:S397–S405

[24] Hohaus C, Ganey TM, Minkus Y, Meisel HJ. Cell transplantation in lumbar spine disc degeneration disease. Eur Spine J. 2008; 17 Suppl 4:492–503

[25] Haufe SM, Mork AR. Intradiscal injection of hematopoietic stem cells in an attempt to rejuvenate the intervertebral discs. Stem Cells Dev. 2006; 15 (1):136–137

[26] Pettine KA, Murphy MB, Suzuki RK, Sand TT. Percutaneous injection of autologous bone marrow concentrate cells significantly reduces lumbar discogenic pain through 12 months. Stem Cells. 2015; 33(1):146–156

[27] Black LL, Gaynor J, Gahring D, et al. Effect of adipose-derived mesenchymal stem and regenerative cells on lameness in dogs with chronic osteoarthritis of the coxofemoral joints: a randomized, double-blinded, multicenter, controlled trial. Vet Ther. 2007; 8(4):272–284

[28] Ohnishi S, Yanagawa B, Tanaka K, et al. Transplantation of mesenchymal stem cells attenuates myocardial injury and dysfunction in a rat model of acute myocarditis. J Mol Cell Cardiol. 2007; 42(1):88–97

[29] Black LL, Gaynor J, Adams C, et al. Effect of intraarticular injection of autologous adipose-derived mesenchymal stem and regenerative cells on clinical signs of chronic osteoarthritis of the elbow joint in dogs. Vet Ther. 2008; 9(3):192–200

[30] Yoshikawa T, Ueda Y, Miyazaki K, Koizumi M, Takakura Y. Disc regeneration therapy using marrow mesenchymal cell transplantation: a report of two case studies. Spine. 2010; 35(11):E475–E480

[31] Orozco L, Soler R, Morera C, Alberca M, Sánchez A, García-Sancho J. Intervertebral disc repair by autologous mesenchymal bone marrow cells: a pilot study. Transplantation. 2011; 92(7):822–828

[32] Le Maitre CL, Baird P, Freemont AJ, Hoyland JA. An in vitro study investigating the survival and phenotype of mesenchymal stem cells following injection into nucleus pulposus tissue. Arthritis Res Ther. 2009; 11(1):R20

[33] Luo W, Xiong W, Qiu M, Lv Y, Li Y, Li F. Differentiation of mesenchymal stem cells towards a nucleus pulposus-like phenotype utilizing simulated microgravity in vitro. J Huazhong UnivSci Technolog Med Sci. 2011; 31(2):199–203

[34] Risbud MV, Albert TJ, Guttapalli A, et al. Differentiation of mesenchymal stem cells towards a nucleus pulposus-like phenotype in vitro: implications for cell-based transplantation therapy. Spine. 2004; 29(23):2627–2632

[35] Tomita N, Morishita R, Tomita T, Ogihara T. Potential therapeutic applications of decoy oligonucleotides. Curr Opin Mol Ther. 2002; 4(2):166–170

[36] Vadalà G, Studer RK, Sowa G, et al. Coculture of bone marrow mesenchymal stem cells and nucleus pulposus cells modulate gene expression profile without cell fusion. Spine. 2008; 33(8):870–876

[37] Watanabe T, Sakai D, Yamamoto Y, et al. Human nucleus pulposus cells significantly enhanced biological properties in a coculture system with direct cell-to-cell contact with autologous mesenchymal stem cells. J Orthop Res. 2010; 28(5):623–630

[38] Yang S-H, Wu C-C, Shih TT-F, Sun Y-H, Lin F-H. In vitro study on interaction between human nucleus pulposus cells and mesenchymal stem cells through paracrine stimulation. Spine. 2008; 33(18):1951–1957

[39] Hiyama A, Mochida J, Iwashina T, et al. Transplantation of mesenchymal stem cells in a canine disc degeneration model. J Orthop Res. 2008; 26(5):589–600

[40] Mesoblast L. Safety and Efficacy Study of Rexlemestrocel-L in Subjects With Chronic Discogenic Lumbar Back Pain (MSB-DR003) 2016 [updated 11/09/2016]. https://clinicaltrials.gov/show/NCT02412735

[41] Mesoblast L. Safety and Preliminary Efficacy Study of Mesenchymal Precursor Cells (MPCs) in Subjects With Lumbar Back Pain: ClinicalTrials.gov; 2011 [updated 10/12/2016]. http://www.mesoblast.com/clinical-trial-results/mpc-06-id-phase-2

[42] Cellular RdT. Treatment of Degenerative Disc Disease With Allogenic Mesenchymal Stem Cells (MSV) (Disc_allo). 2016.

[43] Coric D, Pettine K, Sumich A, Boltes MO. Prospective study of disc repair with allogeneic chondrocytes presented at the 2012 Joint Spine Section Meeting. J Neurosurg Spine. 2013; 18(1):85–95

[44] Ruan D, He Q, Ding Y, Hou L, Li J, Luk KD. Intervertebral disc transplantation in the treatment of degenerative spine disease: a preliminary study. Lancet. 2007; 369(9566):993–999

[45] Ross R, Mirza AH, Norris HE, Khatri M. Survival and clinical outcome of SB Charite III disc replacement for back pain. J Bone Joint Surg Br. 2007; 89(6):785–789

[46] Hee HT, Ismail HD, Lim CT, Goh JC, Wong HK. Effects of implantation of bone marrow mesenchymal stem cells, disc distraction and combined therapy on reversing degeneration of the intervertebral disc. J Bone Joint Surg Br. 2010; 92(5):726–736

[47] Goldschlager T, Oehme D, Ghosh P, Zannettino A, Rosenfeld JV, Jenkin G. Current and future applications for stem cell therapies in spine surgery. Curr Stem Cell Res Ther. 2013; 8(5):381–393

[48] Somia N, Verma IM. Gene therapy: trials and tribulations. Nat Rev Genet. 2000; 1(2):91–99

[49] Hacein-Bey-Abina S, Von Kalle C, Schmidt, M, et al. LMO2-associated clonal T cell proliferation in two patients after gene therapy for SCID-X1. Science. 2003; 302(5644):415–419

[50] Cavazzana-Calvo M, Thrasher A, Mavilio F. The future of gene therapy. Nature. 2004; 427(6977):779–781

[51] Flotte TR. Gene therapy: the first two decades and the current state-of-the-art. J Cell Physiol. 2007; 213(2):301–305

17 Total Disc Transplantation: Current Results and Future Development

Jason Pui Yin Cheung, Dike Ruan, and Keith D.K. Luk

Abstract

Total disc transplantation has been found in both animal and a preliminary human clinical trial to be successful in restoring biochemical and mechanical properties. Degeneration in the form of disc height reduction is still observed after allograft transplantation. Biological agents and nucleus pulposus (NP) cells may have a role in reducing allograft disc degeneration. A combination of cryoprotective agents with a slow cooling rate, limited incubation time, and liquid nitrogen for storage yields the best overall disc metabolic activity and elastic and viscous modulus. Future studies will utilize the goat model due to the poor availability of bipedal animal models. Future study direction includes fine-tuning of the graft harvesting and preservation procedures, understanding nutritional pathways, and novel imaging options for measuring nutrition transfer across the end plates.

Keywords: allograft, autograft, disc, intervertebral, transplantation

17.1 Historical Perspective

Similar to organ transplantation in other parts of the body, the concept of vertebral transplantation has been present for decades. The first reported transplantation of a functional spinal unit was in 1991.[1] The authors transplanted a fresh frozen vertebra with adjacent intervertebral discs (IVDs) into a canine model and at 18 months, the discs survived and the vertebral body was revascularized. Mobility and stability of the spinal column were maintained in this study. The same group performed a follow-up study with a fresh autograft transplantation in a canine model.[2] In contrast to previous findings, the transplanted discs had distorted morphology and metabolic function contributed by fixations that were too rigid and limited disc nutrition. Similar studies conducted by Katsuura and Hukuda,[3] and Matsuzaki et al[4] were performed on quadrupedal models but encountered the same problems with graft fixation.

Professor Keith D.K. Luk and investigators at the Department of Orthopaedics and Traumatology at the University of Hong Kong have been instrumental in experimenting with total disc transplantation. A similar idea regarding disc transplantation has been developed that also avoids too much constraint on the graft. Studies are based on Rhesus monkeys, which as bipedal animals, are closest to humans in terms of biomechanics. Series of research experiments conducted by the team were performed to verify the animal model and develop protocols in autografting, allografting, and fresh-frozen allografting. Further studies including processing and storage techniques were undertaken. A human clinical trial was conducted as well to test the efficacy and safety of this procedure. The following describes in detail each of these groundbreaking studies and also provides a glimpse of the future of disc transplantation based on current research themes and direction.

17.2 Bipedal Animal Model Experiments

17.2.1 Autografting[5]

The first autograft experiment[5] was performed at the Tangdu Hospital, Affiliated Hospital of the 4th Military Medical University, Xian, China, in collaboration with Dr. Dike Ruan. Fourteen male Rhesus monkeys were used for this study because they were most similar to humans. Osteotomies were made 1.5 mm above and below each L3–4 disc without fracturing the end plates during retrieval. The graft was replaced back into the disc space and anchored to the outer annulus with thread sutures only. The animal was allowed to freely move without any fixation. Serial X-rays were used to measure the disc height and observe for any degeneration. Gradual loss of disc height was noted postoperatively with the lowest dip at 2 months (72.9% of the control disc height) but was stabilized with some recovery to 83.5% at 12-month final follow-up. Animals were euthanized at 2, 4, 6, and 12 months after surgery and the grafted discs were taken from two monkeys for biochemical and histological testing. The native discs that were not transplanted were used as controls. Autografts were retrieved from the animals and underwent biochemical, histological, and biomechanical testing. Due to the small sample size, analysis showed no significant differences between the grafted or control discs in terms of water, proteoglycan, and hydroxyproline contents. In the annulus fibrosus (AF), there was a steady drop in water content up to 6 months postoperatively, but with slight recovery up to 12 months. Hydroxyproline content in the AF was higher in operated discs at 2 to 4 months but was similar to control at 6- and 12-month follow-up. For the nucleus pulposus (NP), water content continued to decrease in both controls and operated discs with time. Both groups also had drops in proteoglycan content at 2 to 4 months postoperatively, but there was an increase at 6 months for the operated discs. Hydroxyproline content was higher in operated discs at all follow-ups.

Viable cells were seen in both the AF and NP on histology. Similarly, these were found in the cartilaginous end plates, and there were no signs of fissuring or cracks in the AF or abnormal vascular infiltration. NF had increased cellularity as compared with controls. Under electron microscopy, notochordal cells were found in the NP but were degenerated with loss of nucleus and abnormally shrunken in size. Mobility was seen across all discs during biomechanical testing in both flexion and extension in the early postoperative period. However, increased deformation was found in the operated discs which indicated increased mobility. At 6 months, loss of mobility was noted at the operated discs.

From this bipedal animal study, it was shown that autograft disc cells are able to recover their biochemical and biomechanical function despite transient ischemia. Viable chondrocytes and notochordal cells could still be observed after transplantation in the cartilaginous end plate and NP.

17.2.2 Allograft Experiment

In a natural follow-up to the experiments on disc autografting, allogenic transplantation was required to assess its applicability clinically because living or cadaveric donors are the main sources of transplanted organs. An allograft experiment was performed by switching the L3–4 discs between two monkeys. The age and size of the monkeys were similar and the operations were conducted by two surgical teams simultaneously to attempt standardization of the operating time and blood loss. Problems of subluxation and dislocation were encountered due to graft size mismatch; thus host and recipient size matching of the grafts with press-fit insertion is important to allow for allograft stability without fixation. The issue of immunogenicity was also raised from this study. No preoperative compatibility was performed for the animals and no immunosuppressants were used in this study.

17.2.3 Fresh Frozen Allograft[6]

As a feasibility study to resolve the issues of preservation, immunocompatibility, and size mismatching, further experimentation was performed with fresh-frozen allografting. Seventeen Rhesus monkeys were used in this study. T10–L7 discs were harvested from two monkeys via osteotomies made 1 to 2 mm above and below each disc. This included a vertebra and its adjacent end plates. For storage, grafts were measured and placed in a dimethyl sulphoxide (DMSO) solution and cooled stepwise to –196°C using liquid nitrogen. Three monkeys were used as controls and the rest of the animals were graft recipients. After removing the disc from the recipient, an appropriately sized graft was thawed and was placed snug-fit into the defect. No immunosuppressant was used in these animals. Bony union of the end plates was obtained successfully without graft subluxation or dislocation. The recipient monkeys were euthanized at 2 to 8 weeks, 6 months, and 24 months for analysis. Radiological, biochemical, and biomechanical testing was performed.

Unlike the autograft experiment, the disc height decreased progressively up to 24 months of follow-up down to 64.9% of control disc height. Secondary degenerative changes with traction osteophytes (▶ Fig. 17.1) were also observed. On pathology, disc degeneration was also evident with indistinct boundaries between the AF and NP. Chronic inflammatory changes were noted early and at 6 months only at the osteotomy site indicating that lymphocyte infiltration did not reach the grafted disc, and no immunoreactivity was noted in the cartilaginous end plate. However, the growth layer of the cartilaginous end plate in all specimens showed partial or complete disappearance and electron microscopy showed nuclear disc cell degeneration with irregular nuclei, karyopyknosis, mitochondrial swelling, and cytolysis. Steady decreases in water and proteoglycan content were also observed from postimplantation 6 to 24 months. For mechanical testing, similar mobility and stability was observed for both grafted and control spinal units.

This study confirmed cryopreserved allografts could retain their cell viability and mechanical properties despite degenerative changes. In addition, minimal immunoreaction was found only at the bone interface; thus the bony end plate should be washed prior to cryopreservation. The survivability of cells after cryopreservation requires further investigation especially after the freezing and drying procedures.[7] Due to the loss of water content, cell shrinkage can damage cellular membranes and intracellular molecules. The optimal cryopreservation technique can allow maximum equilibration of water intra- and extracellularly. Refining the preservation protocol is necessary to maintain normal cellular function and delay the degeneration process. These steps are important for establishing a long-term allograft bank.

17.3 Clinical Trial[8]

With the success of the experimental studies, an ethics committee approved a small-scale clinical trial, which was initiated in 2000. One female and four male subjects received disc transplantations at the Navy General Hospital in Beijing, China. Four of the patients had cervical spondylotic myelopathy caused by single-level degenerative disc herniation, whereas one patient

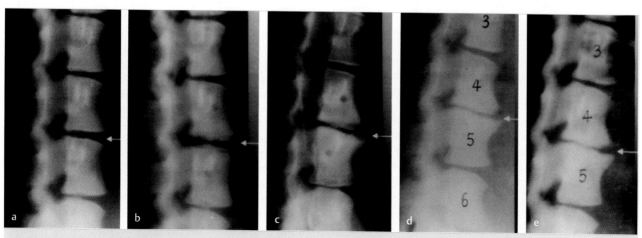

Fig. 17.1 Progressive degenerative changes noted in the allograft disc on radiographs. (a) Prior to transplantation; (b) immediately after transplantation; (c) 6-month follow-up; (d) 12-month follow-up; (e) 22 month-follow-up. (Modified with permission from Spine.[6])

had a traumatic disc herniation with incomplete paraplegia. Four patients had surgery performed on C5–6 and one on C4–5. Grafts were obtained from three previously healthy young female trauma victims within 2 hours from their death. After retrieval, the grafts were placed in a similar solution of 10% DMSO and 10% calf serum (Gibco BRL; Invitrogen, Carlsbard, CA) and were stored at –196°C with liquid nitrogen. Prior to storage, all grafts were sized and these measurements were used in the transplantation for choosing the matched graft size. Peripheral blood and bone specimens were taken and underwent microbial culture and were screened for transmissible diseases including hepatitis B and C, tuberculosis, and human immunodeficiency virus (HIV). No other immunological matching was performed.

Complete discectomy and removal of the posterior longitudinal ligament were performed for cord decompression and preparation of recipient graft bed. Intraoperative measurement of the defect translated to the allograft size chosen for transplantation. The allograft discs were thawed in a 37°C water bath for 30 minutes prior to insertion. Similar to the animal experiments, no internal fixation was required. A neck collar was used as immobilization for up to 6 weeks postoperatively. No immunosuppressing agents were used. Interval flexion-extension radiographs and magnetic resonance imaging (MRI) were performed for assessment.

No complications of graft subluxation or dislocation, or immunoreaction were encountered. One graft was malpositioned too anteriorly but underwent complete remodeling (▶ Fig. 17.2) by the 5-year follow-up. Restoration of the AF and NP was observed indicating disc viability and ability to regenerate. All patients improved with transplantation. The Japanese Orthopaedic Association (JOA) score improved by an average of at least 3 points at the last follow-up. None of the patients experienced significant neck pain and only one patient had loss of disc height upon follow-up radiographs.

Similar to the animal studies, the mean disc height dropped from 5.88 mm to 4.33 mm at 5-year follow-up. Mobility arc of 7 to 11.3 degrees was observed in all but one patient. Spontaneous fusion occurred in the remaining patient and required a revision posterior foraminotomy procedure for residual radiculopathy. The overall arc of motion was reduced compared with the preoperative investigations, and it had also shifted more toward the extension arc. This indicated a reduction in the flexion range and an increase in the extension range. This could be contributed to disc space distraction during graft insertion or over-restoration of the disc space with extension of the spinal segment. The grafts were also placed slightly anterior with a space of 1 to 3 mm posteriorly to avoid recompression of the spinal cord, which might also have contributed to the change in motion arc. On MRI (▶ Fig. 17.3), two patients retained high T2 signal at the NP showing hydrated discs despite the possible cell damage triggered by the freezing process. The remaining three patients with dark discs showed no deterioration or worsening compared with the adjacent levels. No evidence of accelerated degeneration was observed in the other levels.

A longer follow-up was recently published regarding 13 subjects with a similar procedure and an average of 6 years of follow-up.[9] This included 4 of the original subjects at 10 years of follow-up. Disc allografts were still surviving despite degeneration at 10 years and patients were able to undertake usual physiological functions. There were no significant differences in the cervical spine motion, but a mild decrease of the original T2 signal was observed.

At present, no further large-scale clinical studies are being conducted as there are identified problems and deficiencies raised from the pilot study that require further refining in the laboratory. Many projects with regards to allograft preparation, cryopreservation, and surgical technique listed here are underway with the final products yet to be launched. Despite the limitations of clinical studies, there is a novel alternative to allograft disc transplantation. A possible approach is utilizing tissue engineering principles to construct entire spinal motion segments using mesenchymal stem cells (MSCs) and collagen-based biomaterials.[10]

17.4 Storage and Preservation Experiments

17.4.1 Refining Cryopreservation Protocols

To refine the preservation and storage methods for cell survival and delay degeneration, further cryopreservation tests were conducted. The fresh-frozen process can decrease cell viability, proteoglycan, and collagen content. In a study utilizing 72 fresh canine discs, allografts prepared in –196°C liquid nitrogen had higher proteoglycan content and surviving cells than those stored at –80°C in a refrigerator.[11] Storage with liquid nitrogen was found to be most suitable for allogenic disc transplantation based on one-year follow-up results.

To retain the cellular activity and mechanical properties of the disc grafts, manipulation of different cooling rates, immersion solutions, and incubation times are needed. Cryopreservation agents (CPAs) prevent dehydration of the NP by substituting water in the cells with the CPA, thereby minimizing damage caused by the freezing process and also retaining

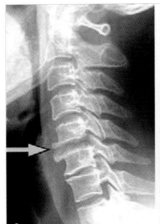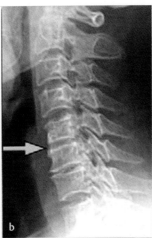

Fig. 17.2 Remodeling of the allograft disc with time. (a) Lateral view of the cervical spine showing a malpositioned C4–5 allograft immediately after surgery. (b) Lateral view of the same disc showing complete remodeling 61 months after surgery. (Modified with permission from the *Lancet*.[8])

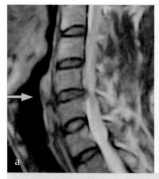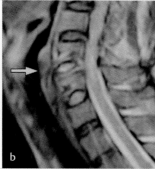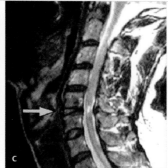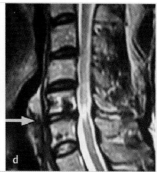

Fig. 17.3 Maintenance of magnetic resonance imaging (MRI) T2 signal with time. (a) Sagittal T2-weighted MRI preoperatively showing a C5–6 disc herniation with cord compression. (b) Sagittal T2-weighted MRI immediately after implantation showing a similar nucleus pulposus (NP) T2 signal as the adjacent C6–7 disc. (c) Sagittal T2-weighted MRI 14 months after surgery showing narrowing of the allograft disc but similar T2 signal as the adjacent C6–7 disc and more hyperintense than the other levels. (d) Sagittal T2-weighted MRI 68 months after surgery showing narrowing of disc height, but the T2 signal in the NP remains similar to C6–7 and more hyperintense than the other levels. (Modified with permission from the *Lancet*.[8])

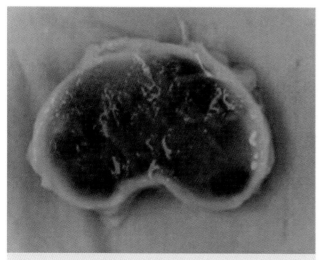

Fig. 17.4 A porcine allograft disc undergoing cryopreservation.

the ability to bind to and absorb water during thawing. A study[12] to optimize disc cell survival by modulating the rate of cooling, concentration of CPA, and duration of incubation was performed on 52 lumbar discs (L2–3 to L4–5) from 22 pigs. Porcine discs (▶ Fig. 17.4) were used in this study due to their size similarities with human discs. Three different cooling rates were tested by immersing disc samples in precooled glass containers filled with 80°C isopropanol, 4°C isopropanol, or in a 16 × 11.5 × 21 cm polystyrene box of 1.6 cm thickness. Three different CPAs were also tested, including 10% DMSO, 10% DMSO with 10% propylene glycol, and 10% DMSO with 0.1% Supercool X-1000 (21st Century Medicine; Fontana, CA). Different precooling intubation time periods between 2 and 4 hours were used. Results showed that a slow cooling rate (–0.3°C/minute), with 10% DMSO and 10% propylene glycol, and a reduced incubation time of 2 hours can improve the overall disc metabolism to 60% of fresh controls (70% of the NP and 45% of the AF).

Further analysis of CPAs and their effects on allograft biomechanical properties was performed.[13] Forty discs (L1 to L6) were harvested from nine pigs. Corneal Potassium Tes 2 solution

(CPTES2) was used as the CPA carrier solution. Different combinations including CPTES2 only, 10% DMSO in CPTES2 solution, and 10% DMSO with 10% propylene glycol in CPTES2 solution were used for testing. The discs were incubated at 4°C for 2 hours and stored after freezing to –80°C with liquid nitrogen for 4 weeks. Thawing with a 37°C saline bath was performed prior to biomechanical testing. Uniaxial compression testing and viscoelastic properties were investigated using compressive loads of up to 200 N. Results showed that cryopreserving allografts using CPAs preserves normal elastic and viscous modulus. Preservation of disc cell viability, integrity of the extracellular matrix (ECM) for water absorption, and maintenance of the intradiscal osmotic pressure was achieved.

17.4.2 Sterilization

Gamma rays are commonly used for sterilization of allograft tissues prior to transplantation. This can cause decellularization of the disc allograft and thus control degeneration by limiting cell proliferation, matrix synthesis, and metabolism.[14,15,16] The appropriate dose for disc sterilization required for disc-banking was unknown. In a study conducted on 30 beagles, spinal columns were harvested on six animals and underwent varying doses of gamma irradiation.[17] In vitro biomechanical testing of the specimens and in vivo transplantation with radiological, macroscopic, and morphological evaluation were performed. For the in vitro study, AF and NP cell viability reduced with increased irradiation dose, but the biomechanical properties did not change. For the in vivo study, X-ray and MRI showed that degeneration relates to the increased dose of irradiation. No subchondral bone or end plate cartilage damage was observed with irradiation of less than 50 kilogray (kGy), but a dose of 18 kGy resulted in significantly less disc height or range of motion loss. Results are useful clinically as gamma irradiation is usually used for tissue banks to reduce bacterial contamination.[18]

This study also presented the possible use of gamma irradiation to decellularize the disc allograft to become a natural scaffold for biological therapies as an adjustable animal model. The disc allograft may be a reliable young, nondegenerated, natural scaffold for cultured endogenous and exogenous cells to be transplanted, survive, and regenerate. However, these are only initial findings and further investigations are warranted.

17.5 Technical Papers

17.5.1 Graft Positioning

Besides optimizing preservation and storage parameters, the technical aspects of grafting was also studied in a goat model.[19] Specifically, the issue with allograft malpositioning and its effect on spine kinematics and possible early failure needed to be addressed. Three goats were disc donors, whereas 15 other goats were assigned into the control, allograft, and malpositioned allograft groups. The entire spinal column of T13 to S1 was harvested en bloc. Osteotomy was performed at the end plates 1 to 2 mm above and below the discs. For storage preparation, the grafts were washed with saline and placed in 10% DMSO and 10% calf serum for 2 hours at 4°C to preserve cellular viability. The discs were then gradually cooled at –15°C for 1 hour, –40°C for 1 hour and –80°C for another hour. The allografts were finally preserved in liquid nitrogen at –196°C until implantation.

For the recipient goats, standard surgical protocol included an L4–5 complete discectomy with preservation of the posterior longitudinal ligament. Compatibly sized disc allograft was transplanted into the disc space. A disc positioned and aligned to the anterior vertebral margin of the excised disc was considered well-aligned. Allografts were malaligned if placed too proud anteriorly by 25% of the allograft's anteroposterior length. Similar to previous experiments, only sutures were used for fixation.

At 6-month follow-up, the T11 to S1 spinal column was harvested en bloc from the euthanized goats for three dimensional (3D) kinematic experimentation. Continuous moment was applied at 0.5 degrees per second in the planes of flexion-extension, bilateral-lateral bending, and axial rotation. Five complete loading cycles were applied with the first four used for preconditioning and the fifth for analysis. Analysis showed a significant difference only in the extension moment. The well-aligned and malpositioned allograft groups both had increased extension as compared with the control group, a finding consistent with the animal experiments and clinical trial.

This study showed that IVD allograft transplantation did not compromise stability or motion even without precise positioning of the graft. The body restores its natural kinematics by remodeling the disc allograft. Despite these promising findings, the loading of quadrupedal animals is likely different from bipedal models. Thus, a goat model is not recommended for analyzing human biomechanics.

17.5.2 Biology of the Allograft

Despite the successes of preliminary allograft IVD transplantation shown by maintenance of spinal motion and stability, degeneration is still observed, manifesting as reduced disc height. To address this issue, studies on the effects of biological treatment were initiated to try to reverse or at least delay the degenerative process.

One such study involving biological treatment to the disc allograft utilized bone morphogenetic protein (BMP)-7, which has known effects on osteocyte and chondrocyte differentiation and metabolism.[20,21] BMP-7 could also stimulate collagen type II and proteoglycan synthesis.[22,23] Previous animal studies have shown that intradiscal injections of recombinant human BMP-7 (hBMP-7) could increase the disc height.[24,25] An experiment on canine cryopreserved IVDs was performed to assess whether hBMP-7 could prevent degeneration of transplanted discs.[26] Three groups of transplanted discs—one with hBMP-7, one with only NP cells, and the third without any supplementation—were observed. Although all groups had reduced disc heights at 24 weeks after implantation, MRI showed that there were delayed signs of degeneration in the hBMP-7 treated discs. In addition, more production of the ECM was observed in these discs. This study showed that despite not preventing degeneration, hBMP-7 did reduce the rate and degree of degeneration in allograft discs.

A similar canine model (▶ Fig. 17.5) was used for human telomerase reverse transcriptase (hTERT) gene-transfected NP cells.[27] Allograft discs from 18 canines were split into three groups: NP injected, NP cells with hTERT, and no treatment. Radiographic, biochemical, histological, and mechanical tests of the lumbar spines were performed at 12 weeks postoperatively. The disc height and NP T2 signal on MRI were observed to be better in both treated groups, with the hTERT group being more superior. Biomechanical stability, NP cell survival, and morphology were also better in the treated groups. This indicated that the degenerative process was reduced in the treated allografts and that hTERT-treated NP cells was superior to NP cells alone. However, this was only up to postoperative 12 weeks; hence longer follow-up studies are required to better understand this mechanism.

17.5.3 Surgical Technique in a Goat Model

Although Rhesus monkeys were used in past experiments, they have become largely unavailable and even restricted from experimentation in some countries. Creation of a quadrupedal model is thus more economical and readily accessible. Goat models are the next preferred model for IVD transplantation due to the similarities of disc geometry and structure to humans.[28,29] The cellular behaviors[30] in the disc and the biochemical and biological changes in the goat disc degeneration model are similar to humans.[31] For technical reasons, the goat is a robust animal and tolerates anesthesia well.[32]

A feasibility IVD transplantation study was conducted on a goat model (▶ Fig. 17.6).[33] From this study, the main difference found between the anatomy of goats and primates is the psoas muscle. Due to its size, a "retro-psoas" approach to the L4–5 disc required anterior elevation of the psoas by dividing its fiber attachments to the anterior surface of the transverse processes. For these preparations, at least 5 mm of vertebral body bone was preserved adjacent to the end plates and as much anterior AF and anterior longitudinal ligament were preserved as possible to avoid over-laxity of the recipient disc slot. At least 2 to 3 mm of bone must be preserved at each end to avoid fracture or dislodgement. In addition, the bony and cartilaginous end

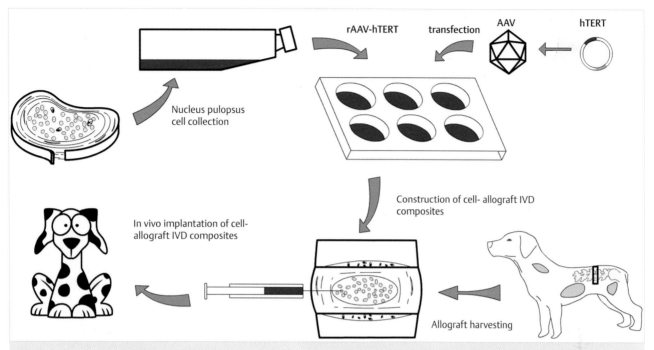

Fig. 17.5 To optimize the effect of allograft total disc transplantation and to avoid further degeneration of the allograft disc, direct injection of activated nucleus pulposus (NP) cells can be performed. This figure highlights the use of human telomerase reverse transcriptase (hTERT)-loaded NP cells in a beagle model. Abbreviations: AAV, adeno-associated virus; IVD, intervertebral disc; rAAV-hTERT, recombinant adeno-associated virus-human telomerase reverse transcriptase.

plates are important for nutrient transfer across the disc and must be included for disc survival.[34] Similar to primates, no internal fixation was required. Successes of this surgical technique allowed further disc allograft transplantation studies to be performed. However, the goat model could never be a perfect model for translation to humans due to the differences in mechanical loading between bipedal and quadrupedal models.

17.6 Future Directions

The clinical application of disc regeneration has yet to be determined. Because disc degeneration is not necessarily symptomatic in most situations, this treatment option should not be offered indiscriminately to all patients with discs that appear degenerated on MRI. The likely future of disc regeneration is as a treatment option offered to patients who experience discogenic pain, neurological problems secondary to nerve impingement by the disc, or instability of the spinal segment. Better understanding of disc degeneration pathology is necessary before disc regeneration can be implemented into our treatment armamentarium. Although the risk of revision surgery and adjacent segment degeneration is still controversial when comparing disc arthroplasty with spinal fusion, arthroplasty is a reasonable choice if motion preservation is desired. Nevertheless, disc regeneration or rejuvenation is a promising concept for disc degeneration in the young and middle aged.

The IVD complex is more than just a peripheral AF and a central NP. The cranial and caudal bony and cartilaginous end plates are important organs for nutritional transfer that must be taken into account in all regenerative strategies. The AF is also deformed and hence, rejuvenation of the NP alone cannot reverse the degenerative process. In disc degeneration, the nutritional pathways through the end plates are jeopardized. The disorganized and distorted microenvironment is not a suitable environment for introducing regenerative cells. There are already scarce nutrients available to the NP cells in a degenerated disc. Introducing more cells will only further competition for resources.[34]

An adjustable role for allograft disc transplantation is for it to take on the role of a biological scaffold. Replacing the diseased nutritional channels with viable channels can reestablish the nutrient support for the host cells or newly inserted stem cells to repopulate and rejuvenate the disc. Thus, further investigations regarding how nutrient pathways are controlled or manipulated are needed to engineer this complex structure. Imaging tools are also required to be able to capture the rate, direction, and flow of nutrients across the end plates, thereby monitoring the microenvironment in the disc allograft.

Nevertheless, successful disc transplantation has been shown in preliminary studies to restore the best mechanical and biological environment for cell survivability. Even in failure to reverse degeneration, the transplanted disc can still provide stability and mobility as evidenced by the previous trials reported here. Kinematics of the functional spinal unit after transplantation has shown that a malpositioned disc will not affect mechanical stability and motion. Furthermore, after remodeling, protection against degeneration is still provided to the adjacent segment. These results can only be applied in the experimental setting as the biomechanical effects of malpositioning have yet to be demonstrated in a human-like model.

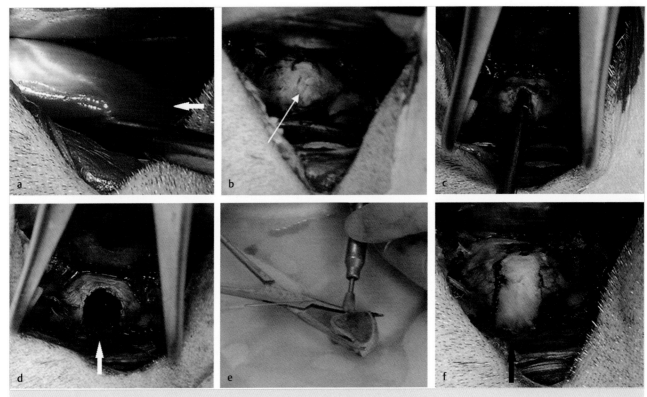

Fig. 17.6 Operative approach to the L-5 disc in a goat model (orientation of figure: left is caudal, right is cranial, top is cranial, and bottom is dorsal). **(a)** The psoas muscle (*white arrow*) is retracted to expose the L4–5 disc. **(b)** After retraction of the psoas, the L4–5 disc can be visualized (*white arrow*). **(c)** Preparation of the recipient bed is performed by removal of the posterior annulus fibrosis, nucleus pulposus, and the cartilaginous and bony end plates. **(d)** The prepared recipient bed here (*white arrow*) will be measured for selecting the correctly sized allograft. **(e)** The compatible frozen allograft is thawed and trimmed to size. **(f)** The allograft (*black arrow*) is placed snug-fit into the recipient bed. (Modified with permission from *European Spine Journal*.[33])

Although most of the studies presented here have shown good preliminary outcomes of autograft and allograft disc transplantation in humans and animals, there are still no large-scale or long-term results of this technique. Procedures including allograft preparation, cryopreservation, and surgical technique still need refining. In addition, questions on issues such as the changes in the host's pain generator and the degenerative processes of a transplanted disc are still unanswered. To take on wider clinical applications, further concerns need to be addressed. These include refining the sterilization techniques to prevent transmissible diseases and availability of suitable donors.

17.7 References

[1] Olson EJ, Hanley EN, Jr, Rudert MJ, Baratz ME. Vertebral column allografts for the treatment of segmental spine defects. An experimental investigation in dogs. Spine. 1991; 16(9):1081–1088

[2] Frick SL, Hanley EN, Jr, Meyer RA, Jr, Ramp WK, Chapman TM. Lumbar intervertebral disc transfer. A canine study. Spine. 1994; 19(16):1826–1834, discussion 1834–1835

[3] Katsuura A, Hukuda S. Experimental study of intervertebral disc allografting in the dog. Spine. 1994; 19(21):2426–2432

[4] Matsuzaki H, Wakabayashi K, Ishihara K, Ishikawa H, Ohkawa A. Allografting intervertebral discs in dogs: a possible clinical application. Spine. 1996; 21 (2):178–183

[5] Luk KD, Ruan DK, Chow DH, Leong JC. Intervertebral disc autografting in a bipedal animal model. Clin Orthop Relat Res. 1997(337):13–26

[6] Luk KD, Ruan DK, Lu DS, Fei ZQ. Fresh frozen intervertebral disc allografting in a bipedal animal model. Spine. 2003; 28(9):864–869, discussion 870

[7] Flynn J, Rudert MJ, Olson E, Baratz M, Hanley E. The effects of freezing or freeze-drying on the biomechanical properties of the canine intervertebral disc. Spine. 1990; 15(6):567–570

[8] Ruan D, He Q, Ding Y, Hou L, Li J, Luk KD. Intervertebral disc transplantation in the treatment of degenerative spine disease: a preliminary study. Lancet. 2007; 369(9566):993–999

[9] Ding Y, Ruan DK, He Q, Hou LS, Lin JN, Cui HP. Imaging Evaluation and Relative Significance in Cases of Cervical Disc Allografting: Radiographic Character Following Total Disc Transplantation. J Spinal Disord Tech. 2016 [Epub ahead of print]

[10] Chik TK, Chooi WH, Li YY, et al. Bioengineering a multicomponent spinal motion segment construct—a 3D model for complex tissue engineering. Adv Healthc Mater. 2015; 4(1):99–112

[11] Wang C, Ruan D, Zhang C, Sun H, Tsui S. Effects of storage temperatures and times on cell viability of cryopreserved intervertebral disc. [Chinese]. Chin J Spine Spinal Cord. 2011; 21:365–369

[12] Chan SC, Lam S, Leung VY, Chan D, Luk KD, Cheung KM. Minimizing cryopreservation-induced loss of disc cell activity for storage of whole intervertebral discs. Eur Cell Mater. 2010; 19:273–283

[13] Lam SK, Chan SC, Leung VY, Lu WW, Cheung KM, Luk KD. The role of cryopreservation in the biomechanical properties of the intervertebral disc. Eur Cell Mater. 2011; 22:393–402

[14] Grieb TA, Forng RY, Bogdansky S, et al. High-dose gamma irradiation for soft tissue allografts: high margin of safety with biomechanical integrity. J Orthop Res. 2006; 24(5):1011–1018

[15] Murrell W, Sanford E, Anderberg L, Cavanagh B, Mackay-Sim A. Olfactory stem cells can be induced to express chondrogenic phenotype in a rat intervertebral disc injury model. Spine J. 2009; 9(7):585–594

[16] Singh VA, Nagalingam J, Saad M, Pailoor J. Which is the best method of sterilization of tumour bone for reimplantation? A biomechanical and histopathological study. Biomed Eng Online. 2010; 9:48

[17] Ding Y, Ruan D, Luk KD, He Q, Wang C. The effect of gamma irradiation on the biological properties of intervertebral disc allografts: in vitro and in vivo studies in a beagle model. PLoS One. 2014; 9(6):e100304

[18] Gamero EC, Morales Pedraza J. The impact of the International Atomic Energy Agency (IAEA) program on radiation and tissue banking in Peru. Cell Tissue Bank. 2009; 10(2):167–171

[19] Lam SK, Xiao J, Ruan D, Ding Y, Lu WW, Luk KD. The effect of remodeling on the kinematics of the malpositioned disc allograft transplantation. Spine. 2012; 37(6):E357–E366

[20] Asahina I, Sampath TK, Hauschka PV. Human osteogenic protein-1 induces chondroblastic, osteoblastic, and/or adipocytic differentiation of clonal murine target cells. Exp Cell Res. 1996; 222(1):38–47

[21] Asahina I, Sampath TK, Nishimura I, Hauschka PV. Human osteogenic protein-1 induces both chondroblastic and osteoblastic differentiation of osteoprogenitor cells derived from newborn rat calvaria. J Cell Biol. 1993; 123 (4):921–933

[22] Chen P, Vukicevic S, Sampath TK, Luyten FP. Bovine articular chondrocytes do not undergo hypertrophy when cultured in the presence of serum and osteogenic protein-1. Biochem Biophys Res Commun. 1993; 197(3):1253–1259

[23] Flechtenmacher J, Huch K, Thonar EJ, et al. Recombinant human osteogenic protein 1 is a potent stimulator of the synthesis of cartilage proteoglycans and collagens by human articular chondrocytes. Arthritis Rheum. 1996; 39 (11):1896–1904

[24] An HS, Takegami K, Kamada H, et al. Intradiscal administration of osteogenic protein-1 increases intervertebral disc height and proteoglycan content in the nucleus pulposus in normal adolescent rabbits. Spine. 2005; 30(1):25–31, discussion 31–32

[25] Masuda K, Imai Y, Okuma M, et al. Osteogenic protein-1 injection into a degenerated disc induces the restoration of disc height and structural changes in the rabbit anular puncture model. Spine. 2006; 31(7):742–754

[26] Chaofeng W, Chao Z, Deli W, et al. Nucleus pulposus cells expressing hBMP7 can prevent the degeneration of allogenic IVD in a canine transplantation model. J Orthop Res. 2013; 31(9):1366–1373

[27] Xin H, Zhang C, Wang D, et al. Tissue-engineered allograft intervertebral disc transplantation for the treatment of degenerative disc disease: experimental study in a beagle model. Tissue Eng Part A. 2013; 19(1–2):143–151

[28] Nisolle JF, Wang XQ, Squélart M, et al. Magnetic resonance imaging (MRI) anatomy of the ovine lumbar spine. Anat Histol Embryol. 2014; 43(3):203–209

[29] Zhang Y, Drapeau S, Howard SA, Thonar EJ, Anderson DG. Transplantation of goat bone marrow stromal cells to the degenerating intervertebral disc in a goat disc injury model. Spine. 2011; 36(5):372–377

[30] Trout JJ, Buckwalter JA, Moore KC, Landas SK. Ultrastructure of the human intervertebral disc. I. Changes in notochordal cells with age. Tissue Cell. 1982; 14(2):359–369

[31] Hoogendoorn R, Doulabi BZ, Huang CL, Wuisman PI, Bank RA, Helder MN. Molecular changes in the degenerated goat intervertebral disc. Spine. 2008; 33(16):1714–1721

[32] Zhang Y, Drapeau S, An HS, Markova D, Lenart BA, Anderson DG. Histological features of the degenerating intervertebral disc in a goat disc-injury model. Spine. 2011; 36(19):1519–1527

[33] Xiao J, Huang YC, Lam SK, Luk KD. Surgical technique for lumbar intervertebral disc transplantation in a goat model. Eur Spine J. 2015; 24(9):1951–1958

[34] Huang YC, Urban JP, Luk KD. Intervertebral disc regeneration: do nutrients lead the way? Nat Rev Rheumatol. 2014; 10(9):561–566

18 What Have We Learned from Mechanical Total Disc Replacement?

Timothy T. Roberts, Colin M. Haines, and Edward C. Benzel

Abstract

This chapter reviews the major lessons derived from the collected experience with cervical and lumbar mechanical disc replacements. Lessons are in three interrelated topics: device design, patient selection, and outcome analysis. Virtually all mechanical discs share identical goals: (1) to eliminate the painful degenerative/dysplastic elements of the joint, (2) to preserve or restore the natural range of spinal motion, and (3) to mitigate stresses on adjacent spinal segments, thereby theoretically limiting adjacent segment disease. Healthy cervical, thoracic, and lumbar vertebrae move with 6 degrees of freedom (DOF), meaning they have the ability to rotate in three planes and translate in three planes. Most physiological movements require combinations of rotation and translation—motions that often occur simultaneously in multiple planes. This is referred to as *coupled motion*. The complexity of coupled spinal motion is difficult to replicate mechanically. This is one of several reasons why intervertebral disc (IVD) replacement has yet to achieve the same clinical success as total hip arthroplasty, a comparatively simple ball-and-socket joint. Mechanical disc designs, both modern and historical, vary greatly in function, material composition, and performance in vivo. Current designs range from relatively constrained (i.e., rotation only, 3 DOF) ball-and-socket prostheses to completely unconstrained elastomeric rubberlike discs that can rotate and translate freely (6 DOF). Each design has its respective advantages and disadvantages. Both clinical and laboratory experience demonstrate that highly mobile unconstrained devices can lead to facet joint overload, whereas highly constrained devices are subject to greater sheer forces that are associated with premature wear and potential failure. Although the optimal device design remains disputed, evidence shows that the careful matching of physiological and mechanical range of motion (ROM) correlates with clinical success. Mismatched motion following arthroplasty procedures is associated with worse outcomes than no motion obtained with fusion procedures. Indications for disc arthroplasty have expanded over the past 2 decades. Today, cervical disc replacements are U.S. Food and Drug Administration (FDA) approved for both one- and two-level myelopathy and/or radiculopathy. Indications for lumbar disc replacements remain comparatively narrow; although studies supporting their safety and effectiveness in both multilevel arthroplasty and arthroplasty-fusion hybrids are emerging. Successful outcomes in disc replacement are highly controversial and are dependent on a range of factors. The most concrete and widely accepted conclusion is that both cervical and lumbar disc arthroplasty can effectively reduce or eliminate preoperative pain and neurological symptoms in both short- and long-term periods. In the cervical spine, the majority of current data seem to support preservation—but not necessarily improvement—of motion at the index level. Spinal segments immediately adjacent to one- and two-level cervical disc replacements may exhibit less postoperative motion than levels adjacent to one- and two-level fusions. Motion data following lumbar disc replacement are comparatively limited and inconsistent. Several short- to mid-term studies suggest that disc arthroplasty reduces the radiographic incidence of adjacent segment deterioration (ASD) in both the cervical and lumbar spines. The degree to which this is clinically significant, however, is intensely controversial. At this time, disc replacement cannot be said to reduce symptomatic adjacent segment disease.

Keywords: degenerative disc disease, mechanical disc replacement, total disc arthroplasty, total disc replacementpinal biomechanics

18.1 Introduction

In its relatively brief history, intervertebral total disc arthroplasty (TDA) has undergone considerable evolution. From its origin as an interpositional ball-bearing spacer to the latest in elastomeric hybrid designs, successes and failures of a diversity of devices continue to direct us toward the so-called Holy Grail of spine surgery: motion preservation in the absence of discomfort and dysfunction.

This chapter reviews the major lessons derived from the collected experience with cervical and lumbar mechanical disc replacements. Lessons are divided into three interrelated topics: device design, patient selection, and outcome analysis. With device design, we review the basics of healthy spinal motion, the biomechanics of various disc designs, and the successes and failures of several notable devices. With patient selection, we review the evolving indications and contraindications for disc arthroplasty, as well as the factors that influence operative successes and failures. Finally, with outcomes, we discuss the short- and long-term effects on symptoms, motion, and adjacent segment degeneration (ASD), and we compare the efficacy of disc arthroplasty with the alternative gold standard, intervertebral fusion.

Despite the considerable range of arthroplasty designs, virtually all mechanical discs share identical goals: (1) to eliminate the painful degenerative/dysplastic elements of the joint, (2) to preserve or restore, to one degree or another, the natural range of spinal motion, and (3) to mitigate stresses on adjacent spinal segments, thereby theoretically limiting ASD.

Total hip replacement is arguably the most successful mechanical arthroplasty procedure performed today. By effectively eliminating the diseased elements of the joint, restoring near-perfect natural joint motion, and relieving stresses on its respective adjacent joints, hip replacements have achieved remarkable success and popularity throughout the world. By many measures, intervertebral disc (IVD) replacement has yet to duplicate the success of hip, knee, and shoulder arthroplasty. The comparatively complex and interrelated motions of the spine make it more difficult to mechanically replicate than the ball-and-socket design of total hip replacement.[1] To an extent, the historical successes and failures of several designs are attributable to an ability and inability to accurately reproduce these natural motions.

18.2 Device Designs

18.2.1 Normal Spine Biomechanics

A basic comprehension of the anatomy and physiology of the IVD is essential to understanding prosthetic disc designs. In the healthy adult spine, the nucleus pulposis (NP) behaves as a gelatinous cushion that resists and transfers compressive forces to the end plates and encompassing annulus. The annulus, by contrast, resists tensile, torsional, and radial forces. Posteriorly, two facet joints govern motion and protect the neural elements. Historically, facet joints are often overlooked as a source of pain and dysfunction. However, isolated facet degeneration may account for up to 20% of all axial back pain.[2]

The *functional spinal unit* (FSU) is a term for the collective motion between two vertebrae. Normal FSU function requires 6 degrees of freedom (DOF): the ability to rotate in three planes (flexion-extension/axial turning/lateral bending) as well as the ability to translate or slide in three planes (sagittal displacement [antero- and retrolisthesis], coronal or lateral displacement, and compression/distraction) (▶ Fig. 18.1). The healthy IVD exhibits all six motions and is thereby termed *unconstrained*. By contrast, the ball-and-socket hip joint is constrained to 3 DOF (flexion/extension, adduction/abduction, and internal/external rotation); a finger interphalangeal joint is highly constrained to 1 DOF (flexion/extension).

Virtually all physiological spinal motions require simultaneous rotatory and translational movement. This means that the center of rotation for any given motion is not a fixed point but one that moves along an axis. When the spine is flexed, the rostral vertebral body translates anteriorly, whereas the NP is displaced posteriorly. The rostral body thus rotates in the sagittal plane around a dynamic fulcrum that shifts posteriorly with the NP. When the spine extends, the rostral vertebral body translates posteriorly, whereas the NP moves anteriorly. These dynamic or instantaneous centers of rotation (ICOR) vary

greatly and depend on the level, plane, direction, and forces associated with motion.[3] During sagittal and coronal plane motions in the cervical spine, for example, the axis of rotation is generally located in the anterior portion of the subjacent vertebral body. During axial rotation, however, it shifts closer to the posterior annulus.[3] With lateral bending of the cervical and lumbar spine, the ICOR shifts to the convexity of motion, that is, leaning to the left rotates the rostral vertebrae around a point on the right side of the disc. During flexion and extension in the lumbar spine, ICORs for L2 through L5 are fairly consistently located around the posterior one third of the disc space, just below the superior end plate of the inferior vertebrae. The ICOR of L5–S1 is more variable but is often located in the posterior one third of the disc halfway between the end plates (▶ Fig. 18.2).[4] Degenerative processes can dramatically alter spinal kinematics in ways that are both difficult to analyze and predict.[3]

To further complicate matters, many motions in the spine are coupled, meaning that for an intended primary motion in one plane, simultaneous motion will occur in another. Coupled motion is perhaps most evident with lateral bending in the cervical and lumbar spines. Laterally bending one's head to the left, for example, is accompanied by ipsilateral vertebral body rotation. The swiveled spinous processes are then palpable to the right of the midline. Bending one's torso to the side, however, couples lumbar lateral bending with *contralateral* vertebral rotation: Laterally bending the torso to the left rotates the vertebral bodies to the right—the spinous processes are then usually palpable to the left of the midline.[3] Virtually all motions of the lumbar spine are coupled. These complex kinematic relationships vary significantly with spinal level, posture, and the presence of joint degeneration or pathologies such as scoliosis.

Coupled motion is guided primarily by the orientation and morphology of the facet joints. Isolated facet degeneration has been shown to alter motion of the FSU.[5] Additionally, the annulus fibers, the anterior and posterior spinal ligaments, the ligamentum flavum, and to a lesser extent the remaining surrounding soft tissues play a role in guiding and restraining motion. The uncovertebral joints of the cervical spine may also guide motion; however, their exact role is disputed.[5]

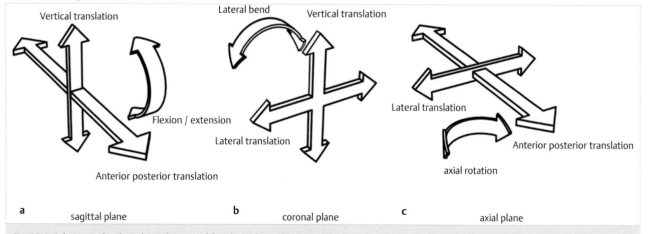

Fig. 18.1 Schematic detailing the 6 degrees of freedom of spinal motion. Each **(a)** sagittal, **(b)** coronal, and **(c)** axial plane has its own rotational and translational motion. Spinal motions are usually coupled, meaning an intended translational or rotational motion along one axis is accompanied by motion in a second axis.

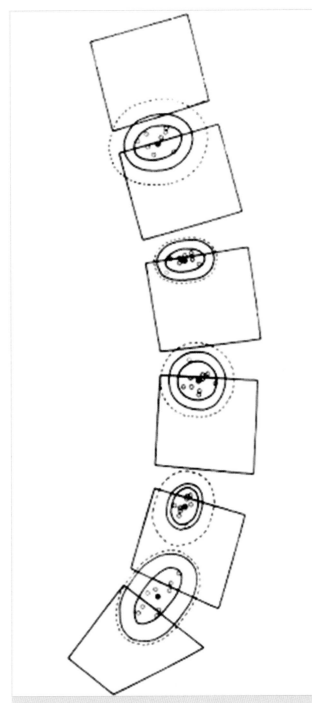

Fig. 18.2 Average instantaneous centers of rotation (ICOR) for flexion/extension in the lumbar spine. ICORs for L2–5 are fairly consistently located around the posterior one third of the disc space, just below the superior end plate of the inferior vertebrae. The ICOR of L5–S1 is more variable but is often located in the posterior one third of the disc halfway between end plates.

Comprehending the basics of spinal motion is essential for the appropriate utilization of prostheses in clinical practice. It is also important from a surgically technical standpoint, as motion restoration requires both appropriate design selection as well as positioning of prostheses. Surgically mismatched motion is

associated with worse outcomes than no motion at all (fusion).[5] Poorly positioned prostheses accelerate degeneration at the index-level facets by up to 2.5 times, as well as at adjacent segments.[5,6] Pars and pedicle stress fractures have also been associated with implant malpositioning.[5] In the lumbar spine, positioning of Mobidisc (LDR Medical, Warsaw, IN) prostheses within 5 mm of individual patients' natural COR were associated with significantly greater improvements in symptoms than those positioned farther than 5 mm from CORs as determined by preoperative flexion/extension radiographs.[6] This finding is supported by in vitro models in which 5-mm anterior or posterior malpositioning of the disc resulted in marked changes to posterior muscular tension as well as forces across the facets and other supporting ligaments.[7]

The coupled and interdependent motions of the FSU are deceptively difficult to replicate mechanically. Further, implantable devices must be sturdy, biocompatible, and durable enough to withstand decades of continuous use. Next, we explore several key prosthetic designs, both historical and modern, and examine the degree to which they foster physiological motion, eliminate pathology, and remain functional in vivo.

18.2.2 Noteworthy Mechanical Disc Designs

One-piece Prostheses

The first human disc replacement was performed by Fernström in the late 1950s. His device consisted of a single stainless-steel ball bearing, which he inserted into diseased lumbar disc spaces.[8] The 10- to 16-mm diameter sphere allowed the superior vertebrae to rotate with 3 DOF, but it did not effectively permit translation. The bearings acted as spacers, allowing indirect decompression of the neural elements, opening of the neural foramen, and appropriate tensioning of the paraspinous musculature.[5]

Fernström's initial success was short lived. In vivo, the steel bearings transferred extreme contact stresses onto adjacent end plates. Many implants failed due to subsidence of the stiff steel into the comparatively soft vertebral bodies. Fernström bearings also resulted in hypermobility at the index level as the devices lacked internal restraints to motion.[9] These early failures emphasized the importance of broader and equal force distribution between vertebrae and were early indicators that supraphysiological ROMs were detrimental.

Over the following decades, researchers investigated a variety of silicon, rubber, and other polymeric-based designs. These devices feature elastic cores that might reproduce the natural cushioning effects of the disc, thereby theoretically preventing subsidence. Several designs claimed to replicate the true 6 DOF of the natural disc. The AcroFlex disc (DePuy-AcroMed; Raynham, MA) consisted of a polyalkene rubber cylinder capped with two titanium end plates. Emerging in the 1980s, it was the first major commercial one-piece or self-contained implant. Its elastic body added 3 degrees of translation to the 3 rotational DOF afforded by ball-bearing or ball-and-socket designs. Although laboratory performance of the AcroFlex was impressive, the few early discs that were implanted garnered lackluster results. Possible carcinogenic properties of the vulcanized rubber led to its withdrawal from the market.[9] Further, Computed tomography (CT) scans at 1- to 2-year follow-up demonstrated premature development of defects in several of the polyalkene rubber cores.[9]

Fixed-bearing Prostheses

Perhaps the simplest variation on Fernström's steel-bearing, ball-and-socket devices pair two metallic end plates with concave and convex hemispherical bearings of various materials (metal-on-metal [MOM], metal-on-polyethylene [MOP], etc.). One of the earliest examples of this design, the ProDisc (Synthes Spine; West Chester, PA), was introduced in Europe in the 1990s. The ProDisc was the first widely used ball-and-socket implant for both the lumbar and cervical spine. It featured 3 degrees of constrained rotational motion (3 DOF). Two large-footprint cobalt-chromium-molybdenum (CoCrMo) plates at each bony interface dispersed axial and sheer loads, mitigating risk of subsidence. Modern versions of the ProDisc feature metal-alloy plates with extensive porous backside-coating to promote bony ongrowth.[10] On the articular side, the superior, concave partial-spherical cup is highly polished CoCrMo that contacts an ultra-high molecular weight polyethylene (UHMWP) partial-spherical convex post.

The major drawback to pure ball-and-socket devices are that their constrained design does not permit translational motion. These 3-DOF devices cannot fully replicate natural coupled spinal motions. In situations where the ICOR is small, such as with the L2–3 and L3–4 IVDs, both the adjacent soft tissues and facets may experience the same excursion and forces with TDA as would the normal spine.[11] However, in segments with larger ICORs, ball-and-socket implants must resist translational motions or catastrophic dislocation (at either the bone–implant or the implant articular interface) will occur. Even in the absence of catastrophic dislocation, large ICORs generate sheer forces at the bone–implant interface that may lead to gradual implant loosening. Further, repetitive and simultaneous axial and sheer forces generate high contact pressures across the artificial articulation, leading to accelerated wear. As discussed, potential for early failure is exacerbated when implants are malpositioned.[12]

Over 15,000 ProDisc devices have been implanted worldwide since 1990 with generally positive results.[10] Short-term clinical success has been reported in more than 90% of patients at an average of 1-year follow-up without major complications.[13] Five-year follow-up from large, randomized control trials (RCTs) of ProDisc-L versus arthrodesis demonstrated that the implant was no less efficacious than circumferential (combined antero-posterior [AP]) fusion in the mid-term.[14] In the United States,

the ProDisc-L received FDA approval in 2006 for implantation in single-level degenerative disc disease (DDD) from L3 to S1.[15]

Another early ball-and-socket design, the Cummins-Bristol disc, utilized two metal-on-metal articulating stainless-steel plates that were anteriorly fixed to each vertebral body with a single AP screw.[16] Early complications involved screw breakage, implant migration, and frequent reports of dysphagia that were attributed to the relatively thick anterior profile of the initial design. Several iterations later, the device was rebranded with a slimmer anterior profile and endowed with multiple points of locking-screw fixation. More significantly, the inferior hemispherical "cup" articulation was elongated to a "trough," thereby introducing a groove in which the superior convex "ball" can translate in sagittal plane.[16] This 4-DOF device was renamed Prestige (Medtronic; Memphis, TN) and has changed relatively little since its redesign. The Prestige is currently approved by the U.S. FDA for investigational device exemption (IDE) use in the cervical spine.

Dual-bearing Prostheses

Dual-bearing TDAs, such as the Charité III (DePuy-AcroMed), feature variations on a mobile biconvex core that is interposed between two concave plates. The prosthesis is essentially two ball-and-socket joints that face one another and share an oblate spheroid-shaped core. Working together, the two rotational joints function in equal but opposite motions to allow the superior plate to translate a small distance. Anterior translation, for example, is achieved with rotational flexion at the inferior bearing and rotational extension at the superior bearing (▶ Fig. 18.3). Several dual-bearing TDAs allow translational motion in the sagittal and coronal planes and therefore possess 5 DOF. To an extent, they can tolerate larger ICORs than fixed-bearing devices.

The relatively unconstrained motion of dual-bearing TDAs is theorized to promote natural motion of the FSU and thus mitigate sheer stresses associated with single-bearing ball-and-socket implants. Recent evidence suggests, however, that motion is not as symmetric or fluid as theorized. In a notable cadaver motion study, the superior bearing was found to undergo more than twice the excursion of the inferior bearing.[12] This correlates with findings from in vivo retrieval studies of Charité implants in which superior bearing surfaces were disproportionately worn.[12] For equal wear to occur, the ICOR must theoretically reside within the center of the biconvex core. Because the natural ICOR for lumbar flexion/extension is

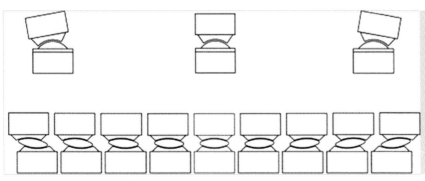

Fig. 18.3 A single-bearing ball-and-socket joint **(top)** exhibiting rotation in a single plane. Ball-and-socket bearings exhibit 3 degrees of freedom (DOF), meaning they can rotate in the coronal, sagittal, and axial planes, but cannot translate. By contrast, this dual-bearing joint **(bottom)** consisting of opposing ball-and-socket joints, can perform biplanar translational motion in addition to rotation with 3 DOF.

typically located in the inferior and posterior aspect of the subjacent lumbar body—a point substantially closer to the rotational center of the superior prosthetic bearing than the inferior—it is reasoned that the superior bearing experiences less resistance and therefore more motion.

Another drawback to early dual-bearing designs is that they lack internal restraint to extremes of motion that would normally be governed by the annulus. Without internal restraint, the facet's joints must serve as the primary restraints to excess translation, resulting in facet loads up to 2.5 times greater those seen in healthy FSUs.[13] Early dual-bearing designs have been associated with failures due to disproportionate rates of facet-generated pain.

In data derived from one FDA noninferiority RCT comparing the Charité (dual-bearing), Kineflex (ball-and-socket; Spinal-Motion, Sunnyvale, CA), and Maverick (ball-and-socket; Metronic Sofamor Danek, Memphis, TN) the authors found the number-one cause of clinical failure at 24 months was facet pain identified through diagnostic injections. Although all prostheses experienced multiple causes of failure, 23% of failures in the Charité group were due to facet pain versus 8.6% and 8% in the single-bearing Kineflex and Maverick groups, respectively.[17] This clinically relevant finding is supported by cadaveric studies in which implantation of L5–S1 Charité dual-bearing discs resulted in greater facet forces, particularly during lateral bending. Its contender, the ball-and-socket ProDisc, alternatively resulted in greater variations in pre- versus postimplantation ICOR.[18]

The Charité III was the first lumbar TDA approved in the United States in 2004, and is the most extensively implanted and studied artificial disc over the past 20 years.[12] It was approved for single-level implantation for degenerative lumbar disc disease.[15] Over 5,000 have been implanted worldwide.

Hybrid Designs

The Bryan disc (Medtronic Sofamor Danek) is a more recent variation on the one-piece elastomeric design. The Bryan disc consists of a saline-bathed polyurethane central disc surrounded by two titanium end plates. The saline solution is purported to both lubricate articulating surfaces, as well as to provide a hydraulic dampening effect.[19] Inside its unibody enclosure, however, the design may share more in common with the dual-bearing Charité. Like the Charité, the Bryan disc is a self-contained dual-bearing device that can both rotate and translate. Compared with polyethylene, the elastic and shock-absorbent polyurethane core may tolerate compressive motion, albeit on a miniscule scale. Some argue, therefore, that the Bryan disc features 6 DOF. The second difference from conventional dual-bearing designs is that the Bryan's internal posts (and potentially outer sheath) provide internal restraint to extremes of motion. This may decrease or eliminate detrimental stresses on the posterior facets. However, the benefits have yet to be clearly demonstrated at the clinical level.

▶ Table 18.1 and ▶ Table 18.2 summarize several device designs for the cervical and lumbar spine, respectively. Select examples of historical and current models are shown in addition to detailing of their respective design parameters, material compositions, and notable advantages and disadvantages.

18.2.3 Bearing Surfaces and Material Selection

In addition to mechanical design, material composition, especially at the bearing surface, is an important factor in functionality and longevity. The two predominant types of bearing surfaces available today are MOM ("hard-on-hard") bearings and MOP ("hard-on-soft") bearings. Both have their respective strengths and weaknesses. Neither has been shown to be clearly superior. Much of the controversy stems from a lack of long-term and high-quality clinical evidence. As such, much of what has been applied to disc prosthetic design has been derived from comparatively robust studies of hip arthroplasty. Polyethylene cross-linking and sterilization processing are two such borrowed concepts.

Hard-on-hard Bearings

Hard-on-hard bearings refer to a variety of metal, ceramic, or composite articulating surfaces. Most commonly, the term refers to identical MOM prostheses such as the CoCrMo-on-CoCrMo found in the Maverick and ProDisc-C for the cervical spine. The foremost advantage of MOM joints is that they generate markedly lower volumes of wear debris than hard-on-soft or MOP bearings. However, MOM bearings generate soluble metal ions that can distribute throughout the joint pseudocapsule, into local soft tissues, and disseminate systemically. Use of MOM bearings in hip arthroplasty is a major source of controversy. MOM hip prostheses have been associated with elevated serum metal ion levels, delayed hypersensitivity immune reactions to metals, localized pseudotumor formation, organ toxicity, and even carcinogenesis. The long-term clinical significance of MOM debris in hip arthroplasty, however, is extremely unclear. Lesser yet is known about MOM debris in spinal prostheses. Bisseling et al studied metal ions in lumbar discs and found serum ions to be considerably lower than those of MOM hip replacements.[20] The authors expressed a low clinical concern for the potential harm of MOM-related wear in spine arthroplasty. Conversely, others have found cobalt and chromium ion levels at 36 months rival those seen in hip replacement.[21] The extent to which intervertebral MOM prostheses generate wear and the extent to which it is clinically significant remains disputed.

What is considerably more clear is that MOM bearings of identical CoCrMo alloys generate less volumetric wear than previously utilized titanium alloys.[22] Titanium bearing surfaces are seldom used in modern arthroplasty due to inferior wear resistance.[23] Titanium alloys, however, are still appropriate for nonbearing surfaces such as back plates and screws and may actually be superior to harder metals for bone-to-implant load transfers.[24] At this time, the majority of MOM implants available utilize CoCr or CoCrMo alloys.

Ceramics are inorganic, nonmetallic solids that possess many desirable features for arthroplasty, including extreme hardness and toughness beyond that of conventional metals, superior smoothness and resistance to wear, and biocompatibility.[23] The extreme hardness of the materials, however, can make them brittle and prone to fracture. Ceramics are also comparatively expensive. They have achieved moderate success in hip arthroplasty, but widespread adoption has been limited due to their

Table 18.1 Characteristics and composition of select cervical disc designs

Bearing(s)	Joint design	DOF	Example	Material	Bearing surface	Notes
Single bearing	Ball-and-socket	3 rotational	ProDisc-C (Synthes Spine)	CoCrMo plates with polyethylene convex articulation	Metal-on-polyethylene	Internal restraint, may protect facets; cannot translate, may be inappropriate for segments with larger ICORs
	Ball-and-socket	3 rotational	PCM (NuVasive)	CoCr plates with polyethylene	Metal-on-polyethylene	As above
	Ball-and-trough	4 (3 rotational, 1 AP translational)	Prestige ST/LP (Medtronic)	ST: stainless steel LP: titanium-ceramic alloy	ST: metal-on-metal LP: ceramic-on-ceramic	Minimal internal restraint to AP translation
Dual bearing	Dual ball-and-socket	5 (3 rotational, 2 AP + lateral translational)	Kineflex C (Spinal Motion)	CoCrMo plates with CoCrMo core	Metal-on-metal × 2	Lacks internal restraint
	Ball-and-socket atop keel-and-trough	4 (3 rotational, 1 AP translational)	Secure C (Globus Medical)	CoCr with polyethylene core	Metal-on-polyethylene core × 2	Moderate internal restraint to AP translation
	Ball-and-socket atop flat sliding bearing	5 (3 rotational + 2 AP + lateral translational)	Mobi-C[b] (LDR Medical)	CoCrMo plates with polyethylene core	Metal-on-polyethylene × 2	Baseplate pegs provide internal restraint to translation
One-piece	Self-contained dual ball-and-socket	5–6[a] (3 rotational, 3 AP + lateral ± axial translational)	Bryan (Medtronic Sofamor Danek)	Titanium concave shells with donut-shaped polyurethane core, contained by wires	Metal-on-polyurethane in saline solution × 2	Wires/peg provide internal restraint; relatively good shock absorption

Abbreviations: AP, anteroposterior; CoCrMo, cobalt-chromium-molybdenum; DOF, degrees of freedom; ICOR, instantaneous center of rotation.

[a]Relative elasticity of polyurethane allows modest compression, therefore arguably 6 DOF.

[b]Currently only U.S. FDA–approved disc for use at both 1 and 2 levels.

high costs, marginal benefits, and association with other undesirable effects such as a tendency in some situations to squeak.[25] In 2014, the FDA approved the Prestige LP Disc (Medtronic), a dual-bearing (4 DOF) cervical prosthesis that utilizes a proprietary titanium-ceramic composite ball-and-trough bearing. Advocates claim superior wear properties over stainless steel and argue that the titanium ceramic has the added benefit of producing less scatter on postoperative magnetic resonance imaging (MRI).[26]

Hard-on-soft Bearings

Hard-on-soft bearings comprise a metal, ceramic, or composite material that articulates with a comparatively soft plastic polymer, usually polyethylene or polyurethane. Under normal circumstances, the softer plastic will not wear down the metal; however, the inverse is not true. Markedly greater particulate volumes of polyethylene are generated per cycle compared with MOM bearings.[23] The clear benefits of hard-on-soft bearings are their low friction properties, proven track record, and lack of associated systemic toxicity.[23]

Whereas system reactions to polyethylene debris are less concerning than systemic exposure to ionic metal debris, local polyethylene wear has drawbacks of its own. In hip and knee arthroplasty, particulate wear is associated with macrophage-mediated osteolysis. Microscopic plastic particles induce inflammatory changes leading to bone resorption and potentially loosening or fracture. The extent to which this occurs in spine arthroplasty is debated; some authors contest that this may be secondary to the local environment, which is devoid of synovial membrane that can produce a macrophage cytokine response.[27] Others state lower joint reactive forces and ranges of spinal motion do not generate enough particular debris to incite significant macrophage response.[23] Various case reports contest that catastrophic wear in unfavorable environments such as subsidence, migration, under-sizing, and adjacent fusion has been associated with osteolysis.[28] High-quality data supporting or opposing use of hard-on-soft bearings in spinal prostheses are currently unavailable.

Many of the material choices for IVD replacement are guided by comparatively well-studied experiences with total hip arthroplasty. Borrowed innovations include the adoption of highly cross-linked polyethylene (HCL) over standard ultra-high molecular weight polyethylene. In HCL polyethylene, gamma radiation is used to break long individual hydrocarbon chains of the plastic and induce cross-links between filaments. This process increases the crystallinity of the plastic, thereby decreasing its propensity to creep (the slow deformation of a loaded material over time) and increasing its resistance to wear. Another borrowed innovation is irradiation sterilization in an oxygen-

Table 18.2 Characteristics and composition of select lumbar disc designs

Bearing(s)	Joint design	DOF	Example	Material	Bearing surface	Notes
Single bearing	Ball-and-socket	3 rotational	ProDisc-L (Synthes Spine)	CoCr plates with convex polyethylene bearing fixed to caudal plate	Metal-on-polyethylene	Internal restraint, may protect facets; cannot translate, may be inappropriate for segments with larger ICORs
	Ball-and-socket	3 rotational	Maverick (Medtronic Sofamor Danek)	CoCr plates (female cranial, male caudal)	Metal-on-metal	As above
Dual bearing	Dual ball-and-socket	5 (3 rotational, 2 AP + lateral translational)	Charité III (DePuy-Spine)	CoCrMo plates with mobile polyethylene core	Metal-on-polyethylene × 2	Lacks internal restraint
	Dual ball-and-socket	5 (3 rotational, 2 AP + lateral translational)	Kineflex (Spinal Motion)	CoCrMo plates backed with titanium for bony ingrowth, CoCrMo mobile core	Metal-on-metal × 2	Lacks internal restraint
	Ball-and-socket atop flat AP-sliding bearing	4 (3 rotational, 1 AP translational)	activL (Aesculap Implant Systems)	CoCr plates with a titanium back-coating and polyethylene core	Metal-on-polyethylene × 2	Features internal restraint to excess AP translation
One-piece	Self-contained rubber polymer	6 (3 rotational, 3 translational)	AcroFlex (DePuy-AcroMed)	Titanium plates attached to polyalkene rubber cylindrical core	n/a	Historical design, withdrawn from market due to premature polyalkene failure and concern for carcinogenic potential
	Single-piece internally restrained ball-and-socket	3 rotational	FlexiCore (Stryker Spine)	CoCr plates	Metal-on-metal	Features internal restraint to excess axial rotation that may relieve facets

Abbreviations: AP, anteroposterior; CoCrMo, cobalt-chromium-molybdenum; DOF, degrees of freedom; ICOR, instantaneous center of rotation.

free environment. The absence of oxygen decreases free radical formation and dramatically improves wear resistance of the polyethylene. Abundance of oxidizing free radicals within plastics is associated with early catastrophic failures. Measures to decrease their propagation, such as the addition of antioxidants such as vitamin E to polyethylene components, are currently emerging.[23]

Limited evidence from a variety of retrieval studies suggests that MOP dual mobile bearing prostheses within the lumbar spine may be more susceptible to wear-related failures than those of the cervical spine. By contrast, fixed or ball-and-socket bearing MOP designs had similarly inferior outcomes in the cervical spine.[29] It must be noted that the in vivo data regarding catastrophic wear are based almost exclusively on small case series or individual studies. A second caveat is that some of this evidence predates several of the modern cross-linking and sterilization processes that have dramatically improved the longevity of polyethylene components. If polyethylene wear is truly accelerated by mobile bearings in the lumbar spine and by fixed bearings in the cervical spine, the phenomenon might be explained by the differences in lumbar versus cervical bearing

sizes, joint reactive forces, local kinematics, and a host of other patient- and design-specific factors. Long-term data are needed before concrete conclusions can be drawn.

18.2.4 Current Designs

Based on lessons dating back to Fernström's bearings, virtually all current disc designs have relatively large footprints with ingrowth or ongrowth surfaces. Fixation at bone–implant interfaces is often bolstered with keels or screws to increase resistance to shear forces. Reports of subsidence in modern implants has been reduced to 0 to 5%.[30]

Debate continues over the superiority of constrained ball-and-socket designs versus unconstrained dual-bearing designs. At this time, variations on both "philosophies" are available for implantation in the cervical spine. Indeed, the optimal selection for disc design may vary on the patient and spinal region. Equally disputed is the superiority of particular combinations of bearing surfaces.

It should be noted that none of the devices currently available can fully replicate all motions of the native healthy disc. It is possible that newer elastomeric- or hydrogel-based compounds —possessing 6 DOF, self-restraint to extremes of motion, and superior longevity and biocompatibility—will constitute the future of disc arthroplasty.

18.3 Patient Selection

18.3.1 Indications

Perhaps more apparent in disc arthroplasty than many other disciplines, patient selection is essential to success. At this time, the FDA-approved indications for cervical disc replacement are mechanically stable degenerative disease at one or two adjacent levels between C3 and C7. Lumbar disc replacement is an alternative to anterior, posterior, or 360-degree fusion for axial pain in a patient with stable single-level DDD.[5] The ideal cervical candidate is one with intractable radicular pain, single-level herniation, and minimal spondylosis. The ideal lumbar candidate must be highly motivated, psychologically stable, with single-level disc disease between L3 and S1 and intact facet joints.[5]

18.3.2 Expanding Indications

In Europe, where surgeons have had more experience with TDA devices, lumbar indications have expanded to include recurrent disc herniation, mild spinal stenosis, and multiple level DDD. The United States has been comparatively measured in its acceptance and approval of the technology; however, stateside indications are expanding. Most recently, the FDA has broadened indications to include two-level adjacent arthroplasty for the Mobi-C (LDR Medical) in the cervical spine. Proponents of multiple-level disc replacements have long since argued that the motion-sparing benefits of arthroplasty are augmented over multiple levels and that multiple-level replacements are together safe and efficacious.[31,32,33] A recent meta-analysis of multiple-level cervical TDA versus single-level cervical TDA found no significant differences in Neck Disability Index (NDI) scores, neck and arm Visual Analog Scale (VAS) scores, reoperation rates, heterotopic ossification (HO) rates, and various parameters of qualities of life between the groups.[34]

Currently, U.S. FDA IDE approval for lumbar replacements are restricted to single-level disease. However, there is growing evidence to support the safe and efficacious use of adjacent two-level lumbar disc arthroplasty. In a study of two-level ProDisc-L in the lumbar spine, investigators demonstrated sustained clinical success and patient satisfaction throughout an average of 9.6 years of follow-up. In the modest 13-patient series, Oswestry Disability Index (ODI) and subjective satisfaction scores remained stable from postoperative baseline at almost 10 years postoperative.[35]

An alternative solution for multisegmental pathologies are hybrid arthroplasty-fusions. Various reports detail the clinical successes of adjacent interbody fusions and TDA in both the lumbar and cervical spines. Authors of a recent RCT comparing adjacent anterior lumbar interbody fusion (ALIF) and lumbar TDA with two-level circumferential fusions (transforaminal lumbar interbody fusions [TLIFs] with posterolateral fusion) found superior outcomes in the hybrid group at three years. Patients receiving hybrid constructs experienced greater postoperative improvements in VAS scores as well as significantly

greater improvements in lordotic alignment. Overall complications were low and did not significantly differ between groups.[36] Hybrid constructs have also been reported in the cervical spine. A meta-analysis of seven clinical studies demonstrated improvements in various validated functional scores from preoperative baseline, as well as appropriate segmental motion at the TDA and successful fusion at respective levels. Complications were rare, and despite the low quality of evidence available, the authors conclude that hybrid cervical constructs may be a safe and efficacious solution to multilevel DDD.[37]

18.3.3 Contraindications

Absolute contraindications to surgery include local or systemic infection, certain metal allergies, major deformity or ligamentous instability, tumor, severe facet arthropathy, and severe neuromuscular conditions. Relative contraindications are disparate and comprise at least 50 different entities published throughout the literature.[38] Circa mid-2000s, commonly cited contraindications include facet arthrosis, central spinal stenosis, lateral recess stenosis, spondylolysis, spondylolisthesis, herniated NP with radiculopathy, scoliosis, osteoporosis, pseudoarthrosis, and deficient posterior elements. As many authors have argued, these and other published lists at the time were both vague and highly exclusive contraindications that precluded TDA for many patients that may well have benefitted from them. As our experience and comfort with TDA has gradually developed, restrictions on their use are slowly loosening.

Moderate-to-severe DDD with significant loss in disc space height (DSH) was historically considered a strong contraindication to TDA. Recent evidence, however, suggests that TDA is effective for all stages of DDD, assuming absence of coinciding facet arthroplasty and an absence of solid intervertebral autofusion. In a long-term prospective study of TDA for lumbar DDD, authors found no correlation between the preoperative degree of DDD and clinical outcomes at up to 50 months postoperative. Interestingly, authors did notice significant improvement in early postoperative VAS scores in patients with higher grades of histological disc degeneration.[39] Whereas diminished DSH in severe DDD may no longer constitute absolute contraindication for TDA, the same study group reports that decreased DSH and limited postoperative segmental ROM are associated with significant decreases in postoperative ROM, especially at the lumbosacral junction. Patient satisfaction, however, was highest in patients with the most severe loss of preoperative DSH.[40]

Disc herniation with radiculopathy and central stenosis was once considered a contraindication for TDA; however, the literature clearly supports its efficacy in the cervical spine for both myelopathy and radiculopathy (see outcomes below). TDA for the relief of single-level radiculopathy or myelopathy is at least equivalent to the gold standard, anterior cervical discectomy and fusion (ACDF), if not superior in several respects (discussed in detail below).[41] A recent systematic review found no differences between outcomes in patients receiving cervical TDA for myelopathy versus radiculopathy.[42] Advanced age is another archaic contraindication[38] that has not been demonstrated to negatively affect outcomes.[42] Alternatively smoking or tobacco use has not been historically cited as a contraindication to surgery. Recent evidence, however, demonstrates NDI outcomes for smokers up to 2 years following cervical TDA.[42]

18.4 Clincal Outcomes

Judging successful outcomes in disc replacement is arguably more difficult than judging fusion procedures alone. In addition to evaluating postoperative pain and neurological symptoms, researchers must quantify motion at index levels, adjacent levels, and overall cervical or lumbar regions. Additionally, researchers have attempted to correlate motion preservation with elusive processes such as ASD. With so many variables at hand, opinions of the true "success" of disc replacements are heterogeneous and often conflicted. Below, the most recent clinical evidence regarding TDA outcomes for pain, motion, ASD, and overall function are reviewed.

18.4.1 Pain and Symptom Relief

The most concrete conclusion supporting disc replacement is that the procedures can effectively reduce or eliminate preoperative pain and neurological symptom in both short- and long-term periods.[43,44,45,46] Most large prospective studies and meta-analyses agree that cervical TDA is at least equivalent to the current gold standard ACDF for symptom relief, with several studies suggesting that certain aspects of TDA may be better than ACDF. In the cervical spine, a 2012 Cochrane review pooled data for 2,400 patients (nine RCTs) and found low-quality but statistically significant evidence that arthroplasty was superior to fusion for the alleviation of arm pain. (Note: Most recent version of this review was withdrawn by the Cochrane Back Group on May 21, 2015, due to "non-compliance with the Cochrane Commerical [sic] Sponsorship Policy." No further information regarding reason(s) for withdrawal are readily available. http://onlinelibrary.wiley.com/doi/10.1002/14651858.CD009173.pub3/abstract)

Small but significant differences were also seen in neck-related functional status and neurological outcomes in favor of arthroplasty. Authors stress that differences seen were "invariably small and not clinically relevant for all primary [neurological] outcomes"; further, there was high likelihood that the small studies included were subject to publishing bias and industry influence.[41] Critics highlight the lack of minimal important difference (MID) between cervical TDA and ACDF in the Cochrane meta-analysis. MID may be defined as the smallest patient-perceived benefit that justifies departure from the gold standard treatment; absence of MID means that whereas some benefits of TDA may have been statistically significant, their clinical benefits are too marginal to justify mass adoption of the technology at this time. Critics have also stressed lack of blinding in all studies and high likelihood of pro-industry bias.[44] Another larger and more recent cervical TDA meta-analysis incorporated 4,516 cases from 19 RCTs. Authors reported superiority of cervical TDA over ACDF for functional outcomes (NDI scores, axial neck pain and neurological pain scores, VAS scores), fewer associated adverse events, and fewer secondary surgical procedures in the short term.[43] It must be stated that this study also reported "serious" risk for bias in each of the outcomes assessed.

Some authors have explored whether TDA success is dependent on its implantation at certain cervical levels. Although few clinical studies directly address this question, prospective evidence in a study of Bryan cervical TDA suggests there is no difference in NDI outcomes between TDA performed at C5–6 versus C6–7.[47] Another study found no significant differences in sagittal or lateral segmental ROM between ProDisc-C TDAs implanted at C3–4, C4–5, C5–6, or C6–7; however, corresponding neurological and disability outcomes were not reported.[48] Multilevel cervical TDA constructs appear to have equivalent, if not superior, effects on pain and neurological symptoms compared with equivalent-level ACDFs. In a mid-term follow-up study of two-level Mobi-C TDAs, TDA patients demonstrated greater NDI improvements, 12-Item Short-Form Health Survey Physical Component Summary scores, patient satisfaction, and overall success than two-contiguous-level ACDF.[49]

In the lumbar spine, a 2012 Cochrane meta-analysis pooled data from six RCTs comparing single-level lumbar fusion with disc replacement. Authors concluded that lumbar TDAs achieved clinically relevant improvements in pain and functional scores from preoperative levels. Compared with interbody fusion, TDAs exhibited greater improvements in VAS and ODI scores at 24 months postoperatively.[45] As with the current cervical meta-data, evidence supporting these statistically significant findings are based on "low-quality" and potentially biased data. The Cochrane review panel concluded that although the benefits of single-level lumbar TDA over fusion were statistically significant, the improvements were modest and applicable to only a select group of patients. Another more recent meta-analysis, which includes several of the same studies utilized by the Cochrane review in addition to more recent data, found similarly improved VAS and ODI scores in TDA over fusion.[50] Authors additionally reported shorter hospitalizations and higher rates of patient satisfaction (patients willing to undergo the same procedures again) in the arthroplasty group. No significant differences were found in complication rates, reoperation rates, or the proportion of patients able to return to work.

Motion

Prosthetic motion in vivo depends on a several factors, including direction and type of motion, design of the prosthesis, location of the implant, and specific patient-related factors such as the preoperative index level ROM, severity of degeneration, and DSH.[42]

Meta-analytical data indicate that single-level cervical TDA affords an average 6.9 degrees of flexion/extension at the index level (95% confidence interval [CI]: 5.5–8.4).[41] This falls within the lower ranges of normal physiological flexion/extension for most levels of the subaxial cervical spine; however, it is probably less flexion/extension than is afforded by C4 5 and C5 6 segments in their prime health.[3] Prospective studies of the Bryan cervical disc found no difference between preoperative and postoperative index-level motion at 4 years after surgery.[30] Investigators of a PCM disc (Nuvasive Inc., San Diego, CA) study, however, found a slight reduction in preoperative ROM (8.0 degrees) and postoperative motion at the index level (6.2 degrees).[51] Overall, many authors opine that preservation—but not improvement—of motion at the index level appears to be the most common outcome following cervical disc replacement.[30]

Motion at levels adjacent to cervical TDA is a related but separate topic of investigation. Compared with motion immediately adjacent to TDA, postoperative motion adjacent to single-level ACDF has been demonstrated to significantly increase, whereas motion adjacent to TDA remains statistically unchanged.[51] Other studies fail to demonstrate significant differences in motion at levels adjacent to single-level TDAs and ACDFs.[30] When constructs are extended to contiguous two-level ACDFs versus two-level TDAs, however, differences in adjacent level motion may be more apparent. A study of patients with one- and two-level Discover (DePuy Synthes; Westchester, PA) TDAs demonstrated significantly less changes in adjacent segment motion versus their respective one- and two-level ACDF comparisons. Authors found greater differences in motion between the two-level TDA versus ACDF comparison than in the single-level comparison.[52]

Segmental cervical alignment may also improve following cervical TDA.[53] Several authors have demonstrated modest improvements in overall cervical lordosis compared with both preoperative alignments and ACDF following implantation.[30,52]

In the lumbar spine, the effects of TDA on pre- versus postoperative index-level motion are variable. Some authors report a slight loss of index-level ROM compared with preoperative motion. Alternatively, data from the 155 patients with ProDisc-L implants suggest that TDA at L4–5 results in a significant 6.3 degree increase in overall lumbar ROM, whereas overall motion in L5–S1 TDAs was not significantly altered at 2 years postoperative.[54] Other studies, still, report no significant changes in index-level, cranial, and caudal adjacent levels, and/or overall lumbar alignment (L2–S1) following single-level lumbar TDA.[55,56] Data detailing the long-term kinematic effects of lumbar TDA are scarce at this time.

Adjacent Segment Disease and Revision Procedures

The beneficial effects of TDA in reducing ASD is perhaps the biggest controversy in spine arthroplasty. Not only are the long-term effects of motion sparing in TDA very difficult to quantify, but so too are the definition and clinical significance of ASD altogether. In fact, a recent notable meta-analysis comparing nonoperative treatments with lumbar fusion for the treatment of chronic low back pain (LBP) concluded that, although fusion patients exhibited greater radiographic changes at adjacent discs, radiographic findings had no influence on patient-reported pain or disability.[57] Therefore, an important distinction to consider is the difference between merely radiographic adjacent segment pathology (RASP) and symptomatic clinical adjacent segment pathology (CASP). Although several well-constructed prospective studies suggest that the long-term incidence of RASP is lower following TDA than fusions,[46,49] a true reduction in clinically significance CASP is markedly more difficult to demonstrate.

Recent meta-analytical data demonstrate that the incidence of cervical RASP following TDA is around 39 to 48% over a range of 24 to 84 months postoperative.[42] Conversely, the incidence of cervical CASP has been found to range from 2.9 to 15.2%.[42,58] Reoperation rates for CASP symptoms are quoted as approximately 0.7% annually.[58] Data are limited, but a recent, large meta-analysis of six RCTs failed to find a significant difference

in revision rates between ACDF and cervical TDA (6.9 vs. 5.1%, respectively).[59]

In the lumbar spine, however, meta-analytical evidence suggests patients who undergo fusions are nearly 6 times more likely to be treated for ASD than those who receive equivalent-level TDA. Data pooled from two RCTs demonstrated 1.2% and 7.0% ASD-related reoperation rates for TDA and fusion groups, respectively ($p < 0.01$).[60]

When considering reoperation rates for all indications, the meta-evidence may slightly favor TDA over fusion. Reoperation or secondary surgical procedures are defined as any revision, implant removal, conversion to fusion (TDA only), implant exchange, or supplemental fixation, noncontiguous levels, and/or the index-level itself. Short-term (2–3 years) meta-analyses demonstrate a significant reduction in secondary surgical procedures for TDA versus ACDF at both revision index levels (2.7% vs. 7.8%, respectively; $p < 0.001$) and at adjacent levels (1.1% vs. 4.1%, respectively; $p = 0.008$).[43] In mid-term meta-analyses (4–5 years), index level reoperations were 4.0% versus 8.3% for TDA versus ACDF, respectively ($p < 0.001$), but were not significantly different for adjacent levels (3.7% versus 5.0%, respectively; $p = 0.25$).[43] Available long-term data are insufficient for meta-analysis. However, data from one large cervical TDA (PCM) versus ACDF study reported that patients who underwent arthroplasty had lower reoperation rates than those who underwent ACDF (3.3 vs. 7.6%, respectively). Results, however, did not achieve statistical significance at the 7-year mark.[46]

Both short- and long-term lumbar reoperations data are sparse compared with the available cervical data. Two meta-analyses of short-term (2-year) data suggest equivalent reoperation rates between TDA and fusion.[50,61] Concrete long-term meta-data for lumbar TDA are currently unavailable.

18.4.2 Complications

In addition to perioperative risks associated with anesthesia and surgical approaches, both cervical and lumbar disc arthroplasty have a unique set complications dissimilar to their equivalent fusion procedures.

HO has been associated a variety of cervical and lumbar procedures; however, the process seems especially common with cervical prostheses. Postoperative development of HO is likely due to increased cutting, milling, and resection of bone.[30] Reported incidences vary greatly. Meta-analysis shows overall HO rate (grade 1–4) to be 27.7%. Rates of high-grade disease (grade 3–4) are quoted at around 7.8%.[42] Neither the presence nor severity of HO, however, has been clearly associated with poor clinical outcomes.[30]

Other complications associated with TDA include wear-related failure and other catastrophic events such as component dislocation. Premature failure due to accelerated polyethylene wear has been reported with polyethylene bearings that predate the now-universal process of gamma inert sterilization and commonly practiced highly cross-linked processing. Both macrophage-mediated osteolysis, secondary to high volumetric polyethylene wear, and pseudotumor formation, secondary to MOM ionic wear, have now been reported with spinal prostheses.[23] It is increasingly apparent that disc arthroplasty may be susceptible to the many wear-related longevity and safety concerns that plague weight-bearing hip and knee arthroplasty.

Catastrophic dislocation, such as those reported with ejection of the central core of dual-bearing prostheses, have been reported. An early Charité design was associated with polyethylene rim fracture[62]; early cervical Cummins-Bristol discs were associated with especially high rates of screw breakage, implant loosening, and migration.[15,16] Such complications, however, are exceedingly rare today and have been mitigated by improvements in device fixation and stability.

18.5 Conclusion

Growing experience with mechanical disc replacement has enforced several lessons on spinal biomechanics, optimal implant design, appropriate patient selection, and expected operative outcomes. Several now-universal design themes have been garnered from early experiences, including large surface areas at bone–implant interfaces and the use of supplemental fixation techniques such as bony ingrowth or ongrowth surfaces, keels, spikes, and screw fixation. Successes with cobalt-chromium and titanium alloy-backed components have led to the abandonment of less durable stainless-steel and titanium bearings. Superior methods of polyethylene cross-linking and gamma inert irradiation have been adopted from total hip arthroplasty. Newer generations of elastomeric or hydrogel compounds may soon achieve an optimum balance of unconstrained motion and inert longevity.

Despite these numerous evolutions, we remain in the relative infancy of mechanical disc replacement. Questions persist as to the optimal choice of 3, 4, 5, or 6 DOF for implants. We have yet to demonstrate longevity of many devices beyond 10 or so years, and we have yet to prove beyond an appropriate doubt that these devices truly reduce the incidence of clinically relevant ASD.

Nevertheless, as we live longer, more active, and physically demanding lifestyles, both patients and providers alike will push for safer, more durable, and natural motion–restoring solutions to degenerative spinal diseases. The brightest days for disc arthroplasty may indeed lie ahead.

18.6 References

[1] Gunzburg R, Mayer HM, Szpalski M, Aebi M. Arthroplasty of the spine: the long quest for mobility. Introduction. Eur Spine J. 2002; 11 Suppl 2:S63–S64

[2] Wang MY. Lumbar facet syndromes and joint arthroplasty. Contemporary Spine Surgery. 2011; 12(3):1–7

[3] Marras WS. Biomechanics of the spinal motion segment. In: Herkowitz HN, Garfin SR, Eismont FJ, Bell GR, Balderston RA, eds. Rothman and Simeone: The Spine. 6th ed. Philadelphia, PA: Elsevier Saunders; 2011:109–128

[4] Pearcy MJ, Bogduk N. Instantaneous axes of rotation of the lumbar intervertebral joints. Spine. 1988; 13(9):1033–1041

[5] Truumees E. Cervical and lumbar disk replacement. In: Rao RD, Smuck M, eds. Orthopaedic Knowledge Update: Spine. 4th ed. Rosemont, IL: American Academy of Orthopaedic Surgeons; 2012:371–393

[6] Lee CS, Lee DH, Hwang CJ, Kim H, Noh H. The effect of a mismatched center of rotation on the clinical outcomes and flexion-extension range of motion: lumbar total disk replacement using mobidisc at a 5.5-year follow-up. J Spinal Disord Tech. 2014; 27(3):148–153

[7] Han KS, Kim K, Park WM, Lim DS, Kim YH. Effect of centers of rotation on spinal loads and muscle forces in total disk replacement of lumbar spine. Proc Inst MechEng H. 2013; 227(5):543–550

[8] Fernström U. Arthroplasty with intercorporalendoprothesis in herniated disc and in painful disc. Acta Chir Scand Suppl. 1966; 357:154–159

[9] Szpalski M, Gunzburg R, Mayer M. Spine arthroplasty: a historical review. Eur Spine J. 2002; 11(2) Suppl 2:S65–S84

[10] Synthes. ProDisc-L. Modular Intervertebral Disc Prosthesis for Stabilizing the Lumbar Spine and Restoring the Physiological Range of Motion. Technique Guide. West Chester, PA: Synthes; 2011.http://synthes.vo.llnwd.net/o16/LLNWMB8/INT%20Mobile/Synthes%20International/Product%20Support%20Material/legacy_Synthes_PDF/036.000.432.pdf. Accessed October 1, 2015

[11] Sears WR, McCombe PF, Sasso RC. Kinematics of cervical and lumbar total disc replacement. Semin Spine Surg. 2006; 18(2):117–129

[12] Patwardhan AG, Havey RM, Wharton ND, et al. Asymmetric motion distribution between components of a mobile-core lumbar disc prosthesis: an explanation of unequal wear distribution in explanted CHARITÉ polyethylene cores. J Bone Joint Surg Am. 2012; 94(9):846–854

[13] Gamradt SC, Wang JC. Lumbar disc arthroplasty. Spine J. 2005; 5(1):95–103

[14] Zigler JE. Five-year results of the ProDisc-L multicenter, prospective, randomized, controlled trial comparing ProDisc-L with circumferential spinal fusion for single-level disabling degenerative disk disease. Semin Spine Surg. 2012; 24(1):25–31

[15] Rosen C, Kiester PD, Lee TQ. Lumbar disk replacement failures: review of 29 patients and rationale for revision. Orthopedics. 2009; 32(8):pii:: orthosupersite.com/view.asp?rID=41919

[16] Le H, Thongtrangan I, Kim DH. Historical review of cervical arthroplasty. : Neurosurg Focus. 2004; 17(3):E1

[17] Pettine K, Ryu R, Techy F. Why Lumbar Artificial Disc Replacements (LADRs) Fail. J Spinal Disord Tech. 2016 [Epub ahead of print]

[18] Rousseau MA, Bradford DS, Bertagnoli R, Hu SS, Lotz JC. Disc arthroplasty design influences intervertebral kinematics and facet forces. Spine J. 2006; 6 (3):258–266

[19] Sasso RC, Martin L. The Brian artificial disc. In: Yue JJ, Bertagnoli R, McAfee PC, An HS,eds. Motion Preservation Surgery of the Spine: Advanced Techniques and Controversies. Philadelphia, PA: Saunders; 2008

[20] Bisseling P, Zeilstra DJ, Hol AM, van Susante JL. Metal ion levels in patients with a lumbar metal-on-metal total disc replacement: should we be concerned? J Bone Joint Surg Br. 2011; 93(7):949–954

[21] Zeh A, Becker C, Planert M, Lattke P, Wohlrab D. Time-dependent release of cobalt and chromium ions into the serum following implantation of the metal-on-metal Maverick type artificial lumbar disc (Medtronic Sofamor Danek). Arch Orthop Trauma Surg. 2009; 129(6):741–746

[22] Hellier WG, Hedman TP, Kostuik JP. Wear studies for development of an intervertebral disc prosthesis. Spine. 1992; 17(6) Suppl:S86–S96

[23] Oglesby M, Fineberg SJ, Singh K. Bearing surfaces in spinal arthroplasty. Contemp Spine Surg. 2013; 14(2):1–8

[24] Hallab N, Link HD, McAfee PC. Biomaterial optimization in total disc arthroplasty. Spine. 2003; 28(20):S139–S152

[25] Walter WL, Yeung E, Esposito C. A review of squeaking hips. J Am AcadOrthop Surg. 2010; 18(6):319–326

[26] Medtronic. 2014. Medtronic Receives FDA Approval for PRESTIGE LP Cervical Disc System [Press Release]. Retrieved from http://newsroom.medtronic.com/phoenix.zhtml?c=251324&p=irol-newsArticle&ID=1952027. Accessed November 1, 2015

[27] Taksali S, Grauer JN, Vaccaro AR. Material considerations for intervertebral disc replacement implants. Spine J. 2004; 4(6) Suppl:231S–238S

[28] van Ooij A, Kurtz SM, Stessels F, Noten H, van Rhijn L. Polyethylene wear debris and long-term clinical failure of the Charité disc prosthesis: a study of 4 patients. Spine. 2007; 32(2):223–229

[29] Veruva SY, Steinbeck MJ, Toth J, Alexander DD, Kurtz SM. Which design and biomaterial factors affect clinical wear performance of total disc replacements? A systematic review. Clin OrthopRelat Res. 2014; 472(12):3759–3769

[30] Sundberg EB, Park K, , Phillips FM. Long-term results of cervical disc replacement. Contemp Spine Surg. 2014; 15(12):1–7

[31] Schulz C, Ritter-Lang K, Gossel L, Dressler N. Comparison of single-level and multiple-level outcomes of total disc arthroplasty: 24-month results. Int J Spine Surg. 2014; 9(14):1–11

[32] Bae HW, Kim KD, Nunley PD, et al. Comparison of clinical outcomes of 1- and 2-level total disc replacement; four-year results from a prospective, randomized, controlled, multicenter IDE clinical trial. Spine. 2015; 40 (11):759–766

[33] Fay LY, Huang WC, Tsai TY, et al. Differences between arthroplasty and anterior cervical fusion in two-level cervical degenerative disc disease. Eur Spine J. 2014; 23(3):627–634

[34] Zhao H, Cheng L, Hou Y, et al. Multi-level cervical disc arthroplasty (CDA) versus single-level CDA for the treatment of cervical disc diseases: a meta-analysis. Eur Spine J. 2015; 24(1):101–112

[35] Balderston, JR, Gertz, ZM, McIntosh, T, Balderon, RA. Long-term outcomes of 2-level total disc replacement using ProDisc-L. Spine. 2015; 39 (11):906–910

[36] Hoff EK, Strube P, Pumberger M, Zahn RK, Putzier M. ALIF and total disc replacement versus 2-level circumferential fusion with TLIF: a prospective, randomized,clinical and radiological trial. Eur Spine J. 2016; 25 (5):1558–1566

[37] Jia Z, Mo Z, Ding F, He Q, Fan Y, Ruan D. Hybrid surgery for multilevel cervical degenerative disc diseases: a systematic review of biomechanical and clinical evidence. Eur Spine J. 2014; 23(8):1619–1632

[38] Wong DA, Annesser B, Birney T, et al. Incidence of contraindications to total disc arthroplasty: a retrospective review of 100 consecutive fusion patients with a specific analysis of facet arthrosis. Spine J. 2007; 7(1):5–11

[39] Siepe, CJ, Heider, F, Haas, E, et al. Influence of lumbar intervertebral disc degeneration on the outcome of total lumbar disc replacement: a prospective clinical, histological, X-ray and MRI investigation. Eur Spine J. 2012; 21 (11):2287–2299

[40] Siepe CJ, Hitzl W, Meschede P, Sharma AK, Khattab MF, Mayer MH. Interdependence between disc space height, range of motion and clinical outcome in total lumbar disc replacement. Spine. 2009; 34(9):904–916

[41] Boselie TF, Willems PC, van Mameren H, de Bie RA, Benzel EC, van Santbrink H. Arthroplasty versus fusion in single-level cervical degenerative disc disease: a Cochrane review. Spine. 2013; 38(17):E1096–E1107

[42] Kang J, Shi C, Gu Y, Yang C, Gao R. Factors that may affect outcome in cervical artificial disc replacement: a systematic review. Eur Spine J. 2015; 24 (9):2023–2032

[43] Zhang Y, Liang C, Tao Y, et al. Cervical total disc replacement is superior to anterior cervical decompression and fusion: a meta-analysis of prospective randomized controlled trials. PLoS One. 2015; 10(3):e0117826

[44] Evaniew N, Madden K, Bhandari M. Cochrane in CORR®: arthroplasty versus fusion in single-level cervical degenerative disc disease. Clin Orthop Relat Res. 2014; 472(3):802–808

[45] Jacobs W, Van der Gaag NA, Tuschel A, et al. Total disc replacement for chronic back pain in the presence of disc degeneration. Cochrane Database Syst Rev. 2012; 9(9):CD008326

[46] Phillips FM, Geisler FH, Gilder KM, Reah C, Howell KM, McAfee PC. Long-term outcomes of the US FDA IDE prospective, randomized controlled clinical trial comparing PCM cervical disc arthroplasty with anterior cervical discectomy and fusion. Spine. 2015; 40(10):674–683

[47] Sasso RC, Metcalf NH, Hipp JA, Wharton ND, Anderson PA. Sagittal alignment after Bryan cervical arthroplasty. Spine. 2011; 36(13):991–996

[48] Park JJ, Quirno M, Cunningham MR, et al. Analysis of segmental cervical spine vertebral motion after prodisc-C cervical disc replacement. Spine. 2010; 35(8):E285–E289

[49] Davis, RJ, Nunley, PD, Kim, KD, et al. Two-level total disc replacement with Mobi-C cervical artificial disc versus anterior discectomy and fusion: a prospective, randomized, controlled multicenter clinical trial with 4-year follow-up results. J Neurosurg Spine. 2015; 22(1):15–25

[50] Rao MJ, Cao SS. Artificial total disc replacement versus fusion for lumbar degenerative disc disease: a meta-analysis of randomized controlled trials. Arch Orthop Trauma Surg. 2014; 134(2):149–158

[51] Park DK, Lin EL, Phillips FM. Index and adjacent level kinematics after cervical disc replacement and anterior fusion: in vivo quantitative radiographic analysis. Spine. 2011; 36(9):721–730

[52] Hou Y, Liu Y, Yuan W, et al. Cervical kinematics and radiological changes after Discover artificial disc replacement versus fusion. Spine J. 2014; 14 (6):867–877

[53] Anderson PA, Sasso RC, Hipp J, Norvell DC, Raich A, Hashimoto R. Kinematics of the cervical adjacent segments after disc arthroplasty compared with anterior discectomy and fusion: a systematic review and meta-analysis. Spine. 2012; 37(22) Suppl:S85–S95

[54] Auerbach JD, Jones KJ, Milby AH, Anakwenze OA, Balderston RA. Segmental contribution toward total lumbar range of motion in disc replacement and fusions: a comparison of operative and adjacent levels. Spine. 2009; 34 (23):2510–2517

[55] Däxle M, Kocak T, Lattig F, Reichel H, Cakir B. [Adjacent segment movement after monosegmental total disc replacement and monosegmental fusion of segments L4/5]. Orthopade. 2013; 42(2):81–89[Article in German]

[56] Johnsen LG, Brinckmann P, Hellum C, Rossvoll I, Leivseth G. Segmental mobility, disc height and patient-reported outcomes after surgery for degenerative disc disease: a prospective randomised trial comparing disc replacement and multidisciplinary rehabilitation. Bone Joint J. 2013; 95-B(1):81–89

[57] Mannion AF, Leivseth G, Brox JI, Fritzell P, Hägg O, Fairbank JC. ISSLS Prize winner: long-term follow-up suggests spinal fusion is associated with increased adjacent segment disc degeneration but without influence on clinical outcome: results of a combined follow-up from 4 randomized controlled trials. Spine. 2014; 39(17):1373–1383

[58] Hilibrand AS, Carlson GD, Palumbo MA, Jones PK, Bohlman HH. Radiculopathy and myelopathy at segments adjacent to the site of a previous anterior cervical arthrodesis. J Bone Joint Surg Am. 1999; 81(4):519–528

[59] Verma, K, Gandhi, SD, Maltenfort, M, et al. Rate of adjacent segment disease in cervical disc arthroplasty versus single-level fusion: meta-analysis of prospective studies. Spine. 2013; 38(26):2253–2257

[60] Wang JC, Arnold PM, Hermsmeyer JT, Norvell DC. Do lumbar motion preserving devices reduce the risk of adjacent segment pathology compared with fusion surgery? A systematic review. Spine (Phila Pa 1976). 2012; 37 (22) Suppl:S133–S143

[61] Nie H, Chen G, Wang X, Zeng J. Comparison of total disc replacement with lumbar fusion: a meta-analysis of randomized controlled trials. J Coll Physicians Surg Pak. 2015; 25(1):60–67

[62] Spivak JM, Stanley T, Balderston RA. Lumbar total disc replacement. In: Herkowitz HN, Garfin SR, Eismont FJ, Bell GR, Balderston RA, eds. Rothman and Simeone: The Spine. 6thed. Philadelphia, PA: Elsevier Saunders; 2011:953–967

19 Regulatory Overview: Obtaining Regulatory Approval of a Biological/Cell Product

Michaela H. Purcell, Penny J. White, and H. Davis Adkisson

Abstract

Physicians and corporate sponsors engaged in the clinical development of biological therapies are faced with a regulatory environment that is continually evolving as new, unique products, particularly those derived of living cells, are introduced. This chapter addresses salient milestones in the historical evolution of this regulatory process, U.S. Food and Drug Administration (FDA) classification of biological products, and the process for studying and approving a new biological treatment in the United States. Additionally, the value of and process by which sponsors can obtain guidance through meeting with the FDA is reviewed. Recommendations for assembling effective quality and regulatory teams are discussed.

Keywords: BLA, cellular therapy, clinical research, development of biological therapy, IND, tissue

19.1 Historical Perspective

The process of regulatory oversight of medicinal products is relatively recent in modern culture. Prior to 1906, all drugs and devices could be sold in the United States as freely as any other marketed commodity. There was no requirement that manufacturers disclose product composition, and therefore preparations could be sold containing inactive, harmless mixtures or very toxic chemicals. Since these early days, a barrage of legislation has ensued. Enactments, which have laid the groundwork for product development, and a brief summary of the most relevant to the regulation of biologics are outlined in the following paragraphs.[1,2,3,4]

In 1902, Congress passed the Biologics Control Act following the death of 22 children from tetanus, 13 of whom received inoculation with contaminated diphtheria antiserum and 9 of whom received contaminated smallpox vaccine. Prior to 1906, there were no central or uniform controls in place to ensure product potency and purity. The Biologics Control Act gave the government control over the processes used to make biological products and the responsibility to ensure their safety for the American public. This authority was assigned to the Hygienic Laboratory of the Public Health and Marine Hospital Service.

In 1906, Congress passed the Pure Food and Drugs Act, which outlawed foods and drugs that were mixed with inferior or impure ingredients (adulterated), or that bore false or misleading claims. However, this law made no reference to biological products. Under another law passed in 1938, the Federal Food, Drug, and Cosmetic Act (FD&C Act) legislated that a biological product was considered to be a drug. Although parts of the 1938 act were applied to biologics, the act did not modify or supersede the provisions of the 1902 Biologics Control Act. After 1938, the appropriate provisions of the 1902 and 1938 acts were used in the regulation of biologics.

In 1930, the Hygienic Laboratory was renamed the National Institute of Health, which became the National Institutes of Health (NIH) in 1948. Biologics control remained part of the NIH until 1972, when it was transferred to the U.S. Food and Drug Administration (FDA), Center for Biologics Evaluation and Research (CBER). Because CBER has unique origins from within the NIH, the regulation of biologics has subtle but impactful differences when compared with the regulation of drugs and devices. This is an important consideration for sponsors who may incorrectly assume that the nuances of drug and device regulation can be extrapolated to biologics, especially in the areas of manufacturing and in the demonstration of clinical safety.

In 1944, Congress passed the Public Health Service Act (PHSA), which covered a broad spectrum of health concerns, including regulation of biological products and control of communicable diseases. Today, the 1938 Food Drug and Cosmetic Act and the Public Health Service Act are the principle laws that govern biologics.

In 1998, the first human embryonic stem (ES) cell was isolated and grown in culture.[5] This discovery ignited unprecedented controversy over the right to harvest and manipulate stem cells, which can potentially be engineered into any cell type in the human body, and may also be genetically altered. Exploration of methods by which human stem cells, both embryonic and adult, may be utilized medicinally to replace diseased cells, prevent the progression of disease, or even prevent disease from occurring, has greatly accelerated. In response, the FDA has quickened its efforts to meet scientific discovery in order to assure the safety and clinical benefit of products comprising living cells. The regulation of cells presents exceptional challenges because each cell type is unique, and may not be easily characterized as compared to a traditional pharmaceutical. Although biologics continue to be developed along a similar path as drugs, the FDA is releasing a quickly evolving set of guidances, unique to living cells and even in some cases specific to cell types. In the following sections, the general "roadmap" by which a biological/cell product can be brought to market is discussed.

19.2 Regulation of Human Cells, Tissues, and Cellular and Tissue-based Products

All therapeutic products are regulated in the United States by the FDA based upon their derivation and mode of action. Human cells and tissue products are regulated under The Code of Federal Regulations, 21CFR 1271.3 (d),[6] which defines human cells, tissues, and cellular and tissue-based products (HCT/Ps) as those articles containing or consisting of human cells or tissues that are intended for implantation, transplantation, infusion, or transfer to a human recipient. The FDA has constructed regulations to prevent the transmission, introduction, and spread of communicable disease through HCT/Ps.

To be exempt from further regulation, the FDA outlines in the regulation the following criteria that must be met:

- Minimally manipulated[7];
- Intended for homologous use;
- Manufacture does not involve combination with other articles except for water, crystalloids, or a sterilizing, preserving, or storage agent that does not introduce additional safety concerns; and
- Either;
a) Does not have a systemic effect and is not dependent on metabolic activity of living cells for its primary function, or;
b) Has a systemic effect or is dependent upon the metabolic activity of living cells for its primary function and is for
  - autologous use,
  - allogeneic use in a first- or second-degree blood relative, or
  - reproductive use.

19.3 Regulation of Biological Products

All products not meeting the definition of an HCT/P will be regulated as a biologic, drug, and/or device and will require premarket approval from the FDA. Biological products (including cell therapies) are derived from living sources (human, animal, or microorganism) and act through a metabolic mode of action. Such products cannot be fully characterized and are regulated within the particular expertise of CBER. CBER regulates cellular therapy products, human gene therapy products, and certain devices related to cell and gene therapy. The directive of CBER is to assure safe collection, manufacture, storage, and usage of biological products.

In contrast, drug products, which can be structurally characterized and interact chemically with the body, are regulated within the Center for Drug Evaluation and Research (CDER). Devices, which function via their physical structure in vivo, fall within the jurisdiction of the Center for Devices and Radiological Health (CDRH).

Though great efforts in providing consistency among these divisions are ongoing, it is wise to understand their inevitable bureaucratic differences. This becomes even more nuanced in situations where one is developing a "combination product." In such cases, more than one agency division will have responsibility for oversight, and it will be internally decided among divisions which entity will take on a lead role as they partner in their evaluation of the product.

19.4 The Investigational New Drug Application Process

Current federal law requires that a drug/biological product be approved for marketing before it can be shipped across state lines. The exemption to this law, by which an investigational drug or biologic can be studied in humans, and shipped across state lines is through the Investigational New Drug Application

(IND) process. It is through this process that the FDA evaluates whether the chemistry and manufacturing controls (CMC), laboratory, and animal studies have demonstrated sufficient safety to allow study in humans.

INDs are submitted by sponsors. Sponsors can be individual investigators, commercial enterprises, or even government agencies. Throughout the clinical investigation of the biologic, the sponsor holds full responsibility for complying with all applicable laws and regulations relative to the product's development. The sponsor may delegate duties to various collaborators, but in the end is the accountable party.

The required content of the IND can be found in the FDA Code of Federal Regulations 312.23.[8,9] An abbreviated summary is provided in ▶ Table 19.1. It should be noted that throughout the investigational life of the product, annual reports are submitted by the sponsor to the FDA to update the contents of the IND and inform the agency of all pertinent information regarding the development history of the investigational product.

Table 19.1 Content of the Investigational New Drug Application (IND)

Section	Content
Cover sheet (Form FDA-1571)	Name of the biologic, all contact information of the sponsor, and if a sponsor has transferred any obligations for the conduct of any clinical study to a contract research organization, full identification of all contractors, and a listing of the obligations transferred; identification of the phase or phases of the clinical investigation to be conducted; and commitment not to begin clinical investigations until an IND is in effect; Institutional Review Board (IRB) oversight and compliance with all other applicable regulatory requirements.
Introductory statements	A statement of all components, route of administration, broad objectives, and planned duration of the proposed clinical investigation(s), previous human experience, with reference to other INDs if pertinent, investigational or marketing experience in other countries that may be relevant to the safety of the proposed clinical investigation(s); rationale for research study, the indication(s) to be studied; estimated number of patients to be administered product and a summary of risks of particular severity or seriousness anticipated on the basis of the toxicological data in animals or prior studies in humans with the investigational product.
Investigator's brochure	Description of the investigational product, summary of toxicological effects in animals and, to the extent known, in humans, and summary of biological disposition in animals and, if known, in

Table 19.1 (continued)

Section	Content
	humans; information relating to safety and effectiveness in humans obtained from prior clinical studies; risks and side effects to be anticipated, and of precautions or special monitoring to be done as part of the investigational use of the investigational product.
Study protocol(s)	Minimum requirements include objectives and purpose of the study, the criteria for patient selection and for exclusion of patients and an estimate of the number of patients to be studied, design of the study and description of control group(s); method for determining the dose(s) to be administered, maximum dosage, and the duration of individual patient exposure to the investigational product; observations and measurements, clinical procedures, laboratory tests, or other measures to be taken to monitor the effects of the investigational product in human subjects and to minimize risk. If pediatric studies are planned, specific information regarding the protection of subjects and informed consent should be given.
Chemistry, manufacturing, and control	Full identification of components of the product, control of raw materials, details of manufacture, the purity, and strength of the investigational product. Purity refers to relative freedom from extraneous matter. Strength refers to potency or the specific ability of the product to yield specific laboratory results that may be logically extrapolated to the assumption of therapeutic effect. If a placebo substance is to be used in clinical investigation, a general description of the composition and manufacture should be provided.
Pharmacology and toxicology	Full description of all laboratory, toxicology, and preclinical studies to date on the basis of which the sponsor has concluded that it is reasonably safe to conduct the proposed clinical investigations
Previous human experience	Previous human experience including clinical study and marketing, either in the United States or other countries, and a list of the countries in which the investigational product has been marketed and withdrawn from marketing for reasons potentially related to safety or effectiveness

19.5 Clinical Investigation of Biologics

Once the IND is approved, human testing of an investigational biologic is undertaken in progressive phases, which are adapted from the drug development process.[10]

19.5.1 Phase I

In Phase I, the primary objective is to study the safety of the product in a relatively small number of subjects. Healthy volunteers can be studied during this period; however, in the investigation of biologics, it is more common for subjects with a targeted disease state to be treated. All adverse events are closely monitored and the potential for toxicity is scrutinized. This may include the assessment of risk associated with escalating dosages.

Depending upon how much is known about the product, and the relative comfort of the FDA regarding safety, it can be helpful in Phase I to treat a very limited number of subjects, monitoring for adverse events for a period of time. Enrollment can then resume, once the absence of immediate, significant risk is confirmed.

In Phase I, it is possible to also assess the preliminary efficacy of the product and to gauge the usefulness of proposed outcome measures; however, the primary focus must be on building sufficient safety information to allow further study of the product in Phase II. It is not customary for subjects enrolled in a Phase I trial to be blinded to treatment or for control groups to be used.

19.5.2 Phase II

Phase II continues with the primary objective of studying the safety of the product. However, it is also during this phase that initial efficacy can be more closely explored, and the prospective capabilities of the product assessed. Importantly, Phase II trials should assume specific utility based upon analysis of Phase I data, feedback on that data from the FDA, and unknown factors that must be well investigated prior to the successful commencement of larger Phase III studies. This early phase of research is the sponsor's opportunity to explore appropriate subject populations, control groups, dosage, and endpoints. It is on the basis of Phase II findings that Phase III studies are statistically powered. Therefore, Phase II studies should be adequately robust to inform the sponsor of key information about the product relative to the proposed indication, to facilitate design of Phase III while minimizing financial risk.

The FDA will generally require evidence of safety and efficacy from at least two adequate and well-controlled clinical trials (as defined by the agency's CFR 314.126) to approve the investigational product for marketing in the United States. It is possible that a Phase II trial can be considered as one of the two adequate and well-controlled trials, but it can be unwise to relinquish the flexibility of Phase II to meet the stringent qualifications of a well-controlled and adequately designed trial.[11]

19.5.3 Phase III

The purpose of conducting Phase III clinical investigations is to meet FDA requirements to "distinguish the effect of a drug (biologic) from other influences, such as spontaneous change in the course of the disease, placebo effect, or biased observation. Reports of adequate and well-controlled investigations provide the primary basis for determining whether there is "substantial evidence" to support the claims of effectiveness for new drugs (biological cellular therapies)." ▶ Table 19.2 summarizes the characteristics recognized by the FDA as meeting these standards.

Table 19.2 Characteristics of an adequate and well-controlled clinical trial

1. Clear statement of the objectives, a summary of the proposed and actual methods of analysis;
2. Use of a design that permits a valid comparison with a control to provide a quantitative assessment of effect. The protocol for the study and report of results should describe the study design precisely; for example, duration of treatment periods, whether treatments are parallel, sequential, or crossover, and whether the sample size is predetermined or based upon some interim analysis. Generally, the following types of controls are recognized:
   a) Placebo concurrent control. The test product is compared with an inactive preparation designed to resemble the test drug as far as possible.
   b) Dose-comparison concurrent control. At least two doses of the drug are compared.
   c) No treatment concurrent control. Where objective measurements of effectiveness are available and placebo effect is negligible, the test drug is compared with no treatment.
   d) Active treatment concurrent control. The test drug is compared with known effective therapy; for example, where the condition treated is such that administration of placebo or no treatment would be contrary to the interest of the patient.
   e) Historical control. The results of treatment with the test drug are compared with experience historically derived from the adequately documented natural history of the disease or condition, or from the results of active treatment, in comparable patients or populations (usually reserved for special circumstances including studies of diseases with high and predictable mortality and studies where the effect of the drug is self-evident (general anesthetics, drug metabolism).
3. The method of selection of subjects provides adequate assurance that they have the disease or condition being studied, or evidence of susceptibility and exposure to the condition against which prophylaxis is directed.
4. The method of assigning patients to treatment and control groups minimizes bias and is intended to assure comparability of the groups. Ordinarily, in a concurrently controlled study, assignment is by randomization, with or without stratification.
5. Adequate measures are taken to minimize bias on the part of the subjects, observers, and analysts of the data. The protocol and report of the study should describe the procedures used to accomplish this, such as blinding.
6. The methods of assessment of subjects' response are well-defined and reliable—in many instances specifically validated for the disease state. The protocol for the study and the report of results should explain the variables measured, the methods of observation, and criteria used to assess response.
7. There is an analysis of the results of the study adequate to assess the effects of the drug. The report of the study should describe the

results and the analytical methods used to evaluate them, including any appropriate statistical methods. The analysis should assess, among other things, the comparability of test and control groups with respect to pertinent variables, and the effects of any interim data analyses performed.

8. For an investigation to be considered adequate for approval of a new drug, it is required that the test drug be standardized as to identity, strength, quality, purity, and dosage form to give significance to the results of the investigation.
9. Uncontrolled studies or partially controlled studies are not acceptable as the sole basis for product approval.

It is possible that a single Phase III clinical trial can be conducted under the guidelines of a Special Protocol Assessment (SPA) in which a thoroughly vetted clinical protocol and statistical design is prenegotiated and agreed by the FDA as adequate to support approval. This option can be useful; however, it should be entered upon thoughtfully with full recognition of its complexity. It can take an extended amount of time to negotiate an SPA with the agency, and once the study is completed, the agency has specific responsibility to evaluate whether agreed conditions have been satisfactorily met.[12]

19.6 Postmarket Clinical Investigations

19.6.1 Postmarketing Requirements

Clinical studies that are conducted after the product has been approved for marketing may be required by the FDA (without the need for sponsor agreement), if the agency determines that there is new risk that has been presented through its commercial use or the commercial use of a related product. The conditions that allow the agency to require postmarket clinical investigations are to

- Assess a known serious risk related to the use of the drug (biologic);
- Assess signals of serious risk related to the use of the drug (biologic);
- Identify an unexpected serious risk when available data indicate the potential for a serious risk.

When one of these conditions is met, FDA may request clinical study(ies) as a Postmarketing Requirement (PMR). The details of such a requirement may be mandated by the FDA and will have specific reporting and execution.

19.6.2 Postmarketing Commitments

Postmarket studies that sponsors have agreed to conduct, and report to the FDA (but are not required) are referred to as Postmarketing Commitments (PMCs). These commitments are publicly disclosed; time lines and periodic progress reports to the agency are expected. However, unlike PMRs, failure to fulfill these obligations does not constitute a violation of federal statute that could result in punitive action.[13]

19.7 Approval to License a New Biological Product

A Biologics License Application (BLA) is a formal written request to the FDA for permission to introduce (or deliver for introduction) a biological product for interstate commerce.[14] The BLA is submitted either by the manufacturer of the product or an applicant who assumes responsibility for full regulatory compliance. The regulations regarding BLAs for therapeutic biological products include 21 CFR parts 600, 601, and 610. The content of the BLA application is voluminous and includes all pertinent details regarding applicant information, product/manufacturing information, preclinical studies, clinical studies, and labeling. The applicant should always keep in mind that unlike a drug, CBER considers that biological/cell products cannot be fully characterized, given that cells produce tens of thousands of different proteins, carbohydrates, lipids and other molecules interacting in extreme complexity. Consequently, a consistent and reproducible manufacturing process must be detailed with evidence to support the consistency in the BLA.

Once submitted, the application is processed through managed review by a Review Committee, which is constituted by the FDA to ensure the appropriate expertise for thorough evaluation of the application. Generally, the purpose of the review is to determine "that the product, the manufacturing process, and the manufacturing facilities meet applicable requirements to ensure the continued safety, purity, and potency of the product." This process examines storage and testing of all cell substrates as well as potency assays, preclinical toxicology, and animal and human studies.

The standard review process may take 1 to 2 years; however, there are certain pathways available for expedited review. At the time of application, Priority Review can be granted to drugs (biologics) that treat an unmet medical need and Orphan Drug Status is granted to drugs (biologics) that treat rare diseases or diseases that have no other available treatments. In addition, a therapy can be designated by the FDA as a Breakthrough product if it is intended alone or in combination with one or more other drugs (or biologics) to treat a serious or life-threatening disease, or condition and preliminary clinical evidence indicates that the drug (biologic) may demonstrate substantial improvement over existing therapies.

19.7.1 Impact of 21st Century Cures Legislation on FDA Approval of Regenerative Cellular Therapies

The 21st Century Cures Act was passed by congress on December 7, 2016 and signed into law by President Obama on December 13, 2016. As part of the Regrow Act contained within this legislation, the FDA agrees to consider accelerated approval of biologic cellular therapies utilizing surrogate markers as primary endpoints, while ongoing studies focus on demonstration of clinical benefit. In other words, a biologic cancer therapy may utilize tumor shrinkage in establishing clinical burden of proof before prolonged survival has been demonstrated. Similarly, a life-threatening disease receiving cellular therapy and demonstrating tissue regeneration may adequately demonstrate substantial improvement over existing therapies. Treatments that go to market as part of the Cures Act are required to be studied further to ensure they provide substantial benefit as they become available to more patients.

19.8 Communication with the FDA

The importance of ongoing collegial communication with the FDA during product development and approval cannot be overstated. The authors have found that collaborative interaction with the agency is the key to negotiating clear expectations, thereby minimizing wasted time and expense. Paramount to skilled communication is the understanding of how the agency has structured specific opportunities for face-to-face meetings.[15,16] These meetings outlined in ▶ Table 19.3 are essential to understanding the concerns of reviewers and allow the sponsor opportunities to lead the discussion of effective solutions.

Table 19.3 Classification of formal meetings with the FDA

Type A	Discussion of an otherwise stalled product program to proceed (critical path) or to address important safety issues	— Products on "clinical hold" — Dispute resolution — Special Protocol Assessments (SPAs) — Postaction meetings (within 30 days of a nonapproval action	Occur within 30 days of FDA receipt of the meeting request
Type B	Discussion (throughout the development process, products which are not stalled and are actively engaged in the development process)	— Pre-IND — Pre emergency usage — End of Phase I — End of Phase II to pre–Phase III — Pre BLA — Postaction meetings (after 3 months of a nonapproval action — Postmarketing requirements (PMRs) — Breakthrough product discussions	Occur within 60 days of FDA receipt of the meeting request
Type C	Format for discussion of all other issues not appropriate for a Type A or B meeting	— Promotional labeling — Advertising	Within 75 days of FDA receipt of the meeting request

Abbreviations: BLA, Biologics License Application; FDA, Food and Drug Administration; IND, Investigational New Drug Application.

In all cases, meetings are requested by the sponsor in writing. The FDA assigns a regulatory project manager to facilitate timing, submission of pre-meeting content, attendance, and follow-up reporting of meeting minutes.

19.9 The Regulatory Team

The Sponsor carries full responsibility for assuring regulatory compliance during the life cycle of the product, both during its development and commercialization. This requires the contribution of experts in the regulation of chemistry, manufacturing and controls, and preclinical and clinical trials, as well as compliance in commercialization.[17]

19.9.1 Manufacturing

Full validation of product manufacture must be accomplished as consistent with the principles of Good Manufacturing Practice (GMP).[18] Diligence must be maintained starting with the actual manufacturing environment through donor screening, cell procurement, all raw materials, processing, storage, packaging, labeling, and distribution.

The sponsor is tasked with ensuring and demonstrating to regulatory authorities a manufacturing process that ensures verification of the identity, strength, quality, purity, and potency of the biological product.

19.9.2 Preclinical Testing

In vivo and in vitro testing must be conducted in accordance with Good Laboratory Practice (GLP).[19] It is largely on the basis of this research that the FDA will determine if a product is safe enough to study in humans. Therefore, the sponsor must include on its regulatory team, individuals who can establish and enforce processes that make certain that acceptable quality in study conduct is maintained. This includes appropriate personnel, laboratory facilities, animal care, equipment, written protocols, operating procedures, and the completion of study reports, which are traceable to meticulously recorded raw data.

19.9.3 Clinical Testing

The FDA has clearly defined the regulatory responsibilities of sponsors during the proper execution of clinical trials in accordance with Good Clinical Practice (GCP) standards.[20] As stated in 21 CFR 312.50 subpart D,[21] "Sponsor personnel are accountable for selecting qualified investigators, providing them updated product information, proper monitoring, adherence to the study protocol, maintaining an effective IND and ensuring that FDA and all participating investigators are promptly informed of significant new adverse effects or risks with respect to the drug."

Although investigators bear the direct burden of ensuring the safety and welfare of each study subject, the sponsor is accountable for the oversight of all clinical investigations.

19.9.4 Commercialization

Diligence must continue during commercialization. The strict adherence to "on-label" marketing and sales is informed though advanced knowledge of FDA regulation regarding promotion of products. All commercial activities including distribution materials, advertising, and physician interaction must include the input of qualified regulatory personnel and all advertising and promotional labeling must be submitted for review to the Advertising and Promotional Labeling Branch of CBER.

19.9.5 Quality Provides Accountability

The assurance of this level of regulatory diligence is provided through the Quality Management System. This function is responsible for identifying risk, documenting procedures, and applying corrective action when appropriate. Quality assurance oversight ensures a trackable process by which regulatory requirements are fulfilled and the safety of the FDA-regulated product is verified.

19.10 Conclusion

Regulatory strategies applied to the development of biological products are continually evolving as groundbreaking, unique products are explored. Best practice demands that sponsors be well educated in the basic animal and human research processes, integrate quality into the manufacturing process, and work closely with the FDA to optimize the possibility of approval and successful commercialization.

19.11 References

[1] Kingham R, Klasa G, Hessler-Carver K. Key regulatory guidelines for the development of biologics in the United States and Europe. In: Wang W, Singh M, eds. Biological Drug Products: Development and Strategies. 1st ed. John Wiley & Sons, Inc.; 2014:75–109

[2] Lipsky MS, Sharp LK. From idea to market: the drug approval process. J Am Board Fam Pract. 2001; 14(5):362–367

[3] Bren L. The road to the biotech revolution: highlights of 100 years of biologics regulation. FDA Consum. 2006; 40(1):50–57

[4] History of Federal Regulation: 1902–Present. fdareview.org 2015

[5] Thomson, JA, Itskovitz-Eldor, J, Shapiro, SS, et al. Embryonic stem cell lines derived from human blastocysts. Science. 1998; 282(5391):1145–1147

[6] Code of Federal Regulations. 21 CFR 1271.3 (d). Human cells, tissues, or cellular or tissue-based products. April 2015

[7] Code of Federal Regulations. Minimal manipulation of human cells, tissues and cellular and tissue-based products. December 2014

[8] Holbein ME. Understanding FDA regulatory requirements for investigational new drug applications for sponsor-investigators. J Investig Med. 2009; 57 (6):688–694

[9] Code of Federal Regulations. 21 CFR 312 Subpart B. Investigational New Drug Application. April 2015

[10] Code of Federal Regulations. 21 CFR 312.12. Phases of an investigation. April 2015

[11] Code of Federal Regulations. 21 CFR 314.126. Adequate and well-controlled studies. April 2015

[12] Guidance for Industry: Special Protocol Assessment. May 2002

[13] Postmarketing studies and clinical trials: implementation of section 505(o) (3) of the federal Food, Drug, and Cosmetic Act. http://www.fda.gov/downloads/Drugs/GuidanceComplianceRegulatoryInformation/Guidances/UCM172001.pdf. April 2011

[14] Code of Federal Regulations. 121 CFR 601. Licensing. April 2015

[15] Formal meetings between the FDA and sponsors or applicants of PDUFA Products. http://www.fda.gov/downloads/drugs/guidancecomplianceregulatoryinformation/guidances/ucm437431.pdf. March 2015

[16] Guidance for industry: formal meetings between the FDA and sponsors or applicants. May 2009

[17] Casaroli-Marano RP, Tabera J, Vilarrodona A, Trias E. Regulatory issues in cell-based therapy for clinical purposes. Dev Ophthalmol. 2014; 53 (53):189–200

[18] CMC and CMP Guidances: Vaccines, Blood & Biologics. 2015

[19] Code of Federal Regulations. 21 CFR 58. Good Laboratory Practice. April 2015

[20] Guidance for industry. E6 good clinical practice: consolidated guidance. http://www.fda.gov/downloads/Drugs/.../Guidances/ucm073122.pdf. April 1996

[21] Code of Federal Regulations. 21 CFR 312.50. General responsibilities of sponsors. April 2015

20 What Makes Biological Treatment Strategies and Tissue Engineering for DDD Interesting to Industry?

Hassan Serhan, Elliott A. Gruskin, and William C. Horton

Abstract

Although traditional therapies of decompression and reconstruction have improved countless lives, they primarily address end-stage disease and do not address the underlying pathophysiology or halt the progression of degenerative disc disease (DDD). Dissatisfaction with mechanical solutions, coupled with large-scale global opportunity, creates an environment where the medical device and pharmaceutical industries are looking to bring forward solutions that are biologically targeted and are relevant more broadly across the continuum of care. Open innovation models are taking root in the medical industry and create opportunities for start-ups to participate in the earliest stages of product development. By this approach, new technologies can be fostered with large company involvement, but remain with the passionate inventors during the early stages of development. However, it must be recognized that to attract the investment of larger device companies, new spine technology developers must factor in a few key areas that are not normally the domain of the small-scale academic labs or enterprises. These include, but are not limited to a clear understanding of the unmet clinical need including the financial or "Triple Aim" aspect on a global basis, the intellectual property that can be protected, the positioning of the new approach relative to the current standard of care, the scalability of the technology with respect to global commercialization, the quality and discriminating capacity of the preclinical data, a progressive risk management strategy for each stage of development, the regulatory pathway from a global vantage point, and the clinical evidence plan.

Keywords: biological repair of degenerative disc, degenerative disc disease (DDD), early intervention DDD, open innovation, Triple Aim

20.1 Introduction

Although traditional therapies of decompression and reconstruction have improved countless lives, these primarily mechanical solutions incompletely address the underlying pathophysiology, and primarily address end-stage disease with little application for either prevention or early intervention. Degenerative disc disease (DDD) particularly impacts the cervical and lumbar spine, accounting for the greatest burden of disability globally, where solutions offer an enormous opportunity for impacting health across large populations and markets globally.[1,2,3] In general, this dissatisfaction with primarily mechanical solutions, coupled with large-scale opportunity, creates an environment where the medical device and pharmaceutical industries are looking to bring forward solutions that are biologically targeted, are relevant more broadly across the continuum of care, and potentially can alter the natural history of this complex disease.

The sources of axial low back pain (LBP) are many including but not limited to soft tissues, neurological, articular, and discogenic. Multiple skeletal abnormalities including compression fractures, spondylosis, spondylolysis, spondylolisthesis, or tumor also are frequently involved. Of all these pathologies, the disc is felt to be the most common link underlying axial and neurological disease, and thus DDD is of great interest as an innovation target. The clinical features of many cases of LBP with DDD are inadequately explained by anatomical abnormalities alone, and the poor sensitivity and specificity of magnetic resonance imaging (MRI) testifies to this problem.[4,5]

A pathophysiological mechanism that may include one or a combination of mechanical and biochemical factors is an alternative explanation that is accompanied by less paradox than a purely structural and mechanical paradigm.[6,7,8,9] Consequently, developing new technologies to treat these spine disorders requires a much deeper understanding of the pathobiology and a broad range of research and development (R&D) competencies that blur the traditional boundaries between device, biological, and pharma enterprises. To address these challenges, industry is more and more turning to multidisciplinary teams, and an open innovation model wherein technologies at various stages of development can be fostered in a risk-adjusted, milestone-based process. A spine company's R&D pipeline can be a mosaic of internal R&D projects, in-licensed technologies, and collaborations with external academic labs or biotech companies, both established and start-up ventures. Successful execution of an open innovation R&D model depends on the ability to identify sound opportunities for investment, assemble the right multifunctional team with appropriate capabilities, and appropriate strategies to sequentially derisk the effort.

One of the most interesting and challenging tasks facing a spine company is determining the value and risks associated with specific opportunities. Evaluating the potential of a disc regeneration technology start-up depends a lot on the value proposition of the treatment. A traditional spinal implant technology, leveraging more familiar and less costly development and regulatory pathways, will have a far different evaluation than a high-risk biological compound company. What evaluations boil down to is the risk involved in the investment as well as the return. Risk can be hard to evaluate because there are so many factors that come into play with biological compounds. For example, investing in a new small molecule or protein to treat DDD may require extensive studies to determine the compounds, their stability, reproducibility, preclinical dose findings, animal safety and efficacy studies, and Phase I to III clinical evaluation. Smaller companies may have difficulty taking on this type of expensive and long-term development.[10] Additionally, reimbursement, intellectual properties, and cost are major concerns with new procedures or treatment pathways and will require a huge investment in longitudinal follow-up and evidence generation. The value proposition, risks, ability to execute, and return on investment are some of the main things industry typically seeks to consider when evaluating internal programs or a start-up with a potential biological solution for DDD. Additionally, when looking at a biological technology, companies will also look closely not only at the technology but also the expertise and breadth of knowledge embodied in the concept. Regenerative or tissue engineering solutions become more attractive when being proposed by a group with deep scientific and development expertise, and a proven track record of successful execution.

20.2 Pathophysiology and Targets for Intervention

Confirming that the biological solution targets a critical pathway of clinical significance is extremely important. There is a strong theoretic basis to support the concept that the clinical features of many patients with lumbar disc conditions may be explained by inflammation caused by biochemical factors alone or mechanical factors, or combined chemical/mechanical factors rather than mechanical factors alone. One such example includes inflammation of neural elements caused by the chemical components of the intervertebral disc (IVD). The recent demonstration of immunohistopathological evidence of an immunocompetent cellular response at the epidural interface of lumbar herniated nucleus pulposus (HNPs) supports the concept of the immunogenic capacity of the nucleus pulposus (NP).[11,12] The identification of high levels of an inflammatory enzyme, phospholipase A2, in lumbar herniated and degenerative discs supports the hypothesis of direct inflammogenic capability of lumbar discs, separate from immunological mechanism.[13] When a biological solution targets a well-established cellular or molecular mechanism, there will be higher levels of corporate interest in investing in the development work.

Although disc regeneration and repair are attractive concepts, the disc has proven to be a harsh and complex environment, and regenerative attempts carry the risk of rebuilding the very "factory" of biochemical pain factors. The lack of understanding of the pain generators in early disc degeneration "black disc" is one of the biggest challenges in determining the best course of treatment and the optimal solutions. There is much that remains to be learned regarding the molecular basis of pain in the setting of degenerative changes within the disc, and then linking those insights to therapies. Addressing the gaps in our understanding of why most degenerative discs are painless while a few are associated with disabling back pain is a challenge. Solutions with well-developed molecular characterization are of great interest to industry when evaluating biologics for DDD. Our growing understanding of the molecular mechanisms behind IVD homeostasis and the molecular events leading to disc degeneration is one example of how basic research may lead to potential new biological therapies for this difficult clinical problem.

Another challenge is the lack of good large-animal models of spontaneous disc degeneration that might mimic the human situation. Most of the animal degenerative disc models are induced by stabbing the disc and creating an "acute herniation" that leads to degenerative changes. As we know acute sharp trauma is not the common cause of the black disc degeneration or herniation. Companies look carefully at the preclinical models that have been well validated and used to characterize a potential biologic to assess potential safety and efficacy.

Another challenge is the unique biomechanical environment of the human spine, given our upright posture. Hence, companies often pilot human clinical trials to explore the effects of a proposed treatment such as the reimplantation of autologous disc cells and/or the use of recombinant growth factors as potential treatment modalities for symptomatic disc degeneration.[14,15,16] These human data will be of great interest to industry; however, without double-blinded, randomized clinical studies, or other high-quality human data the results of such pilot studies will be cautiously interpreted.

Because current diagnostics (MRI, discography, etc.) for DDD have challenges with both sensitivity and specificity[17,18,19] DDD tissue engineering solutions ideally should be developed simultaneously with new early-stage diagnostic tools that enable better understanding of the pain source and indication. Areas of interest include diagnostics that might elucidate pathophysiology, mechanical integrity, pain markers such as cytokines, and genetic analysis to enable optimal patient selection and dosing strategy. This will allow optimization of potential clinical benefit and reduction of potential harm—both of which are critically important to industry in derisking the technology for approval, clinical acceptance, and reimbursement.

20.3 The Quest for Less Invasive Interventions

Of the minimally invasive procedures currently available for the treatment of lumbar disc prolapse (i.e., percutaneous endoscopic discectomy, radiofrequency ablation, laser decompression, chemonucleolysis, etc.), chemonucleolysis represents a true minimally invasive method with the longest period of clinical use. However, clinical complications—including late-onset myelopathy, discitis, spastic paraplegia, sensory loss, and bladder incontinence—as well as the moderate clinical outcome and the narrow selection of patients, are among the reasons for limiting the expansion of this biological treatment.[20] The response of industry and the markets to these complications speaks to the industry focus on safety with all these biological solutions. However, these less-invasive procedures remain of great interest because surgical complication rates correlate with the extent of surgical interventions and a "needle-based" regenerative or biological procedure may be more attractive to patients than traditional minimally invasive surgical interventions. There is a need for alternative cost effective needle-based, outpatient procedures for the treatment of DDD, although some traditional spinal implant industry partners may cautiously consider their ability to effectively penetrate a new market with new unfamiliar providers. These therapies could even be office-based, which represents a point of care more familiar to pharma than to medical device companies, with attendant reimbursement concerns.

20.4 Translational Research Challenges

Successful translational research is actually a rare event. More often, projects are initiated and fail to deliver on their promise. This phenomenon, often referred to as the "Valley of Death," is particularly acute in the spine area where the pathophysiology of the disease is complex and the potential interventions are not clearly related to understood mechanisms. Consequently, companies must adopt a number of strategies to mitigate the risks associated with translational research. In the first instance, innovators and companies benefit from as early a collaboration as possible. This can start with a clear delineation of the clinical need followed by an exploration of how the new potential solution can add value. The design of the product must have value built in to it, and it must use components and processes that can ultimately be scaled up and commercialized with high quality and reasonable costs. The underlying preclinical data must be in adequate model systems that contribute to the regulatory approval process; the design and methods must capture intellectual property that will ensure exclusivity in the market place; and a clinical evidence plan must be practical ensuring timely enrollment and a cost effective design. Finally, each stage of development must discharge risk to attract the escalating expenditures required as the technology moves through the development process. Only through very early collaboration with companies can innovators obtain a clear line of site to the parameters necessary to negotiate the Valley of Death.

20.5 Intellectual Property

A strong intellectual property (IP) position can be one of a start-up company's most valuable assets, and a weak or poorly defined IP position could be its greatest liability. According to Frank Becking, an IP counsel and co-founder of PantheraMed-Tech, "an effective IP portfolio must be managed actively with value-driven goals in mind throughout the development cycle—from idea conception to company acquisition and beyond."[21]

IP rights protect technology and products from infringement and can be a key strategic asset of a small company in positioning for acquisition. Therefore, it is critical to structure the IP portfolio with expanding claims in mind and it should be positioned to navigate away from infringement or other technology intrusion. Becking[21] offers medical device entrepreneurs these five tips for maximizing the value of their IP portfolio:

1. Control access to sensitive information: Don't disclose without a confidentiality agreement. Even with confidentiality agreements in place, until you have filed for a patent any disclosure risks your potential rights and future prospects.
2. Make sure your company owns its IP: This might seem obvious but it is easy to overlook key steps, such as putting in place and enforcing agreements that ensure that work produced by employees and independent contractors becomes the property of the company.
3. Don't neglect country-by-country protection: IP protection opportunities differ around the globe. Select stateside IP counsel that has existing relationships with expert foreign counsel who can advise on how best to navigate international waters.

4. Actively avoid third-party IP entanglement: Too often, corporates focus on the patentability of their own IP. Understanding and tracking third-party patents and the progress of their pending claims may have greater effect on IP value and ultimately corporate valuation.
5. Formulate an IP enforcement strategy: It is important to monitor other competitor's IP filings to ensure that your IP rights are not being infringed. Venture-capital–funded start-ups are extremely opposed to engaging in litigation. Working with experienced IP counsel is a key to understanding and pursuing your enforcement goals.

A view toward pursuing patents to establish barriers and litigating others is too basic. IP can be a critical piece of the company success, but IP activity can only play its supporting role when thoughtfully handled through the development and business cycles.

20.6 Regulatory Pathway

Whereas products are regulated independently by regions, either individual countries or collectives, the growing trend is toward a requirement for substantial efficacy and safety data. A clear understanding of how product design can dictate the regulatory pathway is an important aspect of new technology development and can influence a company's decision to take on a particular new product development project.[22,23] In general, new products that have a clear device function, that is substantially equivalent to a product that is already marketed can be taken through the regulatory pathway and into the marketplace with general controls and preclinical data in relevant animal models.[24] However, the latest developments involving more complex systems such as cell-based approaches and combination drug devices will require expensive, lengthy, and high-risk clinical trials. Exacerbating these inherent risks is the emerging reality that clinical trial designs that offer evidence of noninferiority to existing products have become less and less attractive given the pricing pressures expected for new technologies. Clinical value above and beyond the existing standard of care, coupled with lower costs is expected.

Embarking on a clinical trial program in spine surgery is particularly problematic and this accounts for the scarcity of products that get approved through this pathway. In the first instance, the etiology of DDD is poorly understood. Therefore, a clear structure-activity relationship that can guide successful product development isn't possible. Solutions are arrived at based on hypotheses and much of the underlying evidence is empirical. To make matters worse, there are very limited preclinical models that are validated to deliver a readout that can be directly correlated with a predictable clinical outcome. As a result, every clinical trial attempt is a singular exploration without a clearly predictable likelihood of success. These factors create a very high bar for a company taking on a product that requires this regulatory pathway. Consequently, companies will need to be convinced by a compelling mechanism of action; a robust preclinical data set in a variety of models in a number of species; and a clearly delineated, risk mitigation strategy to take the product through the clinical trial process to detect early safety and efficacy signals. This speaks again to the interest in precise diagnostic and patient-selection approaches to reduce risk of undesired outcomes. More and more, companies are turning to adaptive trial designs as a way of managing these risks.[25] Although the latest technologies have much to offer, the current regulatory trends must be accounted for early in product development.

An exception to this regulatory challenge is the use of autologous cells and tissues. In general, autologous approaches to regenerate tissues are regulated under the U.S. Food and Drug Administration (FDA)'s Human Cells, Tissues, and Cellular and Tissue-Based Products (HCT/P) pathway[26] and similar pathways in other countries and regions. However, this requires that the product meet the following characteristics; it must
- be minimally manipulated;
- be intended for homologous use only;
- not be combined with a drug or device; and
- not have a systemic effect or be dependent on the metabolic activity of living cells for its primary function.

Under the FDA HCT/P and similar pathways globally, products such as a patient's bone marrow aspirate or platelet rich plasma (PR) essentially don't need data to be brought to market.[26] However, the FDA may "change its tune" when it comes to regulating these products in the future, and companies are mindful of the risk of an investment being uprooted by incomplete data or shifting regulatory hurdles. There are several cases involving products that were initially classified as HCT/P but were later reclassified as drugs. The difference between the HCT/P pathway and the drug pathway is a more than $50 million investment,[27] which is certainly a significant barrier to getting some products to market. Understanding the regulatory pathway in the United States and outside the United States, and the reimbursement status of the proposed treatment are the next most important issues to evaluate after IP.

20.7 Health Care Economics

There is a growing realization that the successful health care systems of the future will be those that can simultaneously deliver excellent quality of care at optimized costs while improving the health of their population. Industry partners will be very mindful of how the proposed technology will be accepted, regulated, and reimbursed in all regions of the world where they do business, and will not be interested in DDD solutions that do not bring value. This value equation of improving outcomes while at the same time reducing overall costs is becoming a common goal worldwide, and biologics will have to meet this test to be successful. In the United States this value is known as the Institute for Healthcare Improvement (IHI) Triple Aim[2,8,29] and, we believe, it is the ultimate goal for spine companies, high-performing hospitals, and health systems of the future.

There is abundant interest worldwide in the Triple Aim, since IHI conceived of the framework of the simultaneous pursuit of better health, better health care, and lower per capita costs, a whole array of strategies have opened up for health care reformers. Johnson & Johnson was one of the early adopters of the Triple Aim as it resonates with its credo values.

The Triple Aim is a worthwhile endeavor that, if achieved, will not only save costs across the world's health care systems, but also improve the quality of life for billions of patients. To get there, we need to consider less-invasive technologies such as regenerative therapies for DDD. Therefore, a meaningful advancement in treating DDD should help stop or at least modulate disc degeneration, thus helping the health care systems, governments, and providers (1) improve clinical outcomes, (2) increase patient satisfaction, and (3) contain costs; these three tenets are shared by most global health care reform acts.

20.8 Conclusion

Open innovation models are taking root in the medical device industry and create opportunities for academics, small companies, and start-ups to participate in the earliest stages of product development. By this approach, new technologies can be fostered with large-company involvement, but remain with the passionate inventors during the early stages of development. However, it must be recognized that to attract the investment of larger device companies, new spine technology developers must factor in a few key areas that are not normally the domain of the small-scale academic labs or enterprises. These include, but are not limited to a clear understanding of the unmet clinical need including the financial or Triple Aim aspect on a global basis, the IP that can be protected, the positioning of the new approach relative to the current standard of care, the scalability of the technology with respect to global commercialization, the quality and discriminating capacity of the preclinical data, a progressive risk-management strategy for each stage of development, the regulatory pathway from a global vantage point, and the clinical evidence plan. Addressing a number of these issues will facilitate the collaboration between innovators and large health-care solution providers necessary to bring new spine technologies to the market.

20.9 References

[1] Urban JP, Roberts S. Degeneration of the intervertebral disc. Arthritis Res Ther. 2003; 5(3):120–130

[2] Maniadakis N, Gray A. The economic burden of back pain in the UK. Pain. 2000; 84(1):95–103

[3] van Tulder MW, Koes BW, Bouter LM. A cost-of-illness study of back pain in The Netherlands. Pain. 1995; 62(2):233–240

[4] Luoma K, Riihimäki H, Luukkonen R, Raininko R, Viikari-Juntura E, Lamminen A. Low back pain in relation to lumbar disc degeneration. Spine. 2000; 25(4):487–492

[5] Boden SD, Davis DO, Dina TS, Patronas NJ, Wiesel SW. Abnormal magnetic-resonance scans of the lumbar spine in asymptomatic subjects. A prospective investigation. J Bone Joint Surg Am. 1990; 72(3):403–408

[6] Maroudas A, Nachemson A, Stockwell R, Urban J. Factors involved in the nutrition of the human lumbar intervertebral disc: cellularity and diffusion of glucose in vitro. J Anat. 1975; 120:113–130

[7] Gruber HE, Hanley EN , Jr. Analysis of aging and degeneration of the human intervertebral disc. Comparison of surgical specimens with normal controls. Spine. 1998; 23(7):751–757

[8] Weiler C, Nerlich AG, Zipperer J, Bachmeier BE, Boos N. 2002 SSE Award Competition in Basic Science: expression of major matrix metalloproteinases is associated with intervertebral disc degradation and resorption. Eur Spine J. 2002; 11(4):308–320

[9] Adams MA, McNally DS, Dolan P. 'Stress' distributions inside intervertebral discs. The effects of age and degeneration. J Bone Joint Surg Br. 1996; 78 (6):965–972

[10] Bolander J. How to evaluate a startup company. April 2010. http://www.the-dailymba.com/2010/04/03/how-to-evaluate-a-startup-company/. Accessed January 10, 2017

[11] Inkinen RI, Lammi MJ, Lehmonen S, Puustjärvi K, Kääpä E, Tammi MI. Relative increase of biglycan and decorin and altered chondroitin sulfate epitopes in the degenerating human intervertebral disc. J Rheumatol. 1998; 25 (3):506–514

[12] Lyons G, Eisenstein SM, Sweet MB. Biochemical changes in intervertebral disc degeneration. BiochimBiophys Acta. 1981; 673(4):443–453

[13] Saal JS. The role of inflammation in lumbar pain. Spine. 1995; 20(16):1821–1827

[14] Stanton T. Biologic treatments emerge for IVD. AAOS Now. November 2011. http://www.aaos.org/AAOSNow/2011/Oct/clinical/clinical3/?ssopc=1. Accessed January 10, 2017

[15] Ganey TM, Meisel HJ. A potential role for cell-based therapeutics in the treatment of intervertebral disc herniation. Eur Spine J. 2002; 11 Suppl 2: S206–S214

[16] Alini M, Roughley PJ, Antoniou J, Stoll T, Aebi M. A biological approach to treating disc degeneration: not for today, but maybe for tomorrow. Eur Spine J. 2002; 11 Suppl 2:S215–S220

[17] Frobin W, Brinckmann P, Kramer M, Hartwig E. Height of lumbar discs measured from radiographs compared with degeneration and height classified from MR images. Eur Radiol. 2001; 11(2):263–269

[18] McNally DS, Shackleford IM, Goodship AE, Mulholland RC. In vivo stress measurement can predict pain on discography. Spine. 1996; 21(22):2580–2587

[19] Boos N, Rieder R, Schade V, Spratt KF, Semmer N, Aebi M. 1995 Volvo Award in clinical sciences. The diagnostic accuracy of magnetic resonance imaging, work perception, and psychosocial factors in identifying symptomatic disc herniations. Spine. 1995; 20(24):2613–2625

[20] Bellini M, Romano DG, Leonini S, et al. Percutaneous injection of radiopaque gelified ethanol for the treatment of lumbar and cervical intervertebral disk herniations: experience and clinical outcome in 80 patients. AJNR Am J Neuroradiol. 2015; 36(3):600–605

[21] Becking F. 5 tips to maximize intellectual property portfolio value. Medical Design Technology. April 2015. http://www.mdtmag.com/blog/2015/03/5-tips-maximize-intellectual-property-portfolio-value. Accessed January 10, 2017

[22] FDA. Advancing regulatory science at the FDA: a strategic plan. August 2011. http://www.fda.gov/downloads/ScienceResearch/SpecialTopics/Regulatory-Science/UCM268225.pdf. Accessed January 10, 2017

[23] FDA. Innovation/stagnation: critical path opportunities report. US Department of Health and Human Services 2006. http://www.fda.gov/downloads/ScienceResearch/SpecialTopics/CriticalPathInitiative/CriticalPathOpportunitiesReports/UCM077254.pdf. Accessed January 10, 2017

[24] Mittra J, Tait J, Mastroeni M, Turner ML, Mountford JC, Bruce K. Identifying viable regulatory and innovation pathways for regenerative medicine: a case study of cultured red blood cells. N Biotechnol. 2015; 32(1):180–190

[25] FDA. Guidance for industry: adaptive design clinical trials for drugs and biologics. February 2010. http://www.fda.gov/downloads/Drugs/Guidances/ucm201790.pdf. Accessed January 10, 2017

[26] FDA. Tissue and tissue products. http://www.fda.gov/BiologicsBloodVaccines/TissueTissueProducts/default.htm. Accessed January 10, 2017

[27] Kelly FB, Porucznik MA. Interest in using stem cells in spinal surgery increasing. AAOS Now. September 2014. http://www.aaos.org/news/aaosnow/sep14/cover2.asp. Accessed January 10, 2017

[28] Institute for Health Improvement. Triple Aim for populations. http://www.ihi.org/Topics/TripleAim/Pages/default.aspx. Accessed January 10, 2017

[29] Bucher A, O'Day R. The Triple Aim's missing link: meaningful engagement for patients with chronic conditions. Managed Care Outlook. 2014; 27 (15):1–5

Part V

Outlook

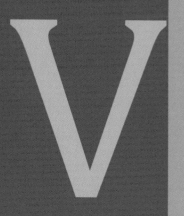

21 What Will the Future Bring? Perspectives From Around the World

Howard An, Tony Goldschlager, Claudius Thomé, Luiz Vialle, Jaime Arias Ruiz, William Omar Contreras Lopez, and Daisuke Sakai

21.1 North America

Many research breakthroughs are covered in this book that have improved our understanding of the biology of the disc, and new biological and less-invasive therapies are being developed to help regenerate the spinal tissues, reduce pain, and restore function. The understanding of the molecular mechanisms of intervertebral disc (IVD) degeneration and the development of the animal models to research them have spurred advancements in designing and testing targeted biological treatments against degenerative disc disease (DDD). Treatments whose strategy is to biologically repair or regenerate the IVD tissues hold great promise for the treatment of discogenic low back pain (LBP) as well as for retarding or even preventing progression of lumbar spondylosis. Biological therapies that focus on introducing viable or genetically modified cells or molecules into the degenerating IVD have the potential to promote matrix repair, restore physiological function, and decrease pain.

The IVD has a unique structure, being composed of a tough outer ring, the annulus fibrosus (AF), and a gelatinous inner core, the nucleus pulposus (NP). The AF, along with the end plates of the adjacent vertebrae, enclose the NP and enable it to resist deformation that would otherwise occur under physiological loading. In a healthy disc, the NP is able to maintain its fluid pressure to balance the high external loads on the IVD because of the abundance of negatively charged proteoglycans. This molecular meshwork of proteoglycans, entrapped in a collagen network, endows the IVD with both compressive stiffness and tensile strength. The progressive loss of the proteoglycan content of the IVD, along with the resulting dehydration of the NP, has been implicated in the pathogenesis of DDD. The loss of matrix homeostasis within the NP is believed to be the result of the combination of both decreased matrix synthesis and increased matrix catabolism. Normal IVD cells synthesize proteoglycans and types I and II collagen, but in the degenerative disc, the synthesis of matrix molecules by IVD cells changes differentially with the degree of degeneration. The viable disc cells decrease in number, most likely due to apoptosis but also due to cell senescence and altered metabolic function. Proteolytic enzymes are found in higher concentrations in degenerative discs compared with normal discs. In addition, there are increased levels of pro-inflammatory cytokines, which are not only implicated in pain but are also thought to result in a further decrease in the rate of extracellular matrix (ECM) synthesis. The future of biological repair or regeneration should address cells, matrix, and pain-related molecules in both the AF and NP to achieve good outcomes over a prolonged period of time. Previous and ongoing research on anabolic growth factors such as osteogenic protein-1 (OP-1), growth and differentiation factor-5 (GDF-5), transforming growth factor β (TGF- β), etc., have shown much promise for their ability to reverse DDD by repairing or regenerating the ECM as well as downregulating the pro-inflammatory factors that are implicated in causing discogenic pain.

Multiple genetic risk factors for DDD have been described. Determining the key genetic markers that are associated with DDD should help in the identification and development of therapeutic molecules for disc repair and regeneration. There have already been several clinical trials using intradiscal protein injection for IVD repair and regeneration, but unfortunately some of these trials have been halted for unknown reasons. With that being said, there have been numerous published papers on cell therapy for IVD repair and regeneration with promising results. In the United States, there are two ongoing Food and Drug Administration (FDA)-approved clinical trials using allogenic juvenile chondrocytes and mesenchymal stem cells (MSCs). The goal of any study for the treatment of DDD should be to achieve a robust and durable regeneration of the disc matrix that is able to withstand the high biomechanical forces seen in the human disc. Because of immune responses and safety concerns, gene therapy itself has not gained traction, and no clinical trials that utilize it are available or planned in the near future.

Despite extensive research on IVD repair and regeneration for the past 3 decades, there is no FDA-approved biological product available for patients suffering from discogenic LBP. Further basic science and clinical trials will definitely bring compounds and even cell therapy into clinical practice. I do not believe that one will necessarily win over the other, however, because DDD is not the same in all patients. For instance, some patients with specific genetic factors may respond to molecular therapy, whereas others with more of a cell deficiency problem may respond better to cell-based therapy. Some patients may have significant discogenic pain with minimal cell and matrix loss, and therefore certain molecules may be more appropriate to address their pain by reducing inflammatory factors rather than causing matrix restoration. Whereas there is still much research to be done in this area, I do believe that the future is bright for the millions of people suffering with LBP and that continued research efforts will yield exciting new therapies for treatment of DDD.

– Howard An

21.2 Australia

It is an honor to present the Australian perspective on biological approaches to spinal disc repair and regeneration. The future is exciting; however, this is only because of the great contributions of the past. I would like to briefly outline some of these contributions as these illustrate the path travelled and a roadmap of where we are likely heading.

Much of our current understanding of the IVD, including its biochemistry, structure, and the role of the notochordal cell comes from Professor Ghosh's work in Sydney, Australia.[1] It is through understanding these facts that regenerative therapies can be developed; however, it is necessary to have animal models with which to test such therapies. In the 1990 Volvo Spinal research award, Osti et al described the surgical induction of an annular "rim lesion" in an ovine model[2] that simulated the known pathology of human disc degeneration. This seminal work, which was carried out in Professor Robert Fraser's laboratory in Adelaide, Australia, has not only contributed to our basic understanding of the underlying molecular mechanisms of disc degeneration, but also provided us with an animal model that has been used for numerous preclinical studies to evaluate stem cells and other biological therapies for the promotion of disc regeneration.

In this regard, the identification of mesenchymal precursor cells (MPCs) by Australian investigators[3,4] as the earliest and most clonogenic cell-line has provided a readily available source of stem cells that are now under commercial development by the Australian company Mesoblast Ltd. for the treatment of disc degeneration and other degenerative disorders. MPCs are perivascular cells found in all vascularized tissues in the body, including bone marrow, dental pulp, and adipose tissue. MPCs are the precursors of all multipotential fibroblastoid colony-forming units (CFU-F), which give rise to all the mesenchymal lineage stem cells and which can differentiate under appropriate stimuli into bone, fat and cartilage. MPCs have specific surface markers such as STRO-1, VCAM-1 (CD106), STRO-3, STRO-4 (HSP-90b), or CD146 that facilitate their extraction and purification using the principles of antibody immunoselection.[3,4]

Two important advantages of these cells are that their numbers can be greatly expanded in culture while maintaining their undifferentiated phenotype, and can be used allogenically because they are immunologically tolerated when transplanted into unrelated recipients.[5]

MPCs have been tested in the ovine models of disc degeneration. In the initial study, discs were injured by the intradiscal injection of the enzyme chondroitinase-ABC (C-ABC) and then rescued with the MPCs.[6] Assessment of the disc response to treatment using magnetic resonance imaging (MRI), biochemistry, and histological studies, as well as radiography to assess the disc height index, revealed improvement in the discs injected with MPCs compared with controls. The authors concluded that the injection of MPCs into degenerate IVDs could contribute to the regeneration of a new ECM. Oehme et al showed similar results using a modified Osti annular injury ovine model.[7]

A Phase II clinical study whereby MPCs were injected into the degenerate IVDs of patients with chronic discogenic LBP had positive results at 12 months, which included a reduction in pain scores, increase in functional endpoints, and a decreased need for analgesia and secondary interventions compared with placebo controls.[8] A Phase III study is now under way, and if the safety and efficacy outcomes are positive then this modality of treatment could revolutionize the treatment of discogenic back pain, one of the most common causes of disability worldwide.[9]

In the pipeline are some other exciting therapeutic developments. Several preclinical studies have now shown that the viability and chondrogenic potential of MPCs are enhanced when formulated with the agent pentosan polysachharide (PPS).[7,10,11] This agent not only suppresses some of the mediators of disc matrix degradation but also upregulates endogenous cell anabolic activities and acts synergistically with MSCs to enhance matrix regeneration.[7,10,11]

Finally, I believe that novel biological approaches aimed at augmenting and enhancing current surgical techniques will have a significant future impact.[12,13] Microdiscectomy is one of the most common surgical procedures performed, and although it is generally successful at alleviating radicular pain, it is detrimental to disc repair. Oehme performed a study demonstrating that MPCs with PPS when administered in a scaffold at the time of microdiscectomy restored disc height, disc morphology, and NP proteoglycan content.[7] We have also demonstrated that a similar MPC, PPS, and scaffold combination can produce cartilaginous tissue following anterior cervical discectomy,[11] in an attempt to preserve cervical motion in a biological manner. This may reduce the problem of adjacent segment disease. Further work is presently in progress to improve the implants used for this novel approach.[11]

In conclusion, Australia has made and continues to make a significant contribution in spinal disc regeneration. In my opinion, the two main areas of likely success in the not too distant future are the treatment of discogenic back pain by cellular injection and specifically targeted regenerative medical techniques focused at enhancing current surgical practice.

– Tony Goldschlager

21.3 Europe

Predicting or anticipating the future has always been a difficult if not impossible task. Our knowledge in medicine has increased exponentially in recent decades and this has been closely linked to information technology (IT), methodological advances, and novel fields such as molecular biology. Translating this explosion of data into treating patients, however, continues to be a challenging endeavor. Current approaches in spine surgery, for example, mostly imply the crude resection of tissue or the metal-based fixation of physiologically mobile elements. Industry pushes the development and marketing of new implants often without solid scientific proof, which has been a source of criticism for both the industry and involved surgeons in recent years. Most spine specialists are convinced that the future will bring biological solutions and that future generations will joke about our current mechanistic concepts, particularly for the abundant degenerative diseases of the spine.

The literature reveals, and this book by Roger Härtl and Lawrence Bonassar perfectly summarizes, the different biological options for repair and regeneration of the human disc. Genes, proteins, growth factors, stem cells, and many other approaches demonstrate encouraging experimental results. Nevertheless, there are many obstacles for translation into clinical practice and these obstacles will determine what the future will bring:

1. Limited knowledge: Although many details and pathophysiological mechanisms of spinal and especially disc degeneration have been unraveled, dramatic knowledge gaps persist. The causal and chronological association between end plate changes and intradiscal degeneration as well as many other fundamental questions are still a matter of debate.

2. Physiological aging: Spinal degeneration itself does not seem to be pathological, but rather a natural phenomenon of aging. Only painful degeneration and morphological substrates such as disc herniations pose a clinical problem, which greatly hinders the use of prophylactic approaches. How do we identify pathological degeneration early, as truly "curing" degenerative diseases calls for preventive measures before symptoms occur?

3. Chronicity of the disease: In contrast to other areas in medicine the outcome of any spinal intervention can only be determined after a long-term follow-up of many years. This is true for current treatment options such as spinal instrumentation, but even more so for regenerative approaches, which may take many years for noticeable effects.

4. Regulatory challenges: As pointed out by Purcell, White, and Adkisson (Chapter 19), there is a long road to travel from a biological therapeutic idea and its experimental confirmation to a medicinal product. Both regulatory challenges and the necessity for long-term follow-up discourage investors, and as we all know, financial support is crucial for success in research.

5. Multifactoriality of the disease: Outcome, namely pain at long-term follow-up, determines the success of any spinal intervention. Pain, however, is a multifaceted phenomenon, influenced by many psychosocial factors in our complex society and by other segments of the spine neighboring the treated region, which greatly bedevils studies in spine surgery.

Regardless of these barriers in translating spinal regenerative approaches into clinical medicine, I am optimistic that the approaches presented in this book will find their way into treatment standards for our patients. My department is currently involved in a study on autologous chondrocyte transplantation after lumbar disc surgery and in numerous experimental efforts in repairing disc tissue as well as AF. I personally believe that the early clinical achievements will be focused on lumbar disc surgery—a very common problem in often only mildly degenerated segments. A first milestone will be the biological repair of annular ruptures in these cases. This would be possible by generating simple collagenous scar tissue and may thus be less complicated than creating chondrocytic disc tissue. Reestablishing annular integrity seems to be a prerequisite for nucleus replacement or augmentation, which will follow thereafter. A cell-free chemotactic solution may be the first step for disc regeneration, until (stem) cell advances allow precise and safe tissue engineering. Although still rarely studied, total disc transplantation could be realized in the near future. Gene therapeutic approaches do and will face regulatory and safety issues, so that spine care will drastically lag behind oncological diseases in this regard.

The second wave of progress may be focused on arthritic changes of the spine. Symptoms of facet joint or end plate degeneration will be reduced by biological regenerative measures. Spinal instability will not be cured to physiological motion, but restabilized by induction of fibrosis comparable to natural stiffening of the spine with age.

Prophylactic interventions for the healthy on the other hand will have a long way to go because we first have to unravel the differences between physiological (age-associated) and pathological (painful) degeneration. To reliably predict the latter currently seems to be an unresolvable problem.

Regardless of the numerous obstacles we need to overcome, I am convinced that these developments will take place, and they will require the close collaboration between basic scientists and clinicians. I personally see Europe in an excellent position for research in regenerative spinal care given that regulatory issues, albeit cumbersome, may continue to be less problematic

than in North America, and demographic changes will focus research more and more on age-related diseases in comparison with the developing world.

– Claudius Thomé

21.4 South America

We all are dying; our degeneration process is slowly killing us, day by day. The lumbar spine is not an exception. Degenerative conditions of the lumbar spine are extremely common. Degenerative spinal diseases such as lumbar IVD disease and lumbar spondylosis have an enormous social impact on patients and their families, as well as a devastating economic impact on health care budgets.[14]

As summarized in this book, the stimulation of the biological disc repair process in the treatment of DDDs could produce an amelioration of pain and restructuring of the degenerated disc, introducing a new approach to modulate the course of disease. Improved transfection efficiency and duration of the action with the injection of growth factors will create a new category of therapy for DDDs.[15]

Biological IVD replacement has been subdivided based on the two different tissues types, the NP and the AF. The biological solutions for NP and AF replacement are still more illusion than fact. However, whereas tissue engineering has just scratched the tip of the iceberg, more satisfying solutions are yet to be added to the biomedical pipeline.[16]

In summary, recent efforts to develop engineered tissues for partial or total disc repair and regenerative medicine strategies have resulted in promising outcomes in vitro and in small animal models. However, these strategies have significant challenges in scaling to a clinically relevant solution. Numerous studies have demonstrated success using cell-based therapies to treat disc disease, and these successes are in the early stages of translation into the clinic. Although not widely available, it is likely that stem cell therapies will become a treatment option for some patients with disc disease in the near future.

The target of tissue engineering strategies is to generate and remodel the ECM of NP tissue using the biological activity of cells. The regenerated tissue should function properly in an environment that is subjected to continuous mechanical perturbation throughout the lifetime of an individual. Regeneration of NP involves complex processes of cell matrix interactions. Biomaterial scaffolds provide structural support for NP regeneration and serve as a carrier for stem cell and gene vector delivery. Though biomaterial scaffolds will provide an initial permissive environment for grafted cell growth; cells should be able to maintain their phenotype and restore a healthy NP tissue with mechanical function. Because of the complexity of the regeneration process of the NP, the combination approach of biomaterials, gene vectors, and stem cells may be a practical solution for NP repair. Recent studies have advanced the strategies of biological therapy through biomaterial implantation, stem cell grafting, and gene therapy approaches. However, researchers need to overcome many challenges before these methods can successfully treat degenerated discs clinically.

Though a number of synthetic and natural materials have been tested for NP cell growth or implantation in the disc, they need to be improved in their material properties such as biocompatibility, stiffness, mechanical strength, and degradation products in order to effectively restore the properties of a healthy disc. The availability of a suitable cell source also limits biological disc repair, because it is difficult to obtain autologous NP cells and stem cells. In gene therapy, the low transfection efficiency of nonviral vectors has limited their application. However, the application of viral vectors is limited by their immunogenicity and a high risk of insertional mutagenesis that may induce neoplasia. Despite many years of research, the etiology of the molecular process of NP degeneration remains poorly understood. Improved understanding of the molecular mechanisms that lead to the degenerative change will provide new clues for the emergence of new strategies for NP regeneration.

Finally, the economics of cell-based therapies will need to be determined. Costs of current spinal treatments are enormous and increasing. For stem cell therapies to be utilized on a large scale, allogenic administration of "off-the-shelf" stem cells, such as MPCs, is required. We consider the autologous route not viable for pragmatic and economic reasons. The costs of cellular therapies will need to be weighed against cost savings in terms of increased work productivity and avoidance of more invasive and expensive procedures. Whether or not patients, insurance providers, institutions, and public health providers will absorb the increased direct costs of cell-based therapies is yet to be established.

– Luiz Vialle, Jaime Arias Ruiz, and
William Omar Contreras Lopez

21.5 Asia

I feel privileged to comment on what is happening and going to happen in the future of intervertebral disc (IVD) research in Asia. Currently, academia is overflowing with medical research articles that come out of Asia, in which the demographic has changed over the last decade. Nowadays, China is second only to the US in terms of English scientific publication output, and by 2019, it is estimated to take over the lead from US, Europe, and Japan. Although there are still many problems like misconduct, fabrication etc., it is likely that the global research scene will be strongly affected by China and India, the emerging giants of world higher education.[17]

In addition to original articles, papers using statistical techniques like meta-analysis are also abundant. Meta-analysis and systemic reviews published by Chinese authors in various topics both in clinical and basic science have shown a 200-fold increase from 2001 to 2011.[18] The foundation for this phenomenon is most likely due to the culture in Asian academia, which becomes uncontrollably competitive, and the number of papers published is the most important bench-mark for scientists' and clinicians' promotion. Despite these changes in the players of the global research scene, significant advancements in the knowledge of spinal research have been achieved in the past decade from Asia, and this trend will is likely to increase in the years to come. For example, a variety of long non-coding RNA (lncRNA) and microRNA (miRNA) have been identified that regulate degenerative changes within the IVD extracellular matrix (ECM) such as degradation, inflammatory responses, apoptosis

and angiogenesis.[19] Basic research associated with pain that originates from the IVD has also been intensively investigated in Asia.[20] Stem cells from various regions of the IVD tissue have been identified by Asian research groups, and these discoveries will presumably continue.[21,22]

Lastly, there is an emerging interest in the application of regenerative medicine in spine clinics. While several cell-based products have already been used in clinical trials, no product has been fully approved by the US Food and Drug Administration (FDA), European Medicines Agency (EMA) or the Japanese Pharmaceuticals and Medical Devices Agency (PMDA). This is likely due to the fact that the process of getting a cell-based product to market is very long. In order to overcome this long time lag, the Japanese government has passed a new law in November, 2014, to establish steps for the safe practice of regenerative and ethical administration of regenerative medical technologies, as well as a manufacturing permit system.[23] This law will help to accelerate the clinical development process of regenerative medicine, by treating regenerative medicine products in a similar manner to orphan drugs. This means that the approved product will typically skip the Phase III trial and obtain marketing authorization after demonstration of safety and minimal signs of efficacy after a solid Phase I and II trial. With this game-changing act of the regulatory authority, it is suspected that other regulatory authorities in various regions of the globe will follow, and most likely that regenerative treatment products will be available for spinal diseases in the near future.

– Daisuke Sakai

21.6 References

[1] Ghosh P. The Biology of the Intervertebral Disc. CRC Press; 1988:1

[2] Osti OL, Vernon-Roberts B, Fraser RD. 1990 Volvo Award in experimental studies. Anulus tears and intervertebral disc degeneration. An experimental study using an animal model. Spine. 1990; 15(8):762–767

[3] Simmons PJ, Torok-Storb B. Identification of stromal cell precursors in human bone marrow by a novel monoclonal antibody, STRO-1. Blood. 1991; 78(1):55–62

[4] Gronthos S, Graves SE, Ohta S, Simmons PJ. The STRO-1 + fraction of adult human bone marrow contains the osteogenic precursors. Blood. 1994; 84 (12):4164–4173

[5] Ghosh P, Goldschlager T, Itescu S.. Back pain—a clinical challenge addressed by Mesoblast using their Mesenchymal Precursor Cells. Nature Outlook. 2013 Nov 14:7475

[6] Ghosh P, Moore R, Vernon-Roberts B, et al. Immunoselected STRO-3 + mesenchymal precursor cells and restoration of the extracellular matrix of degenerate intervertebral discs. J Neurosurg Spine. 2012; 16(5):479–488

[7] Oehme D, Ghosh P, Shimmon S, et al. Mesenchymal progenitor cells combined with pentosan polysulfate mediating disc regeneration at the time of microdiscectomy: a preliminary study in an ovine model. J Neurosurg Spine. 2014; 20(6):657–669

[8] Bae HW, Amirdelfan K, Coric D, et al. A Phase II study demonstrating efficacy and safety of mesenchymal precursor cells in low back pain due to disc degeneration. Spine J. 2014; 14(11):S31–S32

[9] Vos T, Flaxman AD, Naghavi M, et al. Years lived with disability (YLDs) for 1160 sequelae of 289 diseases and injuries 1990–2010: a systematic analysis for the Global Burden of Disease Study 2010. Lancet. 2012; 380 (9859):2163–2196

[10] Oehme D, Ghosh P, Goldschlager T, et al. Disc regeneration using STRO-3 + immunoselected allogeneic mesenchymal precursor cells combined with pentosan polysulfate. Spine J. 2014; 14(11):S86

[11] Goldschlager T, Ghosh P, Zannettino A, et al. Cervical motion preservation using mesenchymal progenitor cells and pentosan polysulfate, a novel

chondrogenic agent: preliminary study in an ovine model. Neurosurg Focus. 2010; 28(6):E4

[12] Goldschlager T, Oehme D, Ghosh P, Zannettino A, Rosenfeld JV, Jenkin G. Current and future applications for stem cell therapies in spine surgery. Curr Stem Cell Res Ther. 2013; 8(5):381–393

[13] Goldschlager T, Jenkin G, Ghosh P, Zannettino A, Rosenfeld JV. Potential applications for using stem cells in spine surgery. Curr Stem Cell Res Ther. 2010; 5(4):345–355

[14] Oehme D, Goldschlager T, Rosenfeld JV, Ghosh P, Jenkin G. The role of stem cell therapies in degenerative lumbar spine disease: a review. Neurosurg Rev. 2015; 38(3):429–445

[15] Zhao CQ, Wang LM, Jiang LS, Dai LY. The cell biology of intervertebral disc aging and degeneration. Ageing Res Rev. 2007; 6(3):247–261

[16] Chan SC, Gantenbein-Ritter B. Intervertebral disc regeneration or repair with biomaterials and stem cell therapy—feasible or fiction? Swiss Med Wkly. 2012; 142:w13598

[17] China's medical research integrity questioned. Lancet. 2015; 385(9976):1365

[18] Ye XF, Yu DH, He J. The rise in meta-analyses from China. Epidemiology. 2013; 24(2):335–336

[19] Chen WK, Yu XH, Yang W, et al. lncRNAs: novel players in intervertebral disc degeneration and osteoarthritis. Cell Prolif. 2016; [Epub ahead of print]. DOI: 10.1111/cpr.12313

[20] Ohtori S, Inoue G, Miyagi M, Takahashi K. Pathomechanisms of discogenic low back pain in humans and animal models. Spine J. 2015; 15(6):1347–1355

[21] Sakai D, Nakamura Y, Nakai T, et al. Exhaustion of nucleus pulposus progenitor cells with ageing and degeneration of the intervertebral disc. Nat Commun. 2012; 3:1264

[22] Liu LT, Huang B, Li CQ, Zhuang Y, Wang J, Zhou Y. Characteristics of stem cells derived from the degenerated human intervertebral disc cartilage endplate. PLoS One. 2011; 6(10):e26285

[23] Minestry of Health. Labor and Welfare. Translated English Overview of 'The Act on the Safety of Regenerative Medicine' - 2014. http://www.mhlw.go.jp/english/policy/health-medical/medical-care/dl/150407-01.p. Accessed Dec 14, 2016

Appendix A: Abbreviations

2D	two-dimensional
3D	three-dimensional
3R	replacement, reduction and refinement
ACDF	anterior cervical decompression and fusion
ADAMTS	the disintegrin-like and metalloprotease with thrombospondin motif 1
ADCT	autologous disc chondrocyte transplantation
AF	annulus fibrosus
ASD	adjacent segment degeneration
bFGF	basic fibroblast growth factor
BLA	Biologics License Application
BMAC	bone marrow aspirate concentrate
BMI	Body Mass Index
BMP	bone morphogenetic protein
BMP-7	bone morphogenetic protein-7
BMSC	bone marrow stem cell
BrdU	bromodeoxyuridine
CA	confidentiality agreement
C-ABC	chondroitinase-ABC
CASP	clinical adjacent segment pathology
CBER	Center for Biologic Evaluation and Research
CDA	confidential disclosure agreement
CDMP2	cartilage morphogenetic protein-2
CDRH	Center for Devices and Radiological Health
CILP	cartilage intermediate layer protein
CoCrMo	cobalt-chromium-molybdenum
CT	computed tomography
DDD	degenerative disc disease
DNA	deoxyribonucleic acid
DOF	degrees of freedom
DSH	disc space height
DTI	diffusion tensor imaging
DWI	diffusion-weighted imaging
EBM	evidence-based medicine
ECM	extracellular matrix
ES	embryonic stem
FDA	Food and Drug Administration
FSU	functional spinal unit
GAG	glycosaminoglycan

GCP	Good Clinical Practice
GDF-5	growth and differentiation factor-5
GDF-6	growth and differentiation factor-6
GLP	Good Laboratory Practice
GMP	Good Manufacturing Practice
HA	hyaluronic acid
HA-pNIPAM	hyaluronic acid (HA) grafted with poly(N-isopropylacrylamide) (pNIPAM)
HCL	highly cross-linked polyethylene
HCT/P	human cells, tissues, and cellular and tissue-based products
HO	heterotopic ossification
HPSC	hematopoietic precursor stem cells
HSC	hematopoietic stem cell
ICOR	instantaneous center of rotation
IDE	investigational device exemption
IFN-γ	interferon-γ
IGF	insulin-like growth factor
IGF-1	insulin-like growth factor-1
IHI	Institute for Healthcare Improvement
IL	interleukin
IL-1	interleukin 1
IL-RA	interleukin receptor antagonist
IND	Investigational New Drug Application
IP	intellectual property
iPSC	induced pluripotent stem cells
IVD	intervertebral disc
JOA	Japanese Orthopaedic Association
Link N	link protein N-terminal peptide
LMP-1	LIM mineralization protein-1
MAC	mesenchymal stem cells
MAVRIC	multiacquisition variable resonance image combination
MID	minimal important difference
MMP	matrix metalloproteinase
MOM	metal-on-metal
MOP	metal-on-polyethylene
MRI	magnetic resonance imaging
MSC	mesenchymal stem cell
NDA	nondisclosure agreement
NDI	Neck Disability Index
NIH	National Institutes of Health
NP	nucleus pulposus
ODI	Oswestry Disability Index

OP-1	osteogenic protein-1
OPDQ	Oswestry Low Back Pain Disability Questionnaire
PDGF	platelet-derived growth factor
PIA	proprietary information agreement
PLGA	polylactic glycolic acid
PMCs	Postmarketing Commitments
PMRs	Postmarketing Requirements
pNIPAM	poly(N-isopropylacrylamide)
PRF	platelet rich fibrin
PRP	platelet rich plasma
QBPD	Quebec Back Pain Disability Scale
RASP	radiographic adjacent segment pathology
RCT	randomized controlled trial
rhGDF-5	recombinant human GDF-5
ROM	range of motion
SA	secrecy agreement
SEMAC	slice-encoding metal artifact correction
SF 36	Short Form Health Survey (36 items)
SOX9	SRY (sex determining region Y) box 9
TDA	total disc arthroplasty
TDR	total disc replacement
TE	echo time
TE-IVD	tissue engineered intervertebral disc
TGF	transforming growth factor
TGF-β	transforming growth factor β
TIMP-1	tissue inhibitor of metalloproteinase 1
TNF-α	tumor necrosis factor-α
UHMWP	ultra-high molecular weight polyethylene
UTE	ultrashort time-to-echo
VAS	Visual Analog Scale
VAT	view-angle-tilting
VEGF	vascular endothelial growth factor

Appendix B: Terminology

Chapter 2 Pathophysiology of Disc Disease: Disc Degeneration	
Afferent neuron	Sensory neuron that carries signals from sensory receptors/organs back to the brain/spinal cord
Annulus fibrosus (AF)	The outer fibrous portion of the intervertebral disc (IVD) rich in organized type I collagen
Chemokines	Cytokines that promote cellular chemotaxis
Degenerative disc disease	Breakdown of the IVD tissue that may be painful or nonpainful
Discogenic pain	Pain originating from the IVD
End plate	Hyaline cartilage layer of tissue that is on either end of the IVD
Extracellular matrix (ECM)	Macromolecular components of the tissue that surround and are secreted by the cells
Notochordal cells	Cells originally derived from the notochord, an embryonic structure that gives rise to the nucleus pulposus, that are thought to have regenerative potential but disappear from the disc during adolescence
Nucleus pulposus (NP)	The gelatinous inner portion of the IVD rich in proteoglycan and type II collagen

Chapter 3 Imaging of the Healthy and Diseased Spinal Disc	
Diffusion tensor imaging (DTI)	A technique that evaluates both the magnitude and direction of diffusion. DTI has mainly been applied in the central nervous system to evaluate white matter tracts. In theory, DTI could be used to evaluate the degree of anisotropy, or the extent to which diffusion is greater in one direction, in interrogating the biochemical structure of the intervertebral disc (IVD).
Diffusion-weighted imaging (DWI)	A technique that assesses the magnitude of diffusion of water molecules and mobile protons to distinguish between different pathological entities
MAVRIC	The multiacquisition variable resonance image combination technique acquires multiple three-dimensional (3D) fast spin-echo image datasets at different frequency bands, offset from the resonant proton frequency. It then combines these datasets to produce an image with reduced susceptibility artifact.
SEMAC	The slice-encoding metal artifact correction technique utilizes robust slice encoding to correct metal artifacts by extending a view-angle-tilting (VAT) spin-echo sequence with additional z-phasing encoding.
T1-rho	A quantitative spin-lock sequence that employs a lower Larmor frequency to permit the detection of low-frequency physiochemical interactions between water and extracellular matrix (ECM) molecules. T1-rho is particularly useful for determining proteoglycan content.
T2* mapping	A quantitative technique traditionally employed to assess the composition of articular cartilage but one that can also provide information about the interaction of water molecules and the collagen network of the intervertebral disc (IVD).
Ultrashort time-to-echo (UTE)	A type of T2* mapping technique that acquires much shorter echo images (echo time [TE] ~ 0.3 ms), compared with conventional T2* mapping techniques, and thus provides the ability to capture very short T2 values of fibrocartilage. This may be helpful in evaluation of the cartilaginous end plates and possibly the annulus fibrosus (AF).

Chapter 4 Biomechanics of the Healthy and Diseased Spine	
Clinical instability	The loss of the ability of the spine to maintain its patterns of displacement under physiological loads
Disc aging	The physiological process of alteration of the morphology and composition of the intervertebral disc (IVD) due to aging
Computational model	A mathematical representation of a mechanical problem (e.g., an experimental test) able to replicate the response of the object of interest, solved by means of a computer. Computational models are nowadays widely used to simulate the biomechanical behavior of the spine.
In vitro test	An experimental investigation in which a spine specimen (human or surrogate, either an animal or artificial model) is subjected to standardized loads or motions to investigate its biomechanical response
Motion segment, or functional spine unit	The set of two adjacent vertebrae, the IVD in-between, and relevant spine ligaments
Neutral zone	The amplitude of the spinal motion that can be achieved with a minimal load, in a specific motion plane (flexion-extension, lateral bending, axial rotation)
Radiological instability	Hypermobility of the motion segment, either translational or rotational, observed by means of radiological methods

Range of motion	The amplitude of the spinal motion (from one extreme to the other extreme) under the effect of physiological loading, in a specific motion plane (flexion-extension, lateral bending, axial rotation). A high range of motion corresponds to a high spine flexibility and to a low spine stiffness
Structural failure	A pathological process (either traumatic or degenerative) in which some components of the tissue lose their structural integrity. Examples are annular tears and end plate fractures.

Chapter 7 Disc Regeneration: In Vitro Approaches and Experimental Results

Bioreactor	Any machine that aims to better mimic physiological conditions in vitro by replicating important features of the native microenvironment. As opposed to standard in vitro conditions consisting of an incubator and media, cells, engineered tissues, and live discs can also be cultured in a bioreactor where standard conditions are maintained and then supplemented with other inputs; common inputs include mechanical forces and varying oxygen tension.
Cell phenotype	The specific set of characteristics that distinguish one cell type from another. Example: The nucleus pulposus (NP) cell phenotype is defined by the production of type II collagen and aggrecan as well as an ability to function in a mildly acidic and oxygen-depleted conditions
Cell source	The larger pool of cells in their original anatomical location from which cells can be isolated for in vitro experiments. Example: Mesenchymal stem cells (MSCs) can be isolated from the larger pool of cells found in the bone marrow of the iliac crest.
Composite disc constructs	The combination of engineered NP and annulus fibrosus (AF) tissues into a single construct, either for the development of an engineered total disc replacement (TDR) or for the investigation of co-culture of these or other cell types
Fully differentiated cells	Any cell that has reached its terminal differentiation state. Examples: AF cell, NP cell, chondrocyte, skin fibroblast.
Hydrogel	A cross-linked, hydrophilic (water-absorbing) network of a natural or artificial polymer. Examples: agarose, hyaluronic acid (HA), polyethylene glycol.
Embryonic stem (ES) cells	Any cell isolated from the embryonic stage of development that has pluripotent differentiation potential
Induced pluripotent stem cells (iPSC)	Cells, typically skin fibroblasts, that are induced into a pluripotent state through a cocktail of genetic signals. This recent technological advance has therapeutic potential for the musculoskeletal system as fibroblasts from the skin can be induced into pluripotency and subsequently differentiated into a chondrocyte- or NP-like phenotype with the appropriate growth factors.
In vitro model systems	Any method that, in a laboratory setting, replicates aspects of the physiological environment for the purposes of evaluating how cell responds to a controlled stimulus
Material substrate	The physical environment in which cells are seeded on, or encapsulated in, for in vitro culture. Examples: tissue culture plastic, various polymers and hydrogels
Mesenchymal stem cells (MSC)	Progenitor cells isolated from any tissue of mesenchymal origin (frequently bone marrow and adipose tissue)
Monolayer culture	The process by which cells are grown on a petri dish and form into planar layers (layers one cell in thickness). Also referred to as two-dimensional (2D) culture.
Multipotent stem cells	Progenitor cells with the ability to differentiate into cells with multiple (but limited) phenotypes. Example: hematopoietic stem cells (HSCs) generate multiple blood cell lineages.
NP progenitor cells	See Notochordal cells in terminology list for Chapter 2, above.
Organ culture	The process by which live discs are freshly isolated from recently deceased animals/humans and then cultured in vitro to evaluate the biological processes of live cells within the disc microenvironment. Disc organ culture often includes a bioreactor system to control external variables such as, for example, dynamic mechanical loads.
Pellet culture	A process in which cells are allowed to aggregate, typically at the bottom of a conical tube, to enable cell proliferation and synthesis of extracellular matrix (ECM) to form spheroids. This is considered a three-dimensional (3D) culture process.
Pluripotent stem cells	Progenitor cells with the ability to differentiate into cells with phenotype from any of the three germ layers (mesoderm, endoderm, ectoderm). Example: ES cells.
Progenitor cells	Parent cells that can, during cell division, give rise to (or differentiate into) cells of a specified phenotype. Example: MSCs differentiate into cells with a chondrocyte-like phenotype when supplied with the appropriate chondrogenic growth factors.
Scaffold	Any biomaterial substrate such as a polymer hydrogel that cells are seeded onto or into and grown in culture

Stem cell potency	The categorization of a stem cell's ability to parent differentiated cells with either a wide or limited range of phenotypes. Examples (in order of potency): totipotent, pluripotent, multipotent, unipotent.
3D culture	The process by which cells are encapsulated in biomaterials such as polymers and hydrogels, or allowed to aggregate as 3D masses, and then grown in culture. Examples: the encapsulation of NP cells in agarose, the aggregation of chondrocytes as pellets.

Chapter 8 Intervertebral Disc Whole Organ Cultures

3R	"Replacement, reduction, and refinement" are the guiding principles for a better use of animal research. For further information: https://www.nc3rs.org.uk/the-3rs
Bioreactor	Single or multiple chamber system that allows the culture (i.e., of whole intervertebral discs [IVDs]) under defined biochemical and loading
Chemotaxis	Cell migration in response to a biochemical stimulus (e.g., cytokines)
HA-pNIPAM	Thermoreversible hydrogel composed of hyaluronic acid (HA) grafted with poly(N-isopropylacrylamide) (pNIPAM), which is a liquid at room temperature and a gel above 32°C
Loading	Static or dynamic application of a mechanical load
Whole organ culture	In vitro culture of a living whole organ such as the IVD (with or without loading)

Chapter 13 Treatment of Degenerative Disc Disease/Disc Regeneration: Stem Cells, Chondrocytes or Other Cells, and Tissue Engineering

Adult stem cell	An undifferentiated cell found in a differentiated tissue that can renew itself and (with certain limitations) differentiate to yield all the specialized cell types of the tissue from which it originated
Allogenic	Two or more individuals (or cell lines) are stated to be allogenic to one another when the genes at one or more loci are not identical in sequence in each organism.
Autologous transplant	Transplanted tissue derived from the intended recipient of the transplant. Such a transplant helps avoid complications of immune rejection.
Bone marrow	The soft, living tissue that fills most bone cavities and contains hematopoietic stem cells (HSCs), from which all red and white blood cells evolve. The bone marrow also contains mesenchymal stem cells (MSCs) that a number of cells types come from, including chondrocytes, which produce cartilage.
Bone marrow stem cell	One of at least two types of multipotent stem cells: HSC and MSC
Chondrocytes	Cartilage cells
Differentiation	The process whereby an unspecialized early embryonic cell acquires the features of a specialized cell such as a heart, liver, or muscle cell
Ectoderm	The upper, outermost of the three primitive germ layers of the embryo; it gives rise to skin, nerves, and brain.
Embryonic stem (ES) cells	Primitive (undifferentiated) cells from the embryo that have the potential to become a wide variety of specialized cell types
Endoderm	Lower layer of a group of cells derived from the inner cell mass of the blastocyst; it later becomes the lungs and digestive organs.
Hematopoietic stem cell (HSC)	A stem cell from which all red and white blood cells evolve
Mesenchymal stem cells (MSCs)	Cells from the immature embryonic connective tissue. A number of cell types come from MSCs, including chondrocytes, which produce cartilage.
Mesoderm	The middle layer of the embryonic disc, which consists of a group of cells derived from the inner cell mass of the blastocyst. This middle germ layer is known as gastrulation and is the precursor to bone, muscle, and connective tissue.
Multipotent stem cells	Stem cells that have the capability of developing cells of multiple germ layers
Pluripotent stem cell	A single stem cell that has the capability of developing cells of all germ layers (endoderm, ectoderm, and mesoderm)
Precursor cells	In fetal or adult tissues, these are partly differentiated cells that divide and give rise to differentiated cells. Also known as progenitor cells.
Primary germ layers	The three initial embryonic germ layers—endoderm, mesoderm, and ectoderm—from which all other somatic tissue-types develop
Somatic cell	Any cell of a plant or animal other than a germ cell or germ cell precursor

Stem cell	A cell that has the ability to divide for indefinite periods in culture and to give rise to specialized cells
Totipotent	Having unlimited capability. The totipotent cells of the very early embryo have the capacity to differentiate into extra embryonic membranes and tissues, the embryo, and all postembryonic tissues and organs.

Chapter 17 Total Disc Transplantation: Current Results and Future Development

Allograft	Transplantation of discs from a nonidentical donor of the same species
Arc of motion	The total range of motion (ROM) of the cervical spine inclusive of flexion and extension ranges
Autograft	Transplantation of discs from the same person
Bipedal	Animals such as monkeys that move with the two rear limbs
Cryopreservation	Process of cooling harvested discs to prevent damage to the disc material by enzymatic or chemical activity necessary for storage
Dislocation	The disc has completely separated from the disc space
Extension arc	The extension range of motion of the cervical spine
Immunocompatibility	The grafted disc and the recipient are compatible without any immunoactivity that may cause rejection
Japanese Orthopaedic Association (JOA) score	Objective assessment score for severity of cervical myelopathy, which includes the four main domains of upper and lower extremity motor function, sensory function, and bladder function
Karyopyknosis	Indicating a transplanted disc that has undergone degeneration where irreversible condensation of chromatin occurs in the nucleus of cells
Osteotomy	Bone cut necessary to prepare a grafted disc or to prepare the recipient bed to receive the transplanted disc
Press-fit insertion	The disc is placed snug-fit into the disc space providing better stability.
Quadrupedal	Animals such as goats that move with four limbs
Subluxation	The disc has partially separated from the disc space.
Traction osteophyte	During disc bulges, the annulus fibrosis (AF) at its bony attachment of the vertebrae causes osteophyte formation at the level of the end plates both on the anterior and lateral sides of the vertebrae.

Chapter 19 Regulatory Overview: Obtaining Regulatory Approval of a Biological/Cell Product

Biologics License Application (BLA)	BLA is a request for permission to introduce, or deliver for introduction, a biological product into interstate commerce, and through which the FDA can determine if the safety and efficacy of an investigational product has been sufficiently established for marketing purposes, and furthermore, that the product label is appropriate for widespread public usage.
Breakthrough Product	This designation is intended to expedite the development and FDA review of investigational products that treat a serious condition, and preliminary clinical evidence demonstrates substantial improvement over available therapy.
Center for Biologic Evaluation and Research (CBER)	CBER is the center within FDA that regulates and provides public information about biological products for human use under applicable federal laws.
National Institutes of Health (NIH)	NIH is the U.S. federal medical research agency, which comprises 27 institutes and centers, each having specific research agendas, often focusing on particular diseases or body systems.
Good Clinical Practice (GCP)	These international guidelines have been adopted by the FDA as legally enforceable regulations outlining the responsibilities and expectations of all participants in the conduct of clinical trials, including investigators, monitors, sponsors and institutional review boards, ensuring the quality of clinical data used to describe the safety and efficacy of an investigational product in humans.
Good Laboratory Practice (GLP)	These regulations promulgated by the FDA have the force of law, and pertain to the conduct of nonclinical laboratory studies (including studies in animals) that support or are intended to support applications for research in humans or marketing permits for products regulated by the FDA. These regulations are intended to assure the quality and integrity of the nonclinical safety data submitted.
Good Manufacturing Practice (GMP)	These regulations, which are enforceable by law, require that manufacturers, processors, and packagers of drugs, medical devices, some food, and blood products take proactive steps to ensure product potency and purity. GMP regulations require a quality approach to manufacturing, enabling companies to minimize or eliminate instances of contamination, mix-ups, and errors.
Investigational New Drug Application (IND)	IND is the process by which the sponsor submits to the FDA all known chemistry, manufacturing and controls, and preclinical data (including studies in animals) regarding an investigational drug or biologic in order to obtain FDA's permission to study in humans and ship investigational product across state lines.

Orphan Drug Status	This designation is given to investigational products intended to treat rare diseases, effecting fewer than 200,000, and/or for which a small commercial market is demonstrated to exist. Under this designation, the sponsor qualifies for various incentives intended to offset the cost of development.
Phase I clinical research	Phase I is the initial introduction of an investigational new product into humans, in which the primary goal is to study its safety in a small number of subjects, who may include healthy volunteers.
Phase II clinical research	Phase II includes controlled clinical studies conducted to evaluate the effectiveness of the investigational product for a particular indication or indications in subjects with the disease or condition under study, and to determine its common short-term side effects and associated risks.
Phase III clinical research	Phase III studies are intended to gather the additional information about effectiveness and safety that is needed to evaluate a product's overall benefit-risk relationship as compared with an appropriate control, and to provide an adequate basis for marketing approval and product labeling.
Postmarketing Commitments (PMCs)	PMCs include studies that a sponsor had agreed with the FDA to perform, but however are not enforceable by statutes or regulations.
Postmarketing Requirements (PMRs)	PMRs include studies and clinical trials that sponsors are required to conduct under one or more statutes or regulations.
Sponsor	An individual, company, institution, or organization that takes responsibility for the initiation, management, and/or financing of a clinical trial
U.S. Food and Drug Administration (FDA)	FDA is the federal agency governed by the U.S. Department of Health and Human Services, which is responsible for protecting the public health by assuring the safety, effectiveness, quality, and security of most of our nation's food supply, products that give off radiation, human and veterinary drugs, vaccines, other biological products, and medical devices.
Chapter 20 What Makes Biological Treatment Strategies and Tissue Engineering for DDD Interesting to Industry?	
Confidentiality agreement (CA)	Also known as nondisclosure agreement (NDA), confidential disclosure agreement (CDA), proprietary information agreement (PIA), or secrecy agreement (SA). A legal contract between at least two parties that outlines confidential material, knowledge, or information that the parties wish to share with one another for certain purposes, but wish to restrict access to or by third parties
FDA's Drug Pathway	FDA's Center for Drug Evaluation and Research (CDER)'s best-known job is to evaluate new drugs before they can be sold. CDER's evaluation not only prevents quackery, but also provides doctors and patients the information they need to use medicines wisely. The center ensures that drugs, both brand name and generic, work correctly and that their health benefits outweigh their known risks.
FDA's human cells, tissues, and cellular and tissue-based products (HCT/P) pathway	Human cells, tissues, and cellular and tissue-based products (HCT/Ps) that are regulated by the Center for Devices and Radiological Health (CDRH) as medical devices and those that are regulated by the Center for Biologics Evaluation and Research (CBER)
Institute for Healthcare Improvement (IHI) Triple Aim	IHI's belief is that new designs must be developed to simultaneously pursue three dimensions, called the Triple Aim: improving the patient experience of care (including quality and satisfaction), improving the health of populations, and reducing the per capita cost of health care.
Intellectual property (IP)	Intangible rights protecting the products of human intelligence and creation, such as copyrightable works, patented inventions, trademarks, and trade secrets
Open innovation	Open innovation is a term promoted by Henry Chesbrough; it refers to the use of both inflows and outflows of knowledge to improve internal innovation and expand the markets for external exploitation of innovation.
Valley of Death	A slang phrase used in venture capital to refer to the period of time from when a start-up firm receives an initial capital contribution to when it begins generating revenues. During the death valley curve, additional financing is usually scarce, leaving the firm vulnerable to cash flow requirements.

Index